T0250129

Advances in Smart Healthcare Technologies

Series Editors: *Chinmay Chakraborty, and Joel J. P. C. Rodrigues*

Blockchain Technology in Healthcare Applications: Social, Economic and Technological Implications
Bharat Bhushan, Nitin Rakesh, Yousef Farhaoui, Parma Nand Astya and Bhuvan Unhelkar

Digital Health Transformation with Blockchain and Artificial Intelligence
Chinmay Chakraborty

Digital Health Transformation with Blockchain and Artificial Intelligence

Digital Health Transformation with Blockchain and Artificial Intelligence

Edited by

Chinmay Chakraborty

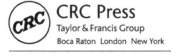

CRC Press
Taylor & Francis Group
Boca Raton London New York

CRC Press is an imprint of the
Taylor & Francis Group, an **informa** business

Cover image: [add credit line if known or TBC if pending]

First edition published 2022
by CRC Press
6000 Broken Sound Parkway NW, Suite 300, Boca Raton, FL 33487-2742

and by CRC Press
4 Park Square, Milton Park, Abingdon, Oxon, OX14 4RN

CRC Press is an imprint of Taylor & Francis Group, LLC

Library of Congress Cataloging-in-Publication Data
Names: Chakraborty, Chinmay, 1984- editor.
Title: Digital health transformation with blockchain and artificial intelligence / edited by Chinmay Chakraborty.
Description: First edition. | Boca Raton : CRC Press, 2022. | Series: Advances in smart healthcare technologies | Includes bibliographical references and index.
Identifiers: LCCN 2021055374 (print) | LCCN 2021055375 (ebook) | ISBN 9781032161181 (hardback) | ISBN 9781032161198 (paperback) | ISBN 9781003247128 (ebook)
Subjects: LCSH: Medical informatics. | Medicine--Data processing. | Blockchains (Databases) | Artificial intelligence.
Classification: LCC R858 .D54 2022 (print) | LCC R858 (ebook) | DDC 610.285--dc23/eng/20211227
LC record available at https://lccn.loc.gov/2021055374
LC ebook record available at https://lccn.loc.gov/2021055375

ISBN: 978-1-032-16118-1 (hbk)
ISBN: 978-1-032-16119-8 (pbk)
ISBN: 978-1-003-24712-8 (ebk)

DOI: 10.1201/9781003247128

Typeset in Times
by SPi Technologies India Pvt Ltd (Straive)

Contents

v

Preface

This book covers the global digital revolution of the post-pandemic era. The population has been overcoming the COVID-19 period; therefore, we need to establish intelligent digital healthcare systems using various emerging technologies like blockchain and Artificial Intelligence (AI). The recent advanced technology helps to promote green and clean modern societies endlessly. The Internet of things (IoT) will be dominating and playing an essential role in the upcoming years in remote health monitoring, and sustainable development through digital transformations. Smart healthcare technology can be defined as using smartphones and electronic technology for good diagnosis of disease, improving treatment of the patients, and enhanced quality of life. The end-to-end clinical data connectivity involves the development of many technologies that should enable secure, reliable, and location-agnostic communication between a patient and a healthcare provider. Smart healthcare can reduce the time, cost, and risk of IoT deployments in healthcare, and gives superior efficiency and patient care. Medical data protection is one of the main challenges nowadays for end-to-end delivery. Internet of Medical Things (IoMT) is the major technological innovation that has included the element of "smartness" in the healthcare industry and also identifies, monitors, and informs service providers about the patient's clinical information with faster delivery-of-care services. Big Data helps to build a smart healthcare system for machine-to-machine and machine-to-home large volumes of medical data processing. The cloud-assisted medical framework is used to enhance the strength of the smart healthcare system because of cost savings, scalability, and system flexibility.

This book focuses on identifying the need for and importance of a gold standard in medical datasets for effective analysis and intelligent diagnostics with blockchain-integrated solutions. Multi-modal approaches for data fusion and IoT and edge computing-based approaches for real-time health monitoring of patients will also be covered here. The book explores the role of blockchain in providing a transparent, faster, secure, and privacy-preserved healthcare ecosystem for the masses. AI is considered here for providing intelligent healthcare system management.

Book Organization

The book consists of 16 chapters in the field of digital smart healthcare systems. A summary of each chapter is presented below.

Chapter 1: Blockchain and Internet of Things in Healthcare Systems: Prospects, Issues, and Challenges

This chapter focuses on the applicability of IoT-based blockchain in the healthcare system. The various technologies used will allow the IoT devices to exchange information about patient's health progress and how they are responding to treatment so their physicians can provide proper monitoring. The issues and challenges of these technologies are inventively discussed and identify the prospects of IoT-based enabled with blockchain in the healthcare sector. The investigation disputes in IoT-based enabled blockchain framework were discussed with a proposed framework for the application of blockchain-enabled IoT-based systems.

Chapter 2: Secure Digital Health Data Management in Internet of Things Using Blockchain and Machine Learning

In this chapter, a two-part novel model is proposed to allay any security and privacy concerns in the Internet of Healthcare Things. The first part analyzes a patient's health parameters using machine learning detecting and discarding anomalous data, and stores the non-anomalous data with findings in a transparent, secure fashion using blockchain. The second part provides a secure way to preserve critical medical records in blockchain using sandboxed Secure Virtual Machines to avoid any of the privacy issues and computational power constraints of current existing solutions, making this model very secure.

Chapter 3: Revolutionizing Healthcare by Coupling Unmanned Aerial Vehicles (UAVs) to Internet of Medical Things (IoMT)

This chapter aims to shed light on coupling different disciplines of IoMT and UAVs in healthcare along with their capabilities, advantages, applications, and challenges, and concludes with some recommendations and future work. This contribution is a noticeable shift from exiting work in the literature, as it provides a panoramic view on the proposed integration between IoMT and UAVs.

Chapter 4: Public Perception toward AI-Driven Healthcare and the Way Forward in the Post-Pandemic Era

This chapter focuses on the general public's understanding and perception of AI-driven smart healthcare systems. To explore if people from different age groups, varied educational qualifications, different incomes, and varying levels of technical literacy will accept this service with the same mindset or it will be different. More numbers of samples have randomly been considered according to the researcher's convenience.

Chapter 5: Security, Privacy Issues, and Challenges in Adoption of Smart Digital Healthcare

This chapter analyzes the architecture and basic protocols used in the smart healthcare system. Then it identifies the security and privacy challenges in a different layer-wise system along with secure computational challenges that want to be addressed to accelerate the deployment and adoption of intelligent healthcare technologies for ubiquitous healthcare access. IoT-based smart healthcare systems have issues of authentication, data integrity, identification and scalability as the smart healthcare system uses heterogeneous devices to collect patient vital information which needs to be processed in real-time.

Chapter 6: Tapping the Big Data Analytics and IoT in the Pandemic Era

This chapter proposes diverse facets of Big Data analytics using IoT and progressions in the healthcare domain. With the conjunction of Big Data and novel technologies such as machine learning, data science, IoT, AI and so on, new enhancements are entirely feasible, which can improve the effectiveness of the healthcare and medical sectors. This massive data contain valuable information that can be applied in a range of contexts such as banking, retail, education, research and so on. The demand for fast and efficient technologies is likely to grow in the post-COVID-19 era.

Chapter 7: The Clinical Challenges for Digital Health Revolution

This chapter discusses the clinical challenges faced by digital health revolutions and the real challenge for clinicians to accept it for transforming healthcare. These days, the whole thing is impacted by the digital revolution—the influence of current expertise on refining the wellbeing of individuals, societies and populations. But these challenges are attainable with time and new technologies like AI, blockchain technology and precision medicine, etc., and multi-departmental research associations.

Chapter 8: An Overview of Artificial Intelligence for Advanced Healthcare Systems

The chapter presents the application of AI-based technologies for recent healthcare systems. The chapter reveals that such combinations with AI techniques are becoming an unavoidable part of the industry helping it to achieve high accuracy, reliability, and high productivity along with cost-effective implementation that will be shortly the driving force of the healthcare industry.

Chapter 9: Future Trajectory of Healthcare with Artificial Intelligence

This chapter mainly focuses on the application of AI in various healthcare domains like robot-assisted surgery, cancer diagnosis, maintaining a patient database and its importance in simplifying the tasks of many healthcare workers. The AI-assisted healthcare system can support patients, who are admitted to the hospital efficiently through various services.

Chapter 10: Artificial Intelligence and Public Trust on Smart Healthcare Systems
The findings of this chapter discovered a significant relationship between public trust and their willingness to adopt the AI-powered smart healthcare system. The results of this chapter's study conceptually strengthened the present body of literature on the human-computer relationship and will also help policymakers and service providers in crafting future strategies for promoting AI-powered smart healthcare systems in an emerging economy like India.

Chapter 11: Role of Artificial Intelligence-Based Technologies in Healthcare to Combat Critical Diseases
This chapter discusses recent advances in AI technology and its biomedical applications, which have the potential to enhance the healthcare industry by enhancing aspects of healthcare systems. Despite the enormous promise of cutting-edge AI-based research and innovation in the realm of healthcare, the ethical issues induced by its applications have been addressed.

Chapter 12: Parkinson's Disease Pre-Diagnosis Using Smart Technologies: A Review
This chapter discusses the pre-diagnosis of Parkinson's disease using modern health technologies. The machine learning algorithms were applied for each biomarker and measured the performance score. Then, drawing from the achievements and limitations established in past research, the chapter concludes with some important challenges that must be addressed before AI techniques can be deployed in clinical settings to assist medical practitioners in robust decision-making for Parkinson's disease diagnosis.

Chapter 13: Emerging Technologies to Combat the COVID-19 Pandemic
This chapter describes the main research related to the use of emerging technologies to ensure a safe working environment for caregivers and manage the COVID-19 situation. Therefore, it is vital to consider measures or tools to help to fight COVID-19 and save patients as well as healthcare workers. This chapter presents the contribution of various technologies in the healthcare sector, where such innovative technologies would contribute positively to both treatment and protection. To note, the discussed technologies here are aligned with the fourth industrial revolution.

Chapter 14: The Role of Machine Learning and Internet of Things in Digital Health Transformation
This chapter provides a review on the role of machine learning and IoMT in smart cities and is mainly focused on the roles of AI, IoT and blockchain in digital health transformation. Future research directions are suggested at the end of the chapter. It was found that ML and IoT approaches had a remarkable contribution to the development of smart cities. Moreover, blockchain can provide an effective

solution to overcoming the security challenges of IoT. In addition, secure health-care digital systems can be achieved via integrating IoT with blockchain. Fog computing technology can be integrated with IoT systems to minimize the latency of e-healthcare.

Chapter 15: Effective Remote Healthcare and Telemedicine Approaches for Improving Digital Healthcare Systems

This chapter discusses the patient disease identification, monitoring, and treatment and proper care with personal assistance including follow-ups and medicine delivery. Hence, easy to use, trustable, and significant use of AI-based telemedicine can reach any remote place where patients hesitate to seek medical professionals due to social stigma. This chapter also explores the different applications of the model with existing techniques. Prospects are also highlighted.

Chapter 16: Legal Implication of Blockchain Technology in Public Health

This chapter highlights the legal implication of blockchain methods in healthcare systems with robust privacy and data protection mechanism. The healthcare industry caters to important transactions, which entail protective smart contracts requiring updated and faster financials. Each healthcare area can get in-radar technology, providing more immediate solutions for a vast population.

At last, we would like to extend our sincere thanks to authors from the industry, academia, and policy experts to complete this work for aspiring researchers in this domain. We are confident that this book will play a key role in providing readers a comprehensive view of intelligent secured health informatics and developments around it and can be used as a learning resource for various examinations, which deal with cutting-edge technologies.

About the Editor

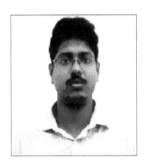 **Dr. Chinmay Chakraborty** is an assistant professor in the Department of Electronics and Communication Engineering, BIT Mesra, India, and a post-doctoral fellow of Federal University of Piauí, Brazil. His primary areas of research include: wireless body area networks, Internet of Medical Things, point-of-care diagnosis, m-health/e-health, and medical imaging. Dr. Chakraborty is co-editing many books on smart IoMT, healthcare technology, and sensor data analytics with CRC Press, IET, Pan Stanford, and Springer. Dr. Chakraborty has published more than 150 papers at reputed international journals, conferences, book chapters, more than 30 books, and more than 20 special issues. He received a Young Research Excellence Award, Global Peer Review Award, Young Faculty Award, and Outstanding Researcher Award.

Contributors

Kazeem Moses Abiodun
Landmark University
Omu Aran, Nigeria

Arij Naser Abougreen
Electrical and Electronic Engineering
    Department
University of Tripoli
Libya

Ayodele Ariyo Adebiyi
Computer Science
Landmark University
Omu Aran, Nigeria

Emmanuel Abidemi Adeniyi
Computer Science
Landmark University
Omu Aran, Nigeria

Marion Olubunmi Adebiyi
Computer Science
Landmark University
Omu Aran, Nigeria

Faris A. Almalki
Department of Computer Engineering,
    College of Computers and
    Information Technology
Taif University
Taif, Saudi Arabia

Marios Angelides
Brunel Design School
Brunel University London
Uxbridge, UK

Dayo Reuben Aremu
Computer Science
University of Ilorin
Ilorin, Nigeria

Joseph Bamidele Awotunde
Computer Science
University of Ilorin
Ilorin, Nigeria

Chinmay Chakraborty
Electronics & Communication
    Engineering
Birla Institute of Technology
Mesra, Ranchi, Jharkhand, India

Mohammad Yasser Chuttur
University of Mauritius
Mauritius

Susmit Das
RCC Institute of Information
    Technology
Kolkata, India

Ajitabh Dash
Jaipuria Institute of Management Indore
MP, India

Spandan Datta
Pune Institute of Business
    Management
Pune, Maharastra

Yashikha Dhiman
TCS
Ahmedabad, India

Anubha Dubey
Independent researcher and analyst
Noida, Uttar Pradesh, India

Leila Ennaceur
National Engineering School of Gabes
Gabes University
Tunisia

Debasish Jena
Department of CSE
IIIT Bhubaneswar
Odisha, India

Ashish Joshi
THDC Institute of Hydropower
    Engineering and Technology
Uttarakhand, India

Jayanta Ghosh
West Bengal National University of
    Juridical Sciences
Kolkata, India

Sreyashi Karmakar
RCC Institute of Information
    Technology
Kolkata, India

Nilesh Tejrao Kate
Pune Institute of Business Management
Pune, Maharastra

Ashish Kumar
Department of Chemistry
Lovely Professional University
Phagwara, Punjab, India

Siddharth Mishra
Department of Hospital Administration
All India Institute of Medical Sciences
Bhubaneswar, India

Bhabendu Kumar Mohanta
Department of CSE
Koneru Lakshmaiah Education
    Foundation
Green Fields, Vaddeswaram, Andhra
    Pradesh, India

Ramkrishna Mondal
Department of Hospital Administration
All India Institute of Medical Sciences
Bhubaneswar, India

Ardhendu Sekhar Nanda
National Institute of Securities
    Markets and Maharashtra National
    Law University
Mumbai, India

Akarsh K. Nair
Indian Institute of Information
    Technology
Kottayam, Kerala

Azina Nazurally
University of Mauritius
Mauritius

S. Niveda
Department of Electronics and
    Communication Engineering
Sri Ramakrishna Engineering
    College
Coimbatore, India

Soufiene Ben Othman
PRINCE Laboratory Research,
    ISITcom, Hammam Sousse
University of Sousse
Tunisia

Isha Pant
THDC Institute of Hydropower
    Engineering and Technology
Uttarakhand, India

EbinDeni Raj
Indian Institute of Information
    Technology
Kottayam, Kerala

Himadri Nath Saha
Surendranath Evening College
Calcutta University
Kolkata, India

Hedi Sakli
EITA Consulting
Montesson, France

A. Siva Sakthi
Department of Biomedical
    Engineering
Sri Ramakrishna Engineering College
Coimbatore, India

Jayakrushna Sahoo
Indian Institute of Information
    Technology
Kottayam, Kerala

S. Srinitha
Department of Electronics and
    Communication Engineering
Sri Ramakrishna Engineering College
Coimbatore, India

Abhishek Srivastava
Pune Institute of Business
    Management
Pune, Maharastra

Aditee Swain
Department of Computer
    Applications
Utkal University
Bhubaneswar, India

Abhinay Thakur
Department of Chemistry
Lovely Professional University
Phagwara, Punjab, India

Apurva Saxena Verma
Researcher computer science
Bhopal, MP, India

.

1 Blockchain and Internet of Things in Healthcare Systems

Prospects, Issues, and Challenges

Kazeem Moses Abiodun and Emmanuel Abidemi Adeniyi
Landmark University, Omu Aran, Nigeria

Joseph Bamidele Awotunde
University of Ilorin, Ilorin, Nigeria

Chinmay Chakraborty
Birla Institute of Technology, Mesra, Ranchi, Jharkhand, India

Dayo Reuben Aremu
University of Ilorin, Ilorin, Nigeria

Ayodele Ariyo Adebiyi and Marion Olubunmi Adebiyi
Landmark University, Omu Aran, Nigeria

CONTENTS

DOI: 10.1201/9781003247128-1

1

1.1   INTRODUCTION

The healthcare industry is directly connected with people's social welfare and lives, so it is a critical concern for both developing and developed countries. In the healthcare sector, research and development should be a continuous process of making life easier by fighting the many health and illness problems. The innovation and latest breakthroughs in machinery have made it easy to witness the improvement in the healthcare sector. The healthcare and medical sectors' current capabilities can be enhanced by using cutting-edge and innovative computer technologies. These technologies can aid doctors and medical professionals in the initial detection of a variety of ailments. These powerful computer technologies can also greatly increase the precision of identifying diseases in their initial periods. The various technologies used will allow the IoT devices to exchange information about patient health progress and how they are responding to treatment to their physicians for proper monitoring. IoT makes the connection of humans to humans possible, human to things, and things to other things [1]. Blockchain technology's uniqueness is its ability to store data immutably without relying on a central authority.

Various developing and innovative computer technologies are already being applied with spectacular outcomes in other industries. IoT, blockchain, machine learning, data mining, NLP, computer vision, the clouds, and many other technologies are among them. The Internet of Things (IoT) refers to the notion that everything is linked to the Web. Vehicles, household equipment, people and other digital objects as well as applications, sensors, drive systems, and connectors that enable data to be connected and collected, and distributed, are all included in this category. Kevin Ashton is known as the "Father of the Internet of Things", which refers to Internet connectivity that extends from devices like PCs, computers, mobile phones, and there are several physical technologies and daily things not available on the Internet. Wireless connectivity, clouds, sensors and security are the most common technologies employed in the IoT. The four parts of the IoT lifecycle are as follows:

1. Data is collected using sensors on devices;
2. The collected data is saved in the cloud for analysis;
3. The gadget then receives the examined data; and
4. The equipment responds appropriately.

[2]

IoT is useful in a variety of fields, making our lives easier. Agribusiness, smart retailers, autonomous driving and healthcare, smart buildings, smart cities are the most common IoT applications. Security is an important part of any technology, and it is fundamental to the successful operation of IoT networks. Secrecy and authenticity of data, IT communication protocols, user confidence and reliance and the implementation of confidentiality principles techniques are some of the active projects for improving IoT security. The IoT security issue develops as a result of poor program design, which leads to vulnerabilities, which is a major cause of network security difficulties. Proper IoT initialization is achieved in IoT architecture physically to prevent an illegitimate recipient from accessing the system. The five levels of IoT architecture are perceptual layer, logical layer, Internet layer, middleware layer, application layer and business layer. Each level has its own set of aims and challenges. Integrity and Reliability are the three cornerstones of a secure network in IoT. (CIA).

Vulnerabilities in IoT can be classified into four categories, according to multiple research papers: physical assault, intrusion software, networking strike and attack cryptography. The physical attack could take several forms, including (a) node tempering, in which the attacker modifies the compromised node to obtain the encryption key; (b) attack of the IoT system, in which the attacker physically damages the IoT system thereby causing a Denial of Service (DOS) attack; (c) injection of malicious code, which allows the attacker to take complete IoT system management; (d) RF Disturbance to radiofrequency signals is used for RFID communications in which the intruder provides random noise over radio frequency signals; (e) the hacker employs psychological manipulation to acquire the client of an IoT system with sensitive data for his purposes; (f) attack to sleep impoverishment, in which nodes are shut down.; and (g) jamming of nodes in WSNs, the attacker can distract wireless communication by using a jammer. Among the software attacks are (a) phishing attacks, where the attacker creates a false website to gain the user's personal information; (b) virus attacks, which can harm the system by propagating harmful code via The Internet and email files, and without the assistance of individuals, the virus may reproduce itself; (c) malicious files used to access the system; and (d) the denial of service (DOS) assault which prevents users to access the system.

Another concern is network assaults, which comprise but are not restricted to (a) traffic investigation attacks, in which the intruder accesses, analyzes; (b) spoofs RFID transmissions to spoof the assailant, modify the data and provide the system with erroneous information (the method receives incorrect data that has been tampered with by the attacker); (c) sinkhole attack, which is one of the most popular types of attack (the assailant introduces a harmful node within the system and that many nodes are identified in one component of the system); and (d) assault of Sybil: the assailant inserts a wormhole attack within the system and the network node adopts numerous node identities. An encryption attack could be the source of yet another security breach. The primary goal of this violence is to gain the private key, which is required to communicate between two devices. The different types are (a) side-channel: in this attack, the attacker provides some additional information when transferring the information from user to server or vice versa; (b) cryptanalysis assaults: the assailant decrypts data from a reading form without knowing the key throughout this assault; and (c) middleman assault:

the assailant monitors data by interfering with connectivity among nodes in the literature, there are a number of security suggestions. Conversely, because of current difficulties such as centralization, single point of failure and so on, security remains a source of concern in IoT networks. As a result, a novel and developing innovation known as 'blockchain' can be utilized in conjunction with IoT to improve IoT security. By addressing the problems in IoT, blockchain's strong technologies may be applied to increase its performance and make it a more robust connection and centralized concerns in current security processes, and introduce the notion of decentralization through the blockchain system [3].

Blockchain is a decentralized point-to-point system without the need a someone else for transactions and communication [4]. All of the transactions are self-contained and separate from one another. The blockchain is the technology that underpins the popular and revolutionary concept of cryptocurrencies. Cryptocurrency is thought to be extremely safe and unhackable. The same blockchain technology can be applied to other networks to enhance security. The fresh and growing advent technologies in any industry can result in several concerns and challenges. As a result, identifying those concerns and obstacles is critical, particularly in the healthcare industry, where people's lives are closely linked. The prospect of implementing blockchain and IoT in the healthcare industry is addressed in this chapter, as well as numerous new healthcare applications that can be created using these revolutionary technologies. The obstacles and issues associated with the use of these two developing innovations in the healthcare industry are then discussed in depth.

The other parts of this chapter include: Section 1.2 review related works; Section 1.3 discusses the IoT and blockchain integration in healthcare system. Section 1.4 focusses on the challenges, prospect and issues in blockchain and IoT integration for healthcare system. Section 1.5 discusses the proposed framework and how it works. Lastly, Section 1.6 recapitulates the research outcomes and proposal for future work.

1.2 LITERATURE REVIEW

In [5], the authors suggested the blockchain-based IoT Model to better systematically handle transactions performed through healthcare technologies. The MQTT protocol was recommended as the main agent for the architectural connection of biosensors with the IoT system. Furthermore, the architecture included the IPFS (Inter-Planetary File System), which may identify state entries or block modifications when certain transactions are affixed to the nodes, reducing the deduplication of the stored transactions. In [6], the authors presented an interactive environment for an IoT-controlled healthcare system. The suggested architecture is based on the ingestion of generating intelligent wearable gadgets and organic sensor readings, as well as providing patients with clear feedback and simple solutions. In [7], the paper presented an intelligent system in the clinic combining sensor performance with human sensors responses for speedier and timelier patient counselling. The proposal encourages the use of RFID, WSN, and wearable devices that operate on one channel to perform tasks such as intelligent detecting the patient's ecosystem, patient allotments based on the criteria for doctor selection, patient monitoring and reporting cantered on model estimation. The authors in [8] designed a platform for the transmission of health information that outstrips the present approach by allowing for pseudonymity and safeguarding customer identity whose information is published and used by clinical study centres. The study also developed the notion of a Consensus Mechanism to 'prove interoperability' that enabled system-based companies to perform seamless and more effective operations completely based on compatibility inside the system. In addition, the researcher introduced a multi-architecture at different stages – the web service, which clinicians will use to submit and preserve the medical records, the cloud middleware, to preserve information from web fetching services via the REST API system and to call on Smart Contracts to perform the prescribed enrolment.

In a similar work, authors in [9] used the ACP Method that is deployed on the public blockchain, provides a parallel health service. The framework describes the use of the Concurrent Medical System centred on the medicinal expertise and experience of the medical professionals as well as the use of a scheme of machine learning which dictates the application and parallel strategy of the Virtual Physicians and Virtual Clinicians in the therapy of their clinicians. The second part of the ACP method is the Clinical and Scientific Process Phase in which the four are integrated with the general clinical and test method to be done on patients. In Section 1.3, the Artificial Medical System and the Actual Health Service are implemented in tandem with the engagement of actual physicians with artificial or application physicians. The essential notion of the distributed connection is that the computer investigations for patients are done by artificial or application physicians based on characteristics that have been introduced to the platform and physicians will verify and improve the findings provided by the artificial physicians. A blockchain System comprising a partnership of physicians, clinics, medical offices and patients was also added into the Complete Healthcare System, which may be used for data review and exchange.

In [10], the authors covered the many forms of blockchain designs that are now accessible, as well as the foundations of all sorts of blockchains and how they may be utilized for data management, verification and storing in the medical business. The blockchain collaboration was also highlighted as the answer that originated primarily from the care services storage box. The blockchain technology of the collaboration is a lawful blockchain with identity management by both the node operator and the miners. In addition, the blockchain consortium is centred on the agreement concept of a significant contributor or Ethereum blockchain component. In [11], the authors presented an advanced blockchain architecture for e-healthcare system governance. The work's main focus was the implementation of a system for the seamless and correct exchange of patient data amongst many participants in an extensible and adaptable network approach. Moreover, modern blockchain technology complies with the major auditing methodologies used to guarantee the authenticity and integrities of a document by participants such as insurance providers, clinics and physicians published on the network.

In [12], the study created a healthcare blockchain in which the HIPAA privacy restriction was handled by employing data including population and ethnic features of controlled patients. Furthermore, the experiment demonstrated a blockchain network's generative architecture, which included three sorts of channels: emergency care, referrals and medical staff networks. The authors in [13] designed and developed an innovative strategy for health monitoring, as well as supporting the fundamental telehealth technology is implemented in remote areas when the connection is available is critical. The project resulted in the creation of a portable technology for sensing patients in remote regions. Moreover, the system can function online as well as offline to enable tiny data packs from the devices to be saved in an on-the-job database and subsequently communicated either on-the-job or via the Web to healthcare professionals, contingent on what is most advantageous at the moment. The solution also dealt with the usage of multi-channel doctors, allowing them to take over patient cases from remote sensing centres.

In [14], the information exchange and cooperation blockchain technology has been connected with the Structure of blockchain. The objective of the system presented in the study was to share and collaborate with a group of organizations including patients, doctors, health professionals and health insurance companies. The wearable device of the patient is linked to a server or internet that keeps all patient information. Because vast numbers of data are collected daily, the research proposes that data batches be stored for convenient and faster data acquisition in a Merkle tree design. Patients may publish data with medical and insurance agencies to obtain services or insurance estimates, as appropriate. The work's system was defined as a client centre platform that has been completed by the patient control over whether or not his or her data was shared. The work's system was defined as a user-centric scheme in which the patient had broad control over whether or not his or her data was shared. This type of technology can be extremely useful in medical research as well as the safeguarding and secrecy of individual medical information are paramount.

A remote e-health system comprising healthcare professionals, medical professionals, and patients was proposed in [15]. Under the IoT scenario, sensors have been used for real-time patient medication, with the use of the intelligent contract ecosystem TESTRPC to store medical information on a blockchain. The safety and privacy of healthcare information are essential in practice; a strategy to handle this issue has been presented [16]. In recent times, Ethereum was utilized to fulfil the P5 need for intelligent e-health, which includes the following: (1) participative; (2) custom; (3) accurate; (4) predictive; and (5) preventative [17, 18]. Looked at the patient safety and survivability steps that can be taken on a big scale in the healthcare business by merging IoT with blockchain. A general assessment of blockchain networks ledger technology has been discussed to address the demands of future biomedicine and e-healthcare [19].

Authors proposed the notion of pseudonymized encryption using several rights to enable a patient to view, examine, and change their medical records on an IoT system [20]. With trust being such a difficult topic, [21] presented an architecture, dubbed IoT-Chain, to help patients control their health devices and data using IoT and blockchain. In [22], dyslexic people and their caregivers utilize the IoT-based digital healthcare management solution Dyslexia to use, preserve and access the dyslexic sequence in a multimodal data exchange structure. Agility has been evaluated for a blockchain infrastructure built on software IoT to provide greater flexibility, cost-effectiveness, and privacy for e-healthcare applications [23]. The blockchain-based IoT-centric patient interface was developed to deliver end-to-end patient monitoring services.

The works review revealed scarce key exploration gaps in present IoT–blockchain e-healthcare facilities, which must be recognized and efficiently employed to fully utilize IoT-centric health services. IoT–blockchain systems have not been investigated for medical services, and IoT-enabled systemic use applications with blockchain in e-healthcare have been investigated which were not developed. As a result, this chapter contributes to filling these research gaps, allowing for a growth of similar interest within the research community.

1.3 BLOCKCHAIN TECHNOLOGY AND IOT

Blockchain is a novel expertise that is being used in a variety of networks to maintain its security and stability. In many transactions management systems, distributed ledgers are also given priority and progressively replace the present system. The encrypted ledger is kept on a blockchain, which is a public distributed database [24]. In a centralized architecture, there is a central coordinating mechanism that is linked to each node. This essential coordination system will communicate, pass and authorize all information amongst the nodes. If the central coordinating platform fails, all these dependent components are removed under this platform. As a result, moving away from a unified scheme and near a dispersed scheme is critical. In the distributed network there will be more than one supervisor. There is no centralized authority in a dispersed system because each node is viewed as a coordinator. Each node is connected, and the system does not depend on one coordinator.

A blockchain is made up of a series of blocks, each of which is a collection of all recently completed and validated transactions. Figure 1.1 depicts the broad and detailed structure of the blockchain, which shows the block sequencing and how every packet is encrypted related. Each block stores all of these transaction details, and a consolidated hash code is produced and stored block by block. This transaction is a key element of the blockchain once the transaction is verified, and the chain continues to develop. Blockchain is a technological leader, second only to bitcoin in popularity. The operation of bitcoins on the blockchain can aid in the comprehension of blockchain technology. The authors in [25] invented bitcoin, the first decentralized digital money, in 2009. Bitcoin employs a variety of cryptographic and mathematical ideas to ensure that the generation and managing of bitcoin are both limited and secure. The procedures and cryptographic tools employed are updated regularly. The electronic and extremely secure blockchain is a ledger structure that tracks how much bitcoins are being processed.

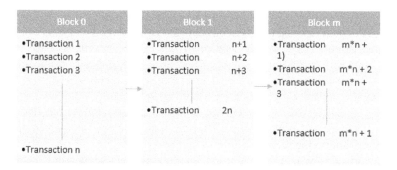

FIGURE 1.1   Structure of the blockchain.

There are several main ideas in the blockchain. Previous hash code is one of them. Every block must have a hash code assigned to it, which serves as a unique identifier for that block. This hash is generated using a sophisticated hashing technique. To be a part of that block, the information about each transaction that occurred must be finalized. The header of a block contains the transaction details in the form of a hex value known as Merkle Root. A block is a critical component of a blockchain recording and completing all transaction history is stored as a permanent database in the blockchain. Blockchain is made up of three different technologies: (1) It secures identities with private key cryptography and employs a hash function to make the blockchain unchangeable; (2) It employs a peer-to-peer (P2P) network, which provides perfect blockchain consistency [26, 27]. Where a person makes a tiny change to a blockchain transaction or block, the modified block cannot be uploaded or shown in blockchain as most people on the networks have an initial blockchain and the block modification can't be included or mirrored in blockchain; and (3) The program that creates the blockchain contains numerous rules and security features. The most popular programming language for creating blockchain smart contracts is called 'Solidity'.

Each transaction that is verified and confirmed when a new block is developed is logged in a blockchain with details on the time, date, parties and cash is sent over. Every user who belongs to the blockchain has its blockchain replica. A difficult math puzzle after solution, the miner checks each transaction in the blockchain, and once the riddle is solved, the transaction is validated and recorded in the ledger.

1.3.1   FEATURES OF BLOCKCHAIN

Decentralization, openness, free software, autonomy, imponderability and anonymity are just a few of blockchain's distinctive and important characteristics, making it a unique and strong solution in an IoT medical organization that guarantees security and dependability [28]. When learning about blockchain, you'll need to know a lot of words. The following are some of the significant capabilities enabled by blockchain technology, as depicted in Figure 1.2.

Features of Blockchain	Decentralized
	Immutable and Non-Repudiable
	Trustless Operation (Consensus)
	Cryptographically Secured
	Digital Ledger
	Distributed
	Transparent and Verifiable
	Chronological and time stamped

FIGURE 1.2   Features of the blockchain.

Decentralized application. The blockchain is built around decentralized apps. It has potential to solve all complications associated with the current centralized approach. The smart contracts are invoked by the user, which makes the decentralized architecture operate. Ethereum is a smart contract-based decentralized platform. It was first proposed in 2013 and then made public in 2015. 'Ether' is the Ethereum Blockchain's value token, which is traded on cryptocurrency exchanges under the symbol ETH. The smart contract includes all of the guidelines that apply to the facility being supplied, including state information and data for smart agreements [29]. A smart agreement is a computerized robotic system for digitally enabling, proving, or imposing the negotiation or performance of a legal contract by bypassing intermediaries and validate the contract immediately using a decentralized platform. Software engineer and encryption expert Nick Szabo coined the term in 1996. Smart contracts, he suggested, with the aid of a distributed ledger, might be established. These are some of the advantages of decentralized apps:

(1) Autonomy: there is no need for a broker or a lawyer because you are the one agreeing;
(2) Trust: in blockchain-based decentralized apps, all documents and data are secured the data will be disseminated using advanced encryption technologies via a distributed platform maintained by a common ledger. If the data is damaged or modified, the members of the Ledger will reject it;
(3) Backup plan: documents are replicated and stored in several locations on the blockchain; and
(4) Reliability: smart contracts are more efficient and less expensive because they avoid the faults that come with physical labour.

Public Distributed Ledger (PDL). Because the data on a blockchain is open to anyone, it provides transparency. As long as you're coupled to the system, you'll be able to see the whole account of dealings that took place since the formation of the blockchain. The user must agree on any modifications to blockchain first. Any changes to the blockchain must be authorized by a majority of the network participants. This is the open portion of the booklet [30]. Hyperledger may be seen as a software component that allows anyone to develop their blockchain service. Only parties directly involved in the transaction were modified and alerted on the ledger on the Hyperledger network.

The Protocol of Consensus. The term "autonomy" comes from the Consensus Protocol. Consensus assures that the most recent block has been accurately put to the chain [31]. Consensus techniques have been implemented for ledger consistency and user security [32]. Table 4 [33] lists a variety of consensus procedures.

Immutable. Immutable refers to something that cannot be altered. It is a key aspect of blockchain that blocks cannot be modified. The concept of proof of work is used to achieve immutability. Mining is used to achieve proof of work, and the miner's job is to modify the nonce. A nonce is a randomly generated value that is smaller than the intended hash value to provide a single hash address for the block. The chances of calculating evidence of work are quite slim. To provide credible proof of labour, many experiments must be conducted. When an attacker gains control of more than 51% of the nodes at the same time, there is only one way to change the block [31].

Anonymity. Anonymity refers to the lack of a name, and it is one of the blockchain's properties. The neutrality of the transmitter and the recipient are the two halves of the anonymity set. When one person provides data to other users, this example works; but it does not expose the user's true uniqueness. Instead, it uses blockchain addresses to communicate with other users. This approach ensures that neither user knows the other's true identity [31, 32].

Improved Security. Because everything on the blockchain is public, the privacy solution is hashing encryption. When compared to traditional systems, blockchain can provide enhanced security and provide certain benefits [33, 34]. To comprehend hashing encryption, we must first comprehend the block's properties. A container is a box that holds transaction information. The block is shared into two sections: the header and the transaction data. The header of a block comprises the transaction details in the hexagonal value known as Merkle Root. Cryptography is performed on the blockchain using the hash function [35].

Traceability. The distribution chain is used to determine the product's origin and track the sequence. The term "traceability" refers to configuration blocks on the blockchain where every block is connected to two adjacent blocks by the hash key [29].

Currency Specifications. A point-to-point network is what blockchain is. The transaction does not necessitate the use of a third party. All transactions are conducted without the involvement of a third party. The transaction is used in cryptocurrency blockchain, and it has a steady flow. All applications in blockchain 2.0 and 3.0 are owned by money [29].

1.3.2 The Internet of Things

The IoT is a collection of special sensors that connect the entire world to the Internet. The term IoT, according to experts, implies the next step in the digital community. The IoT intends to improve academic and commercial institutions' competitiveness. Industry 4.0 [36, 37], which is based on IoT, is about digital transformation, automation and data sharing among multiple providers. Many of our towns are now being transformed into smart cities as a result of our generation's use of IoT. Similarly, several of our learning environments have begun to embrace IoT to transform our campus into a smart campus. For our undergraduate students, a lot of higher learning institutions are currently offering elective IoT-related courses in Computer Ad Engineering. [38]. Urban transformation, waste management facilities, parking spaces, effective traffic management, lighting systems, environmental surveillance, efficient irrigation systems, smart home encroachment revealing systems, banking and other applications are all part of the IoT. Furthermore, social networks have evolved quickly to efficiently enter a wide range of sectors [39–42], and many innovations have been incorporated, with IoT being no exception.

IoT social networks were merged with the Internet to turn the in a simulated actual world. The results of the study suggest the usage of social networking services (SIoT), which allow for the appropriate and productive development of new IoT applications and networking services [43]. The fundamental objective of the social IoT is to integrate devices into the daily lives of people through using social network advantages such as user-friendliness and interconnection. New appealing services must be created to encourage users to connect their devices to others to promote the SIoT project and ensure its long-term viability [44]. Because of continuous breakthroughs in cloud computing, networking, sensors, nanoelectronics, intelligent things and Big Data, IoT advancements will accelerate. The IoT is a component of the Internet that allows people to interact with one another through connecting people and objects, as well as connecting objects with other things.

IoT devices are responsible for ensuring that information and data are transmitted to their targeted receivers through the gadgets. Device-to-device and human-to-device IoT applications allow communication [45]. Every day, the IoT connects millions of domains and devices. IoT technology is used in everyday life to link a variety of everyday items, including cell phones, cars, home lights, electronics web and wearable devices. IoT in healthcare: The medical sector has several concerns and challenges that can be addressed with the help of the IoT [46]. In addition, the IoT has the potential to significantly improve healthcare skills. Inaccurate conventional analyses and other advances like remote access of the patient are feasible due to a lack of actual data, smart cards devices and other advances utilizing IoT in the healthcare sector. IoT could be the solution to all of these issues. IoT can be applied in smart cities, agriculture, industrial automation and control of disasters, to name a few areas. Figure 1.3 depicts some of the applications and sectors where IoT can be used.

1.3.3 BLOCKCHAIN AND IoT TECHNOLOGIES INTEGRATION IN HEALTHCARE

The number of patients in every nation is growing every day, and providing comprehensive medical treatment has become more challenging as a result. With the use of IoT and wearable devices, the quality of medical care has increased in

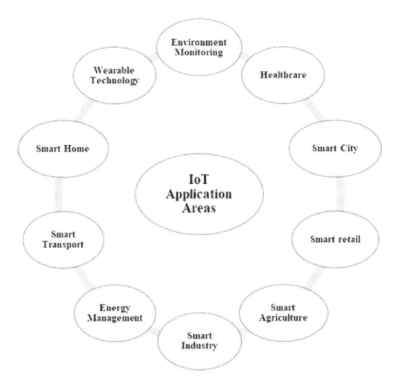

FIGURE 1.3   Application area of Internet of Things.

recent years [47]. The primary method of addressing healthcare issues is remote patient monitoring. Wearable gadgets that gather and transmit data to hospitals, as well as IoT devices, play a critical reload patient surveillance duty [48]. The main aim of these instruments is to provide health specialists with essential information, such as respiratory patterns, blood glucose and blood pressure. [49].

Data gathering equipment in healthcare can be divided into four categories: (i) patient medical sensors; (ii) medical equipment; (iii) wearable devices; and (iv) medical scans equipment. Medical equipment is placed into the human body, the medical equipment wearable: (ii) physicians prescribe this equipment, and wearable medical devices, which are worn on the body. RPM's major goal is to protect data that is being targeted by hackers. Blockchain technology is utilized to safeguard the data. By utilizing the principle of decentralization, blockchain helps to protect data from a variety of threats. Smart contracts on the blockchain also authenticate the data. Healthcare is a type of IoT system that has its own set of needs, such as security of patient data through interconnection and data transmission. The process of sharing data with different sources is referred to as interoperability. The limitation to accomplish interoperability is part of the centralized notion. The IoT is predicated on centralization, with data being stored in the cloud, which is not safe. The security concerns that healthcare apps confront can be overcome by combining blockchain and IoT [50]. Many experiments in blockchain have already been conducted in the field of healthcare [51].

1.3.4 DIGITAL HEALTH TRANSFORMATION USING AI

As a result of its ability to harness the power of large data and acquire expertise for assisting scientific proof clinical decision-making and attaining significance care, artificial intelligence (AI) is quickly growing in healthcare. Professionals in hospitals must grasp the current status of AI technologies and how they may be utilized to maximize the productivity, quality and accessibility of health services, therefore assisting in the digitalization of the healthcare industry. From medical decision assistance at the spot of treatment to patient self-management of chronic diseases at home and therapeutic discovery in the reality, it is clear that AI has started to impact nearly every area of health services.

The smart medical professional requires three main modules: (1) A digitalized channel with enhanced data management, suitable in a cloud service; (2) Technologically sophisticated such as AI and authentic, in-memory insights grounded within enterprise applications; that then incorporates the formation of (3) An intelligent and groundbreaking healthcare software platform are among them. With an integrated approach to innovation and a focus on basic patient needs, the effect of intelligent technology to expedite the execution of real worth care will be transformative for the healthcare sector. So, the doctor–patient connection is going to change from reactive health (a paternalism method is proposed based on clinical symptoms to assessment and treatment) to proactive health (individualized, early warning signs sensors with neutral data collection and pertinent biomarkers as well as forecasting models based on epigenetic predisposition).

Nevertheless, the creation and adoption of AI technology is difficult and expensive. In a bid for AI to be successful, medical associations must address a variety of obstacles. These problems include: insufficient knowledge about what an AI technology can and cannot do; absence of appropriate techniques for implementing various AI technologies into the present healthcare system to help resolve the most urgent concerns that health authorities face today; scarcity of well-trained employees for AI implementation; and lack of integration of AI technologies with previous healthcare institutions [52,53].

1.4 CHALLENGES AND PROSPECTS OF USING BLOCKCHAIN AND IOT IN HEALTHCARE

The following are the primary hurdles in the adoption of blockchain technology and IoT in the healthcare and medical sectors:

1. Security Concerns. Decentralization improves the security of blockchains, but it also has some drawbacks, such as data being published in a public ledger, which can lead to privacy leakage. Blockchain creates

an environment in which people know and trust one another and can safely share data. It may, however, fail in certain circumstances, such as if 51% of the consensus nodes are malevolent. Due to security concerns, many patients may be hesitant to share their personal medical information [54].

2. Scalability and storage. It is impossible to keep track of every single person's information. Documents, photographs and lab reports are commonly included in medical records. The digital preservation of many patients' medical records will necessitate massive storage volume. Medical businesses for each individual kept in a dispersed fashion, with the same record stored in multiple locations, will necessitate a large amount of storage capacity and may have an impact on the healthcare system [55].

3. Standardization. Even though blockchain is a popular technology that has been embraced in numerous nations. In areas and networks involving and cryptocurrency the ideas of security, confidence and trackability, the issue of the standard remains a challenge. Standardization of protocols, technology and other elements is critical. Data types, sizes and formats that can be supplied to the blockchain, as well as data types that may be kept, explicitly specified in the blockchain [56, 57].

4. Interoperability issues. In the blockchain network, healthcare interoperability implies exchanging information with one another. It is the most difficult due to the enormous number of providers and its open nature [58]. There could be a variety of participants, including hospitals, insurance firms, physicians and private doctors, among others. It can be difficult to ensure proper interoperability in the healthcare industry.

5. Sharing of information. Many hospitals, particularly for-profit situations, are hesitant to disclose patient-related and other medical details because they would like to offer various customer prices. Healthcare facilities and insurance are also involved firms may be hesitant to disclose their data because keeping fees-related data to themselves can be commercially advantageous. Building trust between the stakeholders and persuading them to give their data for the sake of an improved healthcare system is critical [59].

6. Patients are hesitant to share their history of medicine. The achievement of these technological advancements in medical and healthcare systems is vital to building credibility with one of the most important stakeholders, patients. Many patients are cautious to share and expose their medical details with third-party organizations in the public domain. As a result, building patients' loyalty in the data protection elements of the medical system blockchain and IoT is critical.

7. Doctors and medical practitioners require technical skills. It might be difficult to convince specialists and other health professionals to switch from paper to technology. Many people find it difficult to switch from paper-based prescriptions to electronic records and prescriptions. In their

daily work, doctors, for example, rarely fill in extraneous fields while filling out forms. Doctors, on the other hand, cannot delete mandatory fields from computerized records. Likewise, using remote monitoring technologies such as blockchain and IoT can increase concerns about their accuracy and efficiency among many clinicians. The precision, efficiency and performance of this technology-driven healthcare will be determined by specialists' skills and training. So, before putting these skills into exercise, doctors must have sufficient training and the necessary abilities to gain confidence in their use.

8. Data possession and responsibilities data possession and responsibility are further obstacles to the integration of blockchain and IoT in the healthcare industry. The main concerns are who holds the data, who permits to share personal health-related data with individuals, and who owns it. Despite all of the problems described above, the benefits of employing blockchain and IoT exceed the disadvantages because they are easily overcome.

The following are the benefits of blockchain and IoT in healthcare:

1. **Privacy/Anonymity:** Blockchain employs public-key cryptography to create a digital identity for transactions. This method conceals the true identity of IoT applications that contain sensitive information.

2. **Reliability:** Data from IoT applications is routed across infrastructure that is owned by multiple businesses [59]. This is essential to track data from IoT applications to advance the facilities that enterprises deliver. Supply chain monitoring has traditionally relied on unified design, but blockchain's distributed ledger provides greater confidence when moving resources (physical or virtual) through infrastructure held by various and varied participants.

3. **Smart contracts:** Some blockchain networks, like Ethereum, have "smart contract" features that allow users to create agreements that will be implemented when certain circumstances are satisfied. One system, for example, is certified to pay if certain settings are met (services delivered). Smart contracts are built into the system.

4. **DDoS mitigation and notification:** Smart contracts and blockchain can be combined to create a collaborative architecture that offers DDoS notification across several domains. For example, utilizing software-defined network technologies, the work in [60] suggests a solution based on smart contracts that broadcast white- or black-listed IP addresses between users and autonomous devices in a public and distributed infrastructure. Furthermore, attackers are prevented from directly installing malware on IoT devices and establishing IoT botnets to conduct enormous DDoS attacks using trustworthy blockchain-based transactions. Checking outbound traffic also stops DDoS messages from spreading from IoT devices.

1.5   PROPOSED FRAMEWORK

Figure 1.4 shows the proposed framework for improving the security of the healthcare system using blockchain technology and at the same time improved data collection from the patient for better record keeping and providing an excellent diagnosis.

The architecture of the proposed system is depicted in Figure 1.5. It has four modules that work together to improve the healthcare system.

MODULE 1: Module 1 is tagged the Medical Information Module, where we have the patient supplying information to the medical practitioner of what he/she is feeling in a secured environment. The module also involved the response of the medical practitioner to the patient.

MODULE 2: This is the Medical IoT devices module that aids the patient in sending vital information to the healthcare provider. We have several examples available like wearable devices and monitoring devices.

MODULE 3: This module provides secured transactions between the patient and the Medical Practitioners using smart contracts so that private data will not be exposed to the general public. Blockchain has to be proved overtime to maintain the security of information among the parties that uses it.

MODULE 4: The cloud module plays a vital role in keeping data secured and makes it easy to retrieve data. It makes data available anytime, anywhere and wherever one needs it.

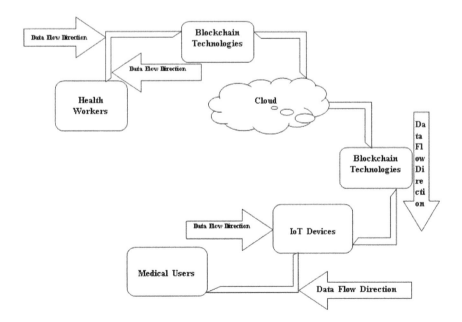

FIGURE 1.4   Blockchain and IoT framework for the healthcare system.

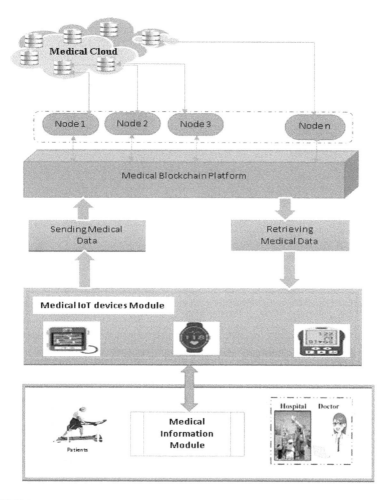

FIGURE 1.5 The proposed blockchain-enabled IoT-based architecture.

The data flow of the healthcare system is shown in Figure 1.6, the patient through the IoT system generates information that is passed through the blockchain and later stored in the cloud. The healthcare provider requests the information from the cloud using the necessary access code and then analyzes the data and gives a response through the same channel to the patient who then acts on the information and once again gives feedback using the same process.

1.6 CONCLUSION

This research looked at how blockchain and IoT technology can be used to improve healthcare systems and services. The IoT-based blockchain healthcare architecture was demonstrated, which allows users to access and manage

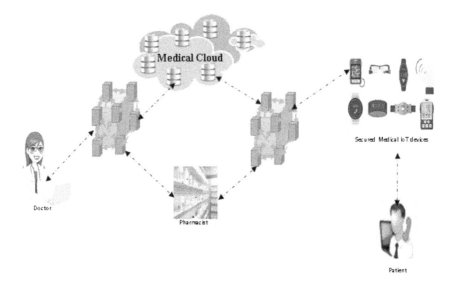

FIGURE 1.6 Data flow application of the blockchain and IoT healthcare system.

healthcare data in a highly trusted, secure, transparent and efficient manner. The idea is to give patients authority and ownership over their medical data, allowing them to share it with whoever they wish in a secure setting. The healthcare ecosystem is predicted to be reshaped by blockchain technology. Not only will the procedure be transparent and secure, but the quality of healthcare will also improve while costs are reduced. Even with these significant advancements in medical and smartphone applications, there are still significant security concerns, as blockchain is not without its flaws. Healthcare, and any other party interested in using blockchain-enabled devices, should invest in additional research in these areas to enhance them, and build a strong ecosystem that can be utilized to increase patient data empowerment.

Future work should look into the scalability of blockchain-enabled healthcare because healthcare is a developing industry, and as our society evolves, scalability is a big concern. As the number of blockchain-enabled applications grows, it will become progressively more difficult to run them as more patients on the system increases. The implementation of the proposed framework will be looked into to see if it has future work in the area of healthcare system to assess the applicability of the proposed framework.

CONFLICT OF INTEREST

There is no conflict of interest.

FUNDING

There is no funding support.

DATA AVAILABILITY

Not applicable.

REFERENCES

1. J. Kizza, *Internet of Things (IoT): Growth, challenges, and security in Guide to Computer Network Security* (pp. 517–531), 2017. Springer, Berlin, Germany.
2. D. Sachin, C. Chinmay, F. Jaroslav, et al., SSII: Secured and high-quality steganography using intelligent hybrid optimization algorithms for IoT, *IEEE Access*, vol. 9, pp. 1–16, 2021, 10.1109/ACCESS.2021.3089357.
3. D. Cinay, L. D. Brian, and C. Chinmay, Generative Design Methodology for Internet of Medical Things (IoMT)-based Wearable Biomedical Devices. In *Int. Congress on Human-Computer Interaction, Optimization and Robotic Applications (HORA'21)* (pp. 1–4), 2021, doi: 10.1109/HORA52670.2021.9461370
4. J. Wang, et al., Blockchain-based data storage mechanism for industrial internet of things, *Intelligent Automation & Soft Computing*, vol. 26, no. 5, pp. 1157–1172, 2020.
5. T. Dey, et al., Health sense: A medical use case of Internet of Things and blockchain. In *2017 International Conference on Intelligent Sustainable Systems (ICISS)* (pp. 486–491), 2017. IEEE. 263
6. D. Budida, and R. Mangrulkar, Design and implementation of smart healthcare system using IoT. In *Innovations in Information, Embedded and Communication Systems (ICIIECS), 2017 International Conference on* (pp. 1–7), 2017. IEEE.
7. S. Sivagami, D. Revathy, and L. Nithyabharathi, Smart healthcare system implemented using IoT, *International Journal of Contemporary Research in Computer Science and Technology*, vol. 2, no. 3, (pp. 1–11) 2016.
8. A. Theodouli, S. Arakliotis, K. Moschou, K. Votis, and D. Tzovaras, On the design of a Blockchain-based system to facilitate Healthcare Data Sharing. In *2018 17th IEEE International Conference On Trust, Security And Privacy In Computing And Communications/12th IEEE International Conference On Big Data Science And Engineering (Trust Com/BigDataSE)* (pp. 1374–1379), 2018, August. IEEE.
9. J. B. Awotunde, R. O. Ogundokun, S. Misra, E. A. Adeniyi, and M. M. Sharma, Blockchain-based framework for secure transaction in mobile banking platform, *Advances in Intelligent Systems and Computing*, 1375 AIST, pp. 525–534, 2021.
10. Z. Alhadhrami, et al., Introducing blockchains for healthcare. In *Electrical and Computing Technologies and Applications (ICECTA), 2017 International Conference on* (pp. 1–4), 2017. IEEE.
11. W. Liu, S. Zhu, T. Mundie, and U. Krieger, Advanced blockchain architecture for e-health systems. In *e-Health Networking, Applications and Services (Healthcom), 2017 IEEE 19th International Conference on* (pp. 1–6), 2017. IEEE.
12. T. Ahram, Blockchain technology innovations. In *Technology & Engineering Management Conference (TEMSCON)* (pp. 137–141), 2017. IEEE.
13. A. K. Gupta, C. Chakraborty, and B. Gupta, Secure transmission of EEG data using watermarking algorithm for the detection of epileptic seizures, traitement du signal, *IIETA*, 38(2), 473–479, 2027, doi:10.18280/ts.380227
14. X. Liang, J. Zhao, S. Shetty, J. Liu, and Danyi Li, Integrating blockchain for data sharing and collaboration in mobile healthcare applications. In *Personal, Indoor, and Mobile Radio Communications (PIMRC), 2017 IEEE 28th Annual International Symposium on* (pp. 1–5), 2017. IEEE.

15. H. L. Pham, T. H. Tran, and Y. Nakashima, A secure remote healthcare system for a hospital using blockchain smart contract. In *Proc. IEEE Globecom Workshops* (pp. 1–6), 2018.

16. K. Manpreet, MBCP: Performance analysis of large scale mainstream blockchain consensus protocols, *IEEE Access*, vol. 9, pp. 1–14, 2021. d: 10.1109/ACCESS.2021.3085187

17. A. Talukder, Proof of disease: A blockchain consensus protocol for accurate medical decisions and reducing the disease burden. In *Proceeding IEEE Smart World, Ubiquitous Intell. Comput., Adv. Trusted Computer, Scalable Comput. Commun., Cloud Big Data Comput., Internet People Smart City Innov.* (pp. 257–262), 2018.

18. K. Amit, et al., A novel fog computing approach for minimization of latency in healthcare using machine learning, *International Journal of Interactive Multimedia and Artificial Intelligence*, pp. 1–11, 2020, doi:10.9781/ijimai.2020.12.004

19. T.-T. Kuo, H.-E. Kim, and L. Ohno-Machado, Blockchain distributed ledger technologies for biomedical and healthcare applications, *Journal of the American Medical Informatics Association*, vol. 24, no. 6, pp. 1211–1220, 2017.

20. S. Badr, I. Gomaa, and E. Elrahmanb, Multi-tier blockchain framework for IoT-EHRs systems, *Procedia Computer Science*, vol. 141, pp. 159–166, 2018.

21. B. Yu, J. Wright, S. Nepal, L. Zhu, J. Liu, and R. Ranjan, IoTChain: Establishing trust in the Internet of things ecosystem using blockchain. *IEEE Cloud Computing*, vol. 5, no. 4, pp. 12–13, Jul./Aug. 2018.

22. Md A. Rahman, E. Hassanain, M. M. Rashid, S. J. Barnes, and M. S. Hossain, Spatial blockchain-based secure mass screening framework for children with dyslexia, *IEEE Access*, vol. 6, pp. 61876–61885, 2018.

23. S. Arindam, Z. A. Mohammad, M. S. Moirangthem, Chinmay C. Abdulfattah, and K. P. Subhendu, Artificial neural synchronization using nature inspired whale optimization, *IEEE Access*, pp. 1–14, 2021. doi:10.1109/ACCESS.2021.305288

24. N. M. Kumar, and P. K. Mallick, Blockchain technology for security issues and challenges in IoT, *Procedia Computer Science*, vol. 132, pp. 1815–1823, 2018.

25. M. B. Hoy, An introduction to the blockchain and its implications for libraries and medicine, *Medical Reference Services Quarterly*, vol. 36, no. 3, pp. 273–279, 2017.

26. T. M. Fernández-Carames, and P. Fraga-Lamás, A review on the use of blockchain for the internet of things, *IEEE Access*, vol. 6, pp. 32979–33001, 2018.

27. Z. Deng, Y. Ren, Y. Liu, X. Yin, Z. Shen, and H.-J. Kim, Blockchain-based trusted electronic records preservation in cloud storage, *Computers, Materials & Continua*, vol. 58, no. 1, pp. 135–151, 2019.

28. Q. Wang, F. Zhu, S. Ji, and Y. Ren, Secure provenance of electronic records based on blockchain, *Computers, Materials & Continua*, vol. 65, no. 2, pp. 1753–1769, 2020.

29. A. Reyna, C. Martín, J. Chen, E. Soler, and M. Díaz, On blockchain and its integration with IoT. Challenges and opportunities, *Future Generation Computer Systems*, vol. 88, pp. 173–190, 2018.

30. J. Cheng, J. Li, N. Xiong, M. Chen, H. Guo, and X. Yao, Lightweight mobile clients privacy protection using trusted execution environments for blockchain, *Computers, Materials & Continua*, vol. 65, no. 3, pp. 2247–2262, 2020.

31. I.-C. Lin, and T.-C. Liao, A survey of blockchain security issues and challenges, *IJ Network Security*, vol. 19, no. 5, pp. 653–659, 2017.

32. Z. Zheng, An overview of blockchain technology: Architecture, consensus, and future trends. In *Proceedings of the 2017 IEEE International Congress on Big Data (BigData Congress)*, IEEE, Boston, MA, USA, December 2017.

33. J. Mattila, */e Blockchain Phenomenon–/e Disruptive Potential of Distributed Consensus Architectures,/e*, Research Institute of the Finnish Economy, Helsinki, Finland, 2016.

34. J. Wang, W. Chen, L. Wang, R. Simon Sherratt, O. Alfarraj, and A. Tolba, Data secure storage mechanism of sensor networks based on blockchain, *Computers, Materials & Continua*, vol. 65, no. 3, pp. 2365–2384, 2020.

35. G.-J. Ra, C.-H. Roh, and I.-Y. Lee, A key recovery system based on password-protected secret sharing in a permissioned blockchain, *Computers, Materials & Continua*, vol. 65, no. 1, pp. 153–170, 2020.

36. L. Atzori, A. Iera, and G. Morabito, The internet of things: A survey, *Computer Networks*, vol. 54, no. 15, pp. 2787–2805, 2010. doi:10.1016/j.comnet.2010.05.010

37. J. B. Awotunde, R. O. Ogundokun, and S. Misra, Cloud and IoMT-based big data analytics system during COVID-19 pandemic, *Internet of Things*, pp. 181–201, 2021.

38. R. O. Ogundokun, J. B. Awotunde, S. Misra, O. C. Abikoye, and O. Folarin, Application of machine learning for ransomware detection in IoT devices, *Studies in Computational Intelligence*, vol. 972, pp. 393–420, 2021.

39. C. Chinmay, Computational approach for chronic wound tissue characterization, *Elsevier: Informatics in Medicine Unlocked*, vol. 17, pp. 1–10, 2019, doi:10.1016/j.imu.2019.100162

40. C. Mhamdi, M. Al-Emran, and S. A. Salloum, Text mining and analytics: A case study from news channels posts on Facebook, *Studies in Computational Intelligence*, p. 740, 2018. doi:10.1007/978-3-319-67056-0_19

41. J. B. Awotunde, C. Chakraborty, and A. E. Adeniyi, Intrusion detection in industrial internet of things network-based on deep learning model with rule-based feature selection, *Wireless Communications and Mobile Computing*, 2021.

42. S. A. Salloum, C. Mhamdi, M. Al-Emran, K. Shaalan, Analysis and classification of Arabic newspapers' Facebook pages using text mining techniques, *International Journal of Information Technology and Language Studies*, vol. 1, no. 2, pp. 8–17, 2017.

43. J. B. Awotunde, R. G. Jimoh, S. O. Folorunso, E. A. Adeniyi, K. M. Abiodun, and O. O. Banjo, Privacy and security concerns in IoT-based healthcare systems, *Internet of Things*, pp. 105–134, 2021.

44. V. Beltran, A. M. Ortiz, D. Hussein, and N. Crespi, A semantic service creation platform for Social IoT. In: *2014 IEEE World Forum on Internet of Things (WF-IoT)* (pp. 283–286), 2014. IEEE. doi:10.1109/WF-IoT.2014.6803173

45. M. K. Abiodun, J. B. Awotunde, R. O. Ogundokun, S. Misra, E. A. Adeniyi, M. O. Arowolo, and V. Jaglan, Cloud and big data: A mutual benefit for organization development, *Journal of Physics: Conference Series*, vol. 1767, no. 1, 2021

46. M. Shabaz, and U. Garg, Predicting future diseases based on existing health status using link prediction, *World Journal of Engineering*, 2021.

47. S. Parvathavarthini, An improved crow search based intuitionistic fuzzy clustering algorithm for healthcare applications, *Intelligent Automation and Soft Computing*, vol. 26, no. 2, pp. 253–260, 2020.

48. V.-S. Naresh, Internet of things in healthcare: Architecture, applications, challenges, and solutions, *Computer Systems Science and Engineering*, vol. 35, no. 6, pp. 411–421, 2020.

49. P. Yu, Z. Xia, J. Fei, and S. Kumar Jha, An application review of artificial intelligence in prevention and cure of COVID-19 pandemic, *Computers, Materials & Continua*, vol. 65, no. 1, pp. 743–760, 2020.

50. T. McGhin, K.-K. R. Choo, C. Z. Liu, and D. He, Blockchain in healthcare applications: Research challenges and opportunities, *Journal of Network and Computer Applications*, vol. 135, pp. 62–75, 2019.

51. F. Ajaz, COVID-19: Challenges and its technological solutions using IoT, *Current Medical Imaging*, 2021.

52. M. K. Abiodun, J. B. Awotunde, R. O. Ogundokun, E. A. Adeniyi, and M. O. Arowolo, Security and information assurance for IoT-based big data, *Studies in Computational Intelligence*, vol. 972, pp. 189–211, 2021.

53. Mckinsey and Company. AI adoption advances, but foundational barriers remain. Survey Report. 2018 (11). Available at: https://www.mckinsey.com/featured-insights/artificial-intelligence/ai-adoption-advances-but-foundational-barriers-remain. Accessed June 6, 2019. Google Scholar

54. M. N. K. Boulos, J. T. Wilson, and K. A. Clauson, *Geospatial Blockchain: Promises, Challenges, and Scenarios in Health and Healthcare*, Bio Med Central, London, UK, 2018.

55. L. A. Linn, and M. B. Koo, Blockchain for health data and its potential use in health it and healthcare-related research. In *Proceedings of the ONC/NIST Use of Blockchain for Healthcare and Research Workshop*, Gaithersburg, MA, USA, September 2016.

56. C. Stagnaro, *White Paper: Innovative Blockchain Uses in Healthcare*, Freed Associates, CA, USA, 2017.

57. T. Kumar, Blockchain utilization in healthcare: key requirements and challenges. In *Proceedings of the 2018 IEEE 20th International Conference on E-Health Networking, Applications and Services (Healthcom)*, IEEE, Ostrava, Czech Republic, September 2018.

58. R. Beck, Beyond bitcoin: The rise of the blockchain world, *Computer*, vol. 51, no. 2, pp. 54–58, 2018.

59. A. D. Dwivedi, G. Srivastava, S. Dhar, and R. Singh, A decentralized privacy-preserving healthcare blockchain for IoT, *Sensors*, vol. 19, no. 2, 2019. [Online. Available: http://www.mdpi.com/1424-8220/19/2/326

60. B. Rodrigues, T. Bocek, A. Lareida, D. Hausheer, S. Rafati, and B. Stiller, A blockchain-based architecture for collaborative DDoS mitigation with smart contracts. In *IFIP International Conference on Autonomous Infrastructure, Management and Security*. Springer, Cham, 2017, pp. 16–29.

2 Secure Digital Health Data Management in Internet of Things Using Blockchain and Machine Learning

Susmit Das and Sreyashi Karmakar
RCC Institute of Information Technology, Kolkata, India

Himadri Nath Saha
Surendranath Evening College, Calcutta University, Kolkata, India

CONTENTS

2.1　INTRODUCTION

The healthcare sector includes different organizations like pharmacies, clinics and hospitals which are equipped with diverse heterogeneous collections of amenities [1]. Healthcare services must ensure the patient's health's data management at a superior level. Yet, in this sector, critical information and data of the patients are scattered among multiple systems in different departments. This is the reason, at the hour of need the data is not easily available. Certain major changes are required

DOI: 10.1201/9781003247128-2

for secure handling of crucial health data and exchange of this information in a secure manner. The various challenges are therefore stimulating a drive for a revolution, and innovation for transformation [2]. With the revolution in the digital world and technological advancements, digitalization is improving processes. Patients' health information can be collected, processed and analyzed using sensing devices for constant monitoring and observation of vital signs. For providing healthcare services the vital data are shared with hospitals and their relevant departments in order to provide necessary services [3]. The efficiency of healthcare services can be improved, all medical data should be managed in a centralized system and sharing is imperative [4]. During the pandemic condition of COVID-19, in order to reduce the risk of infection, guidelines were specified that patient isolation should be conducted and movement restricted, so providing distant e-healthcare service is the need of the hour [5]. The typical client-server and cloud-based medical data management systems suffer from various difficulties which are, a single point of failure, centralized data stewardship, data privacy and system vulnerability. In a new age of technology, the hospitals and medical centres have only been trying to use IoT and cloud computing technologies, but for complete remote healthcare services, absolute implementation of these technologies with superior modern security protocols and architectures such as blockchain is essential [6]. It is of utmost importance that vital health data is transparently shared between the concerned parties in a secure fashion [7]. This data must be tamper-proof to avoid manipulation and needs to have a certification mechanism in place to prevent any kind of unauthorized access, be it accidental or intentional. It is important to ensure and maintain the privacy of the patient [8]. The health data collected by IoT devices are sent to a healthcare provider for the diagnosis of the patient. The IoT paradigm is rapidly advancing and is able to revolutionize the healthcare [9] industries by producing a significant number of improvements in terms of secure communication between patients and doctors, e-health and medical records (EHR/EMR), e-prescription data, and insurance information [8, 10,48,49] However, the computing and storage capacity of IoT devices are very restricted [11, 12]. Cloud computing came to the rescue for IoT devices by boosting their efficiency and reducing the cost in the healthcare system. But being centralized, if once the servers break down, all users are affected. There is a possibility that the data stored in cloud servers could be leaked for commercial profits, as healthcare and medical data are highly sensitive and valuable [13, 14].

Also, the requirement of external third-party verification can cause substantial delays to the medical data preservation process due to common issues like server outages and delayed wait or time-out mechanisms, which has the potential to cause significant issues for the health providers involved especially when multiple end-users are involved. This is where blockchain technology can revolutionize existing systems. It is a distributed ledger technology, the peer-to-peer network of computers termed nodes ensure immutability and not by any centralized authority in order to avoid the risks of a central failure point, it keeps track of all transactions and activities happening throughout the blockchain network. A blockchain consists of data records arranged in order in a block structure that contains transactions secured by complex cryptographic hash algorithms in blocks and uses the hash of the preceding block as the key for every succeeding block. Each block is connected and maintained in the blockchain network.

Due to the range of advantages and secure characteristics of blockchain, a lot of companies and establishments are resolving issues that affect the current medical system such as FACTOM [15]. In the healthcare system, effortless data sharing between healthcare solution providers can help in accuracy in detection and diagnosis, effective treatment, in a cost-effective ecosystem [16]. Moreover, blockchain for the health sector empowers multiple units of the healthcare ecosystem to remain in synchronous and distributed ledger enabling secure sharing of data, and the participants in the system can share information without having to worry about any additional options for data integrity and security [17, 18] it monitors patient health-related data and other activities happening in the system.

Even so, as the security and privacy concerns of storage data within blockchain are still critical challenges [19], we propose a secure scheme for data storage and sharing for healthcare based on a secure consensus algorithm using Virtual Machines to sandbox data from external influence. Health data can be collected from IoT devices or hospitals by every user. Besides, unlike common database systems where one can get access to everything stored, in blockchain health data is stored in encrypted form and no one could have access to the data without the credentials of a trusted party in the network. Due to the anonymous nature of the blockchain systems, there has been a good amount of research for utilizing this feature. But most of the other works which have proposed trust assessment mechanisms, however, are not adaptive to blockchain-based healthcare systems. Such studies and experiments are inadequate to provide much detail as they did not regard managing the diverse facets of health data. In this paper, we are trying to solve the problem of 'data management' in smart healthcare networks in addition to the proposed assessment mechanism that is well-fitting to the blockchain scenario. Compared with a few other existing solutions, our model takes the characteristics of health-related data and the anonymity of blockchain.

Moreover, we perform an implementation. The model is effective from the numerical experiment results. The low computing resource consumption provides a grand level of scalability and ties in directly to cloud computing. It is crucial for blockchain systems to discriminate against malicious users, and particularly for healthcare-related blockchain systems.

The main contributions of this paper are summarized as follows:

- We propose a blockchain-based smart healthcare model for the preserving of privacy of health data and confirm its secure sharing in a transparent fashion.
- Blockchain and AI are deployed to achieve secure and efficient data storage and data sharing.
- In the first part of our model, machine learning is used to train CNN models to check for anomalous data due to various causes including machine faults as well as possible tampering. In CNN suitable estimators are being used to discard anomalous data after its detection.

- The non-anomalous data from IoHT devices is securely stored in the cloud using blockchain technology.
- The second part of our model concerns long-term decentralized storage of health records of patients which is easily accessible with proper credentials.
- Virtual Machine Workstations are used within IoT fog devices to securely encapsulate the health records inside blockchain.

In this paper, we propose the integration of IoT, blockchain and cloud technologies in the medical environment for offering e-healthcare and e-medical services. The model enables a secure manner to monitor the vital signs of the patient in a smart hospital or a remote environment. Secure data storing and sharing is authorized by blockchain technology. We also present recent ongoing operations and case studies of projects for exhibiting the feasibility and usefulness of blockchain technology for various healthcare applications. The successful adoption of blockchain in the medical sector is obstructed by several challenges.

In Section 2.2, we review the related works after discussing the background study. The system model is introduced in Section 2.3. In Section 2.4, the details of the proposed scheme and methodology are described. The analysis of the model and its performance evaluation are given in Section 2.5. Finally, Section 2.6 concludes this paper. Possible future research directions are mentioned in Section 2.6.

2.2 BACKGROUND AND RELATED WORK

Blockchain technology first began from financial applications, namely in the decentralized digital cryptocurrency termed bitcoin [18]. Over time, it was realized how the decentralized and secure nature of blockchain can pave the way for secure decentralized verification as well as data storage and management in various other industrial fields apart from cryptocurrency [20]. Day by day, innovations are advancing and so are the implementation of blockchain in various realms of technology [21]. Blockchain is able to transform various applications due to its advantageous features like decentralization, trustworthiness, secure data storage system, zero exchange transaction fee (removal of intermediaries in distributed applications), and transparent immutable nature [22].

The qualities like unforgeability, immutable, decentralized nature with fault tolerance make it acceptable and appropriate for cybersecurity use cases. Blockchain network, in simple terms, is a distributed ledger network where the nodes in the network communicate and collaborate with one another for trading transactions and data [23]. The blockchain is great for various use cases, as it allows reliable data transactions in a transparent fashion [24]. All transactions executed and processed in the network are recorded and maintained permanently on the blockchain. A full copy of the ledger is conserved on each node of the blockchain network on which it is implemented and, on the validation and authentication of each transaction, these ledgers update continuously [25].

The ledger contains all the blocks that are chained together with a hash mechanism in the blockchain network [26].

There are two parts in each block, out of which the head contains the number of executed and validated proceedings and transactions. In the decentralized network of blockchain technology, a block consists of lots of valid transactions along with its associated attributes. These transactions could be as critical as health records, a financial transaction or communication messages over a network. Different data structures are used in blockchain, for instance, in the Merkle tree data structure, the reverse hash mechanism is used, and the central root hash is saved as the hash of the block. The second part of the block is the block header, in which various header information like the timestamp of the transaction, hash of that block and hash of the previous block is stored. Thus, a chain-like structure is formed, by joining a series of existing blocks together with the help of hash algorithms. The chain becomes more resilient against falsification as the blocks keep adding and the extent of the chain grows. Furthermore, if any attempts are made to alter the data and transaction of a block by the malicious user, it would affect the hashes of all subsequent blocks, and thus it would be visible to everyone present in the blockchain network. Hence it is nearly impossible to change data once stored in the blockchain. The special type of node which is known as the miner node is responsible to generate a block and validate transactions. A basic structure of blockchain is given in Figure 2.1.

A number of consensus algorithms are used to validate new blocks and link them to the genesis blockchain. The consensus process lets blockchain network nodes agree upon adding a new block to the blockchain network [27]. In the bitcoin network, one of the consensus algorithms is called Proof of Work (PoW) in which a mathematical puzzle must be solved by miner nodes to validate and add a block [28]. The difficulty of the mathematical puzzle is generated by a variable called 'nonce', which is short for "number only used once" [29], according to which the time needed to validate new blocks can be changed as per the computation power of the miner nodes [30].

The main motivation for nodes to participate as miners is that they are rewarded for adding new blocks. Blockchain has emerged as an avant-garde growth system. Blockchain technology is suitably applied to the entire industrial sector as the

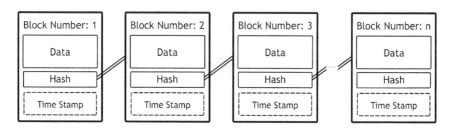

FIGURE 2.1   Basic structure of the blockchain.

fundamental element of a fourth-industrial-revolution enabler [30]. Presently, "blockchain" has become one of the most appreciated and trusted technologies, as it is capable of providing reliable means of securing IoT ecosystems in a distributed fashion due to the combined usage of heavy cryptographic hash functions for message digest and economic modelling, applied to a peer-to-peer network. The most critical barriers as considered for IoT are cybersecurity and privacy [31]. Therefore, to address the vulnerabilities of IoT accurately, it is necessary for a novel secure model due to the rapid development in the domain of IoT. Best practices are capable of combining security-by-design approaches with particular technical countermeasures designed at different technological stacks, as well as novel organizational processes capable of tackling information security for IoT in a much better way.

Currently, blockchain is evolving as a very safe, secure and trustworthy platform for securely sharing data in diverse domains of application like supply chain management, banking, food industry, the Internet, medical, energy and IoT. Moreover, this booming new technology has been developed to break into a variety of data-driven spheres, including the health sector. The blockchain paradigm is used in administering security in different communicating and processing systems. Administering security healthcare programs does not require trusted third parties. In order to prevent any anonymous and unauthorized access of critical data by illegitimate users the principal focus of modern healthcare applications is on the privacy of the patient's medical data and security of the information shared [32]. Trust, authentication and privacy have become the major requirements.

In recent years, administering the blockchain paradigm as a decentralized ledger for monitoring shared information has become a familiar practice [33, 34]. To enhance the quality and security of sharing of health data and preventing any unauthorized interruptions blockchain-assisted authentication and trust-based security are assimilated with medical systems [35, 36]. A rapidly ageing population in several parts of the world along with the dramatic increase in the cost of healthcare in hospitals have led to the awareness of the importance of efficient healthcare systems and fostered several research directions at the integration of healthcare data security preservation. In today's world, Electronic Health Records (EHR), also known as Electronic Medical Records (EMR), are used by every major hospital and healthcare provider for improved care, sources and causes of various new diseases, tracking a disease, research and development of drugs based on patient medical history, studying pattern and ultimately prevention. All these vital applications are based on medical data, which needs to be secure and authentic. However, EHR uses a client-server architecture to store and manage medical data. This crucial medical information is stored on the server of the respective hospitals. In this type of system, it is very difficult for doctors to provide a highly effective treatment plan to a particular patient because the data of the patient is stored at different hospitals and often it may cause delays to access the medical data for various formalities and authentication procedures. To solve this issue in traditional EHR, various organizations developed cloud-based systems to manage and process medical data. However, a centralized server is used to store these highly important medical data of patients and drugs and a centralized system can suffer from a single point failure, cyber-attacks, lack of security and privacy. To provide a solution to the various problems in traditional EHR, research efforts are going on to use blockchain technology to manage and store medical data. An application called MedRec was proposed [37]. It is a data sharing application based on blockchain. With the help of MedRec, doctors share the medical data of the patients on a blockchain network.

MedRec uses medical data as an alternative in order to provide an incentive for mining. However, this approach is a cause of serious privacy issues in the case of the patients, whose data is stored within the blockchain network, as they have no access to this data.

MedRec also uses Ethereum as a base model for blockchain, which is very resource consuming and restricts the number of devices capable of mining blocks to the blockchain. Healthcare data gateways: Found healthcare intelligence on blockchain with novel privacy risk control [38].

A patient's medical data is only permitted to view by healthcare professionals. "A cloud computing solution for patient's data collection in healthcare institutions" a framework was proposed in which data is analyzed and processed by the proposed system itself during data input and the relevant data output. Data collection is achieved by sensors in the system [39].

With the help of sensors, which are directly attached to the various medical equipment, data is collected and stored in the system for analyzing and processing as required. However, in this proposed system, these medical data can only be accessed by medical professionals. In the paper, "A Case Study IoT and Blockchain powered Healthcare", a case was studied in which benefits of IoT and blockchain were explored [40].

They used various IoT devices to monitor and collect real-time medical data of patients. These data were stored in a blockchain network. Scalability in the case of Big Data in terms of blockchain was also studied and illustrated, also various controllability of the blockchain network is also studied. Some significant work has been done in the field of healthcare to monitor patients' health using sensors and IoT in the paper, "Health monitoring using Internet of Things (IoT)" [41] by the authors Dr Himadri Nath Saha, SupratimAuddy, Subrata Pal, Shubham Kumar et. al.

In the work, "Artificial Neural Synchronization Using Nature Inspired Whale Optimization" [42], Arindam Sarkar et al. proposed a faster highly secure Double Layer Tree Parity Machine (DLTPM) model for neural synchronization. In order to develop a secure cryptographic key exchange protocol, whale optimization of weight vectors of neural synchronization is proposed in their work. In the Artificial Neural Networks (ANN), two DLTPM networks having identical configurations are synchronized. Optimal Weight Vector Generation Algorithm and Double Layer Tree Parity Machines Synchronization are employed. The simulation of the model provided wonderful results for defence against potential attacks, in the paper, "A Novel Fog Computing Approach for Minimization of

Latency in Healthcare using Machine Learning" [43]. The paper minimized latency of IoT devices using fog computing and machine learning Algorithm. The proposed model sends real-time data from sensors in healthcare networks to cloud servers in fog with minimum possible latency. The model employed the 'random forest' algorithm in order to diminish over-fitting. IoT devices have low computation capability, so the fog network is kept close to the devices to store, process and analyze the collected health data. Various delays in the network are calculated while data transfer from IoT devices to fog and finally to the cloud. The novel intelligent multimedia data segregation (IMDS) uses k-fold random forest in the fog layer. The results of the proposed model are very promising.

In the most recent work "SDN–IoT empowered intelligent framework for industry 4.0 applications during COVID-19 pandemic" by Anichur Rahman et al. [44]. An intelligent architecture is developed to manage the smart industry using IoT devices while maintaining social distancing. The proposed architecture efficiently handles industries in the difficult times of the pandemic by unified transmission and communication of various units of the service. IoT is the catalyst of Industry 4.0. The Software Defined Networking (SDN) is employed with IoT applications for managing the network along with improving the node balance. For attaining virtualization, saving energy and managing the overall functionalities Network Function Virtualization (NFV) is engaged. The Perception layer is enriched to fit this challenging virus outbreak situation. IoT applications reduce human to human interactions and automatically sense data and are able to track the most affected areas. The model can be evolved by using blockchain technology, which is used in the model proposed by us. So, from what we have seen, while there are existing models for health data management in blockchain [45], these have some concerning privacy issues and lack of transparency in these models as well as the risk of anomalies in the data [46, 47]. Some such models like MedRec require very computational power to use vastly, limiting the scalability of the model and limiting the type of usable devices.

In our model, we have used aid from machine learning to minimize the risk of anomalies and store the data in blockchain in a transparent fashion without compromising on the privacy of the trusted parties.

2.3 PROPOSED MODEL

We are proposing a model which has two parts for 'Secure Health Data Management'. Modern bleeding-edge technologies have been used in this model, in which AI is used to filter out data anomalies and blockchain is used for storage and management of data in a secure fashion. The first part of the model deals with storage of non-anomalous sensory data within blockchain for cloud storage and analytics in a transparent fashion. The anomaly check is performed using machine learning trained Convolutional Neural Network (CNN) with suitable estimators in CNN based feature learning network. The CNN model is trained with expansive datasets of health parameters from various patients as well as healthy individuals to detect anomalies in the sensor data provided. The anomalous data is removed post-detection, followed by cloud storage of the non-anomalous data in block-chain to conserve transparency and privacy throughout the process. The second part of this model deals with the secure storage and data management of health events of individuals in a transparent fashion by taking advantage of the immu-table nature of blockchain technology.

The first part of this model is the 'Secure Sensory Data Management and Storage Model'. Here, various parameters of the body such as body temperature, pulse rate and oxygen saturation are recorded over time. For this, body area net-work sensors are used with edges devices in an IoT network. Within the same IoT network, fog computing devices are set up to which the sensory data from the body area network is sent. A CNN is pre-trained with prepared expansive data sets of various physical parameters in the fog devices using machine learning with suitable estimators like decision tree and support vector machine, as shown in Figure 2.2 [42]. The body area network sensor data is analyzed by this machine learning trained model for normalcy check to detect anomalies. The anomalous data that fails the normalcy check by the machine learning trained model is dis-carded after logging the event.

The non-anomalous body area network sensor data that successfully completes the normalcy check of the machine learning trained model is stored as blocks in a blockchain within the fog devices. The blockchain is mirrored in real-time in the cloud, allowing remote analysis of the data by all trusted parties such as the con-cerned healthcare providers by frontend applications connected to the cloud, thereby enabling remote diagnosis, remote health monitoring etc. The process is completely transparent, and the removal of anomalous data minimizes the possi-bility of data tampering or noise and by use of blockchain, the data is accessible to all trusted parties including the concerned patient. This blockchain implemen-tation uses a robust consensus algorithm with very secure cryptographic hash algorithms to provide Proof of Work for mining of the individual blocks. All health provider entities involved in the healthcare process can readily access these data over the cloud via the blockchain hash key. The whole process is transparent, and the data is accessible to all parties including the end-user and other trusted entities that have the key to the blockchain data at any given time once they are added and verified as trusted entities within the webspace used. The immutable tamper-proof nature of blockchain helps in developing further trust between the various parties involved. The pseudonymous nature of blockchain also conserves the privacy of the person/persons subject to the diagnosis. This method of data management and storage minimizes the possibility of tampering of sensory data both during input by filtering anomalous data using machine learning and post-storage using blockchain as shown in Figure 2.3.

The second part of our proposed model is the 'Secure Medical Record Management and Storage Model'. Here, blockchain is used to preserve and store all health-related events of a patient within the medical IoT network. The decen-tralized nature of blockchain allows the inclusion of new events whenever needed without the need of any third party. Every time, there is a new health event for the same individual, such as a new diagnosis, administration of new medicines, course

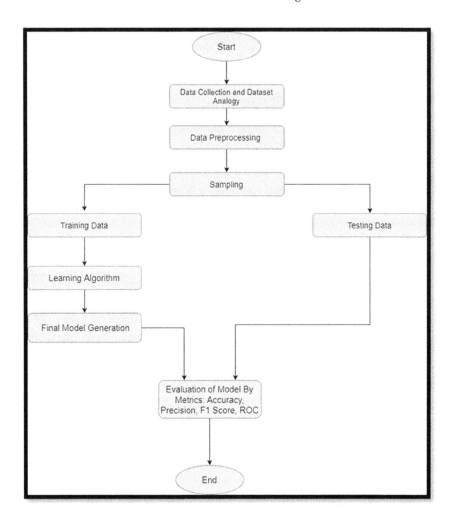

FIGURE 2.2   Machine learning framework for detection of anomalies.

of a new antibiotic or vaccination records, a new block is created and then added
to the blockchain for data preservation. New health events can be registered to add
a new block from secure virtual machine workstations within a fog setup inside
the IoT networks, thereby allowing smart devices of various computational powers to add new blocks without the need for specialized hardware. These secure
virtual machine workstations can be accessed remotely by using a secure client
application on smart devices and then providing secure login credentials provided
to all trusted parties such as medical health provider agents such as doctors, diagnostics labs, etc, as well as the end-user, that is, the concerned patient and other
trusted parties related to the patient. Unlike other existing medical robust systems,

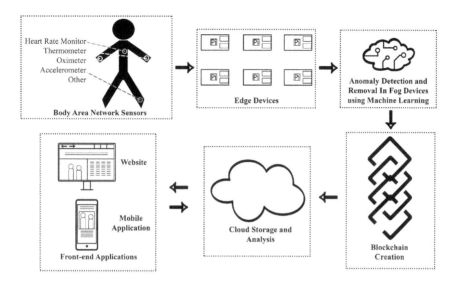

FIGURE 2.3 Secure sensory data management and storage model.

this robust model allows both healthcare providers, the concerned patient and other trusted parties to add new health events as blocks whenever needed. The entire health record of the individual patient will be available within the same blockchain making it very easy to get access to the data whenever needed, saving the parties involved a lot of hassle, while also providing security due to the intrinsic nature of blockchain. Also, separate blockchains are used to store the health data of separate patients, and this data is accessible only to the parties involved to the concerned individual and no one else, unlike other medical record implementations which store the records of multiple patients within the same networks. This is a much better approach and allays privacy concerns of the patients involved. The hashes of each block in the blockchain are cross-verified whenever a new block is added to the blockchain to avoid corrupt blocks being added. The immutable nature of blockchain provides anti-tamper security making this model suitable for the long-term preservation of health data. The blockchain is then mirrored to the cloud, allowing access to the entire health record to any health provider worldwide as long as the hash key of the health event concerned is provided using frontend applications like websites or mobile apps. The entire process is illustrated in Figure 2.4.

2.4 METHODOLOGY

Firstly, for the Secure Sensory Data Management and Storage Model, a variety of Body Area Network Sensors such as Body Thermometer, Accelerometer, Oximeter, are set up and connected to smart IoT devices in an IoT network. The

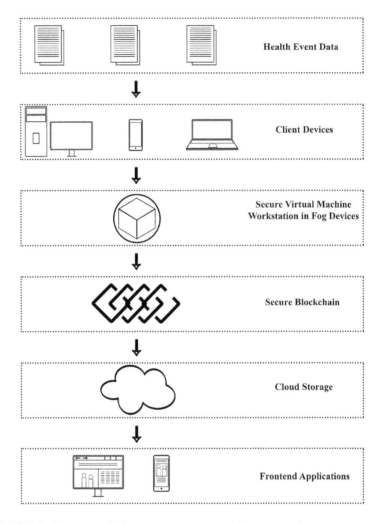

FIGURE 2.4 Secure medical record management and storage model.

raw inputs from these devices are converted to digital float values by the IoT
devices and sent to computationally powerful fog devices within the IoT network
at a pre-determined interval called 'Sensor Communication Interval' that suits the
model to decrease redundancy of data without introducing too much lag. Within
these fog devices, there is a CNN model, which is pre-trained with prepared
expansive categorically organized datasets of various physical parameters from
various patients, as well as healthy people, using machine learning with suitable
machine learning estimators such as artificial neural network, decision tree, support vector machine and random forest. The converted float sensory data over a
fixed period of time from the smart IoT devices are now organized into arrays and

checked for normalcy to detect the existence of anomalies via analysis with various estimators. If anomalies are found within a particular data array, the event is logged in a data log and that particular data array is discarded.

The non-anomalous data arrays are outputted. This output is to be stored in a blockchain and then mirrored to the cloud for analytic purposes. For this, a suitable hashing algorithm is to be chosen that satisfies the required security and bandwidth needs of the software and hardware systems used and a nonce is randomly generated. The consensus algorithm used for mining the block is given in Table 2.1. The target is used to be set that expected computational time per block over a significant number of samples follows the mentioned constraints where the mean is μ and the standard deviation is σ. From the empirical rule of normal distribution, we know:

$$P\left(\mu - 3\sigma \leq X \leq \mu + 3\sigma\right) = 99.73$$

This indicates that 99.73% of observations lie within the range of $\pm 3\sigma$ of μ. Hence, we need to set such a difficulty target difference that $\mu + 3\sigma$ of computational time per block of the samples is very close to the Sensor Communication Interval used but not greater than it. This will give us the highest possible integrity for the implementation without adding any delay in the system. The blockchain is ultimately mirrored to the cloud so that it is accessible to any of the trusted parties involved by the use of frontend applications. The entire process is shown in the form of a flowchart in Figure 2.5.

For the Secure Medical Record Management and Storage Model, mirrorable secure virtual machine workstations are set within the fog devices. The involved parties have to use a secure client application in their respective IoT devices, that authenticates the credentials of the party in question, to enter health event data to be recorded within the blockchain. This data is then sent to the Secure Virtual Machine Workstation within the fog device. Then the data is mined into the blockchain as a new block using the algorithm given in Box 1. Using this approach, the high computational power of the fog device can be used instead of low-powered IoT devices like smartphones and Raspberry Pi-like devices, allowing us to get greater security without compromising on computational time or resources like current solutions. Also, the sandboxed nature of virtual machine makes it nearly impossible for anyone to tamper with the data or compromise the integrity of the blockchain in any way. The blockchain is then mirrored from the fog Device to the cloud, where the data can be viewed by any trusted party using frontend applications. A flowchart of the entire methodology is given in Figure 2.6.

2.5   IMPLEMENTATION AND DATA ANALYSIS

The proposed model is used in a simulation of a healthcare diagnostic lab using the following body area networks sensors – Bluetooth Oximeter and Bluetooth Thermometer to monitor oxygen saturation, pulse rate and body temperature.

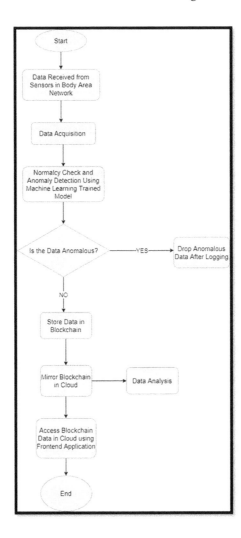

FIGURE 2.5   Methodology of secure sensory data management and storage model.

These sensors are paired to a Raspberry Pi 4 Model B, in which a python application gathers the data from these sensors. This application also supports scripted custom input to override the sensor data, which can be used to simulate anomalous data. The sensor data is converted to float, stored in arrays and sent to the fog device in the IoT network once every Sensor Communication Interval, which is configured to be 10 seconds. We have used 12,000 data samples from the Body Area Network Sensors in this implementation.

Our fog device is a customized machine with 5.0 Ghz 6-Core Intel® Core™ i7-8700K OC, 16GB RAM, Nvidia GeForce GTX 1060. In this device, a neural network has been pre-trained on an open-source dataset from Kaggle on Healthcare

BOX 2.1   CONSENSUS ALGORITHM FOR BLOCK MINING

Block Mining Algorithm
Input Block of Data

Output Chain of Blocks

```
1:  procedure Block Mining
2:  for n = 1 to Range, (incrementing n by +1 uptomaxNonce) do
3:          if Hash Selection(block)<= target then
4:              add(block)
5:          else
6:              nonce_block = Random_nonce()
7:          end if
8:  end for
9:  end procedure
10: end if
11: end procedure
```

Provider Fraud/Anomaly Detection Analysis of 31,650 samples. We have used all the following Estimators: Decision Tree, Logistic Regression, Artificial Neural Network, Support Vector Machine and Random Forest. The training accuracy of these estimators is given in Figure 2.7. Distribution of anomalies within the dataset is given in Table 2.1.

The float data from the Raspberry Pi is subject to normalcy checks by the machine learning model. The testing accuracy of the used estimators is given in Figure 2.8.

The anomalous data arrays are discarded, and the non-anomalous data arrays are exported. This export data is sent as input into the blockchain. We are using Blake2s as the cryptographic hash algorithm, due to the robust security it provides as well as for its well-optimized structure for modern hardware and software. We have used a difficulty target difference of 16, which gives mean computational time per block (μ) of 5.4785 seconds with a standard deviation(σ) of 1.4412 seconds for 1,000 blocks.

So z seconds and $\mu + 3\sigma = 9.8021$ seconds. This perfectly satisfies the conditions in our methodology of $\mu + 3\sigma$ of being as close to Sensor Communication Interval of 10 seconds without being bigger than it to maximize security without introducing lag. The data stored within the blockchain is free from any anomalies and secure from tampering, illegitimate access and other security and privacy issues that typically plague IoT based healthcare implementations. A sample console output from our implementation has been provided in Figure 2.9.

For the medical record model, we are using blockchain to store the medical records of an anonymous volunteer. We are using the same cryptographic hash

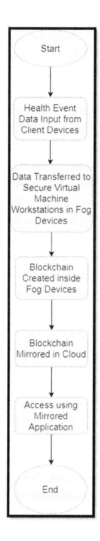

FIGURE 2.6 Methodology of secure medical record management and storage model.

algorithm as the diagnostic model, that is, Blake2s for its robust security provisions and good optimization. We have used a difficulty target difference of 20 here.
A secure Virtual Machine is set up using Oracle VirtualBox and Linux within the
fog device for the purpose of adding health events as blocks in the blockchain.
RDP Port 3389 is used to access this VM from smart IoT devices letting us mine
blocks into the blockchain from low-powered IoT devices like mobile phones.
Here, health event data is added to the blockchain by connecting to the VM from
the android smartphone, Mi A2 and uploaded to the cloud. From the cloud, this
data can be accessed either via the use of terminal or by the use of frontend

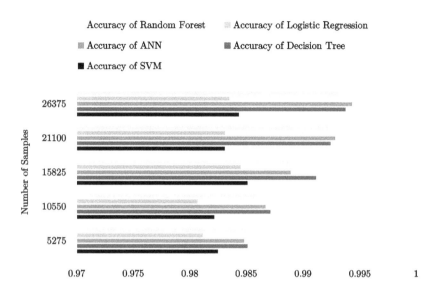

FIGURE 2.7 Training accuracy of various estimators.

TABLE 2.1
Distribution of Anomalies in the Dataset

Anomalies	Frequency Count	% of Total Data	% of Anomalies Data
Noise data	728	2.3002	4.3625
Sensor failure	174	0.5498	9.7098
Malicious data	21	0.0664	1.1719
Manipulated data	419	1.3239	23.3817
Setup failure	103	0.3254	5.7478
Calibration error	347	1.0964	19.3638
Total	1,792	5.6621	100

applications, such as web-apps or smartphone apps. Anyone with the proper credentials can access this data, hence the entire process is transparent. As the data is stored within the blockchain, due to its immutable nature, once stored, this data cannot be modified in any form. Hence the security and privacy of the data is conserved. A sample console output from our implementation is shown in Figure 2.10.

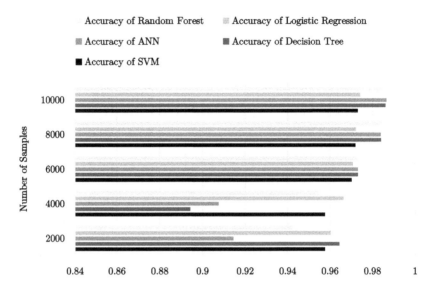

FIGURE 2.8   Testing accuracy of various estimators.

```
--------------------------------------------------------------------
Block Number: 998
Block Data (Oxygen Saturation,  Pulse  Rate, Temperature): [[97.0, 70.0, 96.4]]
Block Hash: f7744ce1fd3a9ad664cd09ee4fe103908024653c9218426e977053095ee973df
Previous Hash: e183f0919a5ccd70a6c99dbdd8550fe843e0e2dc760fd13b1fe2ea13771e7fcb
Nonce: 1507287249
Time Stamp 2021-03-24 13:41:46.542722
--------------------------------------------------------------------
Block Number: 999
Block Data (Oxygen Saturation,  Pulse  Rate, Temperature): [[97.0, 77.0, 96.4]]
Block Hash: e9b849d94802c37e1b2f93b9cc7fd726546115c8db257a7fdfc5ddd8aa9acc09
Previous Hash: f7744ce1fd3a9ad664cd09ee4fe103908024653c9218426e977053095ee973df
Nonce: 2303866936
Time Stamp 2021-03-24 13:41:56.562964
--------------------------------------------------------------------
Block Number: 1000
Block Data (Oxygen Saturation,  Pulse  Rate, Temperature): [[98.0, 68.0, 96.4]]
Block Hash: a0cc7145c80d3ef65b554c4a11b79c50e768a075d78ce07efeb3d8acf5e3c413
Previous Hash: e9b849d94802c37e1b2f93b9cc7fd726546115c8db257a7fdfc5ddd8aa9acc09
Nonce: 2248313800
Time Stamp 2021-03-24 13:42:06.628339
--------------------------------------------------------------------
 Mean Computation Time per Block in ms: 5478.5021585
 Standard Deviation of  Computation Time per Block in ms: 1441.2196352
 Sensor Communication Interval in ms: 10000.0
 Hash Algorithm Used: Blake2s
```

FIGURE 2.9 Secure sensory data management and storage model blockchain implementation.

```
Block Number: 3
Patient ID: 76aacb5a6808b8d1e733de1e50c5da26
Event Type: Symptom Report
Details: Difficulty Breathing
Block Hash: ccd67acd598174aee6558e3147c298d0e4f9e6e59ee5475b53e44417e97951cb
Previous Hash: bd4c2a8bdd162ce86381c0241a18e3bc7d5887f4db648366561a22e8249baa19
Nonce: 2122494963
Time Stamp 2021-03-20 17:48:35.059656
- - - - - - - - - - - - - - - - - - - - - - - - - - - - - - - - - - - - - - - - - - - - - - - - - -
Block Number: 4
Patient ID: 76aacb5a6808b8d1e733de1e50c5da26
Event Type: Diagnosis
Details: Asthma
Block Hash: 0299194888a6e9285e02b423dbbf923e3f29d51964293818d6c95e897ba7b651
Previous Hash: ccd67acd598174aee6558e3147c298d0e4f9e6e59ee5475b53e44417e97951cb
Nonce: 2844033580
Time Stamp 2021-03-20 19:07:49.239176
- - - - - - - - - - - - - - - - - - - - - - - - - - - - - - - - - - - - - - - - - - - - - - - - - -
Block Number: 5
Patient ID: 76aacb5a6808b8d1e733de1e50c5da26
Event Type: Prescription of Drugs
Details: Foracort Inhaler 200, Duration: 3 weeks
Block Hash: 6f07a12b7cb2a2492a01a8410452f38f696e8a5b29ff7a538e00fe6504ff9870
Previous Hash: 0299194888a6e9285e02b423dbbf923e3f29d51964293818d6c95e897ba7b651
Nonce: 1082646277
Time Stamp 2021-03-20 20:10:31.470558
- - - - - - - - - - - - - - - - - - - - - - - - - - - - - - - - - - - - - - - - - - - - - - - - - -
 Computation Time per Block in ms: 80462.9172365
 Hash Algorithm Used: Blake2s
```

FIGURE 2.10 Secure medical record management and storage model blockchain implementation.

2.6 CONCLUSION

In this paper, we have proposed a model for securely managing data in healthcare system using cutting edge technologies like blockchain and AI. Among the two parts of the model, the first part stores non-anomalous data from sensors in the blockchain for cloud storage and analytics in cloud. Using machine learning-trained CNN normalcy check of the data is performed, and find anomalous data. Suitable estimators in CNN are being used to remove anomalous data after its detection. The following part of the model handles the secure storage of health record data. To achieve secure and transparent storage of healthcare data, blockchain technology is deployed. It offers transparency of data and maintains the privacy of the parties involved. Alongside the proposed model, we have discussed the methodology used in detail. Thereafter, we have implemented the model in our lab and provided the details of this implementation with analytics of its performance.

2.7 FUTURE RESEARCH DIRECTIONS

- Privacy and Security in blockchain can be compromised, so it can be improved to maintain crucial healthcare data.

- IoT devices are low power computing devices, so lightweight cryptographic hash functions can be devised to implement blockchain in IoT devices.
- Different Deep Learning and machine learning models can be employed to enhance the security of IoT devices and can help to utilize its potential to collect data using sensors as medical data is crucial.
- A standardized AI-augmented IoT architecture is still not available for healthcare, so a novel can be designed in IoT.
- Low-latency cipher of Blocks in the blockchain network can be implemented in the healthcare domain.
- Trust management can be improved in blockchain.
- A lightweight consensus algorithm can be designed for blockchain for healthcare data.
- Data-driven models can be designed for analysis and improvement of healthcare processes.

CONFLICT OF INTEREST

There is no conflict of interests.

FUNDING

There is no funding support.

DATA AVAILABILITY

Not applicable.

REFERENCES

1. Siyal, A. A., Junejo, A. Z., Zawish, M., Ahmed, K., Khalil, A., & Soursou, G. "Applications of Blockchain technology in medicine and healthcare: Challenges and future perspectives." *Cryptography*, 3(1), 3, 2019.
2. Wang, Ziyu, Luo, Nanqing, & Zhou, Pan. "GuardHealth: Blockchain empowered secure data management and Graph Convolutional Network enabled anomaly detection in smart healthcare." *Journal of Parallel and Distributed Computing*, 142, 1–12, 2020.
3. Wang, Haoxiang. "IoT based clinical sensor data management and transfer using blockchain technology," *Journal of ISMAC*, 2 (3), 154–159, 2020.
4. Dubovitskaya, A., Xu, Z., Ryu, S., Schumacher, M., & Wang, F. Secure and trustable electronic medical records sharing using blockchain. In *AMIA Annual Symposium Proceedings* (Vol. 2017, p. 650). American Medical Informatics Association, 2017.
5. Kaur, H., Alam, M. A., Jameel, R., Mourya, A. K., & Chang, V. "A proposed solution and future direction for blockchain-based heterogeneous medicare data in cloud environment," *Journal of Medical Systems*, 42(8), 156, 2018.
6. Shae, Z., & Tsai, J. J. On the design of a blockchain platform for clinical trial and precision medicine. In *2017 IEEE 37th International Conference On Distributed Computing Systems (ICDCS)* (pp. 1972–1980). IEEE, 2017, June.

7. Sachin D., Chinmay C., Jaroslav F., Rashmi G., Arun K. R., & Subhendu K. P. "SSII: Secured and high-quality Steganography using Intelligent hybrid optimization algorithms for IoT," *IEEE Access*, 9, 1–16, 2021. doi:10.1109/ACCESS.2021. 3089357

8. Al Omar, A., Bhuiyan, M. Z. A., Basu, A., Kiyomoto, S., & Rahman, M. S. "Privacy-friendly platform for healthcare data in cloud based on blockchain environment." *Future Generation Computer Systems*, 95, 511–521, 2019.

9. Ray, P. P., Dash, D., Salah, K., & Kumar, N. "Blockchain for IoT based healthcare: background, consensus, platforms, and use cases." *IEEE Systems Journal*, 1–10, 2020, (in press). doi;10.1109/JSYST.2020.2963840

10. Gupta, A., Chinmay, C., & Gupta, B. "Secure transmission of EEG data using watermarking algorithm for the detection of epileptical seizures." *Traitement du Signal, IIETA*, 38(2), 473–479, 2021, doi:10.18280/ts.380227

11. Griggs, K. N., Ossipova, O., Kohlios, C. P., Baccarini, A., Howson, E. A., & Hayajneh, T. "Healthcare blockchain system using smart contracts for secure automated remote patient monitoring." *Journal of Medical Systems*, 42(7), 130, 2018.

12. Godfrey Anuga, Akpakwu, Silva, Bruno J., Hancke, Gerhard P., & Abu-Mahfouz, Adnan M. "A survey on 5G networks for the internet of things: Communication technologies and challenges." *IEEE Access* 6, 3619–3647, 2017.

13. Gai, Keke, Yulu, Wu, Zhu, Liehuang, Qiu, Meikang, & Shen, Meng "Privacy preserving energy trading using consortium blockchain in smart grid." *IEEE Transactions on Industrial Informatics*, 15(6), 3548–3558, 2019.

14. Gai, Keke, Yulu, Wu, Zhu, Liehuang, Lei, Xu, & Zhang, Yan "Permissioned blockchain and edge computing empowered privacy-preserving smart grid networks." *IEEE Internet of Things Journal*, 6(5), 7992–8004, 2019.

15. Zhang, Chuan, Zhu, Liehuang, Xu, Chang, Sharif, Kashif, Du, Xiaojiang, & Guizani, Mohsen "LPTD: Achieving lightweight and privacy-preserving truth discovery in CIoT." *Future Generation Computer Systems*, 90, 175–184, 2019.

16. Snow, Paul, Deery, Brian, Lu, Jack, Johnston, David, & Kirby Peter, *Factom: Business Processes Secured by Immutable Audit Trails on the Blockchain*, Whitepaper, Factom, 2014.

17. Gai, Keke, Lu, Zhihui, Qiu, Meikang, & Zhu, Liehuang. "Toward smart treatment management for personalized healthcare." *IEEE Network*, 33(6), 30–36, 2019.

18. Khatoon, A. "A blockchain-based smart contract system for healthcare management." *Electronics*, 9(1), 94, (2020).

19. Khezr, S., Moniruzzaman, M., Yassine, A., & Benlamri, R. "Blockchain technology in healthcare: A comprehensive review and directions for future research." *Applied Sciences*, 9(9), 1736, 2019.

20. Manpreet, K., Mohammad, Z. K., Shikha, G., Abdulfattah, N., Chinmay, C., & Subhendu K. P. "MBCP: Performance analysis of large-scale mainstream blockchain consensus protocols." *IEEE Access*, 9, 1–14, 2021. doi:10.1109/ACCESS.2021.3085187

21. Nakamoto, Satoshi "Re: bitcoin P2P e-cash paper." *The Cryptography Mailing List*, 2008.

22. Ruj, Sushmita, Rahman, Mohammad Shahriar, Basu, Anirban, & Shinsaku, Kiyomoto, "Blockstore: A secure decentralized storage framework on blockchain." In *2018 IEEE 32nd International Conference on Advanced Information Networking and Applications (AINA)*, pp. 1096–1103. IEEE, 2018.

23. Akram, Shaik V., Malik, Praveen K., Singh, Rajesh, Anita, Gehlot, & Tanwar, Sudeep "Adoption of blockchain technology in various realms: Opportunities and challenges." *Security and Privacy*, 3(5), e109, 2020.

24. Mohanta, Bhabendu Kumar, Panda, Soumyashree S., & Jena, Debasish. "An overview of smart contract and use cases in blockchain technology." In *2018 9th International Conference on Computing, Communication and Networking Technologies (ICCCNT)*, pp. 1–4. IEEE, 2018.

25. Puthal, Deepak, Malik, Nisha, Mohanty, Saraju P., Kougianos, Elias, & Yang, Chi. "The blockchain as a decentralized security framework [future directions]." *IEEE Consumer Electronics Magazine*, 7(2), 18–21, 2018.

26. Wang, Zuan, Tian, Youliang, & Zhu, Jianming. "Data sharing and tracing scheme based on blockchain." In *2018 8th international conference on logistics, Informatics and Service Sciences (LISS)*, pp. 1–6. IEEE, 2018.

27. Kuo, Tsung-Ting, Kim, Hyeon-Eui, & Ohno-Machado, Lucila "Blockchain distributed ledger technologies for biomedical and healthcare applications." *Journal of the American Medical Informatics Association*, 24(6), 1211–1220, 2017.

28. Ajao, Lukman Adewale, Agajo, James, Adedokun, Emmanuel Adewale, & Karngong, Loveth. "Crypto hash algorithm-based blockchain technology for managing decentralized ledger database in oil and gas industry." *J—Multidisciplinary Scientific Journal*, 2(3), 300–325, 2019.

29. Bamakan, Seyed Mojtaba Hosseini, Motavali, Amirhossein, & Babaei, Alireza Bondarti. "A survey of blockchain consensus algorithms performance evaluation criteria." *Expert Systems with Applications*, 154, 113385, 2020.

30. Szalachowski, Pawel, Reijsbergen, Daniël, Homoliak, Ivan, & Sun, Siwei. "Strongchain: Transparent and collaborative proof-of-work consensus." In *28th {USENIX} Security Symposium ({USENIX} Security 19)*, pp. 819–836, 2019.

31. MacKenzie, Donald. "Pick a nonce and try a hash." *London Review of Books*, 41(8), 35–38, 2019.

32. Ren, Wei, Jingjing Hu, Zhu, Tianqing, Ren, Yi, & Choo, Kim-Kwang Raymond. "A flexible method to defend against computationally resourceful miners in blockchain proof of work." *Information Sciences*, 507, 161–171, 2020.

33. Swami, Mahesh, Verma, Divya, & Vishwakarma, Virendra P.. "Blockchain and industrial internet of things: applications for industry 4.0." In *Proceedings of International Conference on Artificial Intelligence and Applications*, pp. 279–290. Springer, Singapore, 2021.

34. Romaniuk, Ryszard S. "IoT—Review of critical issues." *International Journal of Electronics and Telecommunications*, 64(1), 95–102, 2018.

35. McGhin, Thomas, Choo, Kim-Kwang Raymond, Liu, Charles Zhechao, & He, Debiao. "Blockchain in healthcare applications: Research challenges and opportunities." *Journal of Network and Computer Applications*, 135, 62–75, 2019.

36. Won, J., Seo, S.-H., & Bertino, E. A secure communication protocol for drones and smart objects. In *Proceedings of the 10th ACM Symposium on Information, Computer and Communications Security*, pp. 249–260, 2015.

37. Aloqaily, M., Al Ridhawi, I., Salameh, H. B., & Jararweh, Y. "Data and service management in densely crowded environments: Challenges, opportunities, and recent developments." *IEEE Communication Magazine*, 57, 81–87, 2019.

38. Yazdinejad, Abbas, Srivastava, Gautam, Parizi, Reza M., Dehghantanha, Ali, Choo, Kim-Kwang Raymond, & Aledhari, Mohammed. "Decentralized authentication of distributed patients in hospital networks using blockchain." *IEEE Journal of Biomedical and Health Informatics*, 24(8), 2146–2156, 2020.

39. Zhang, Peng, White, Jules, Schmidt, Douglas C., Lenz, Gunther, & Trent Rosenbloom, S., "FHIRChain: Applying blockchain to securely and scalably share clinical data." *Computational and Structural Biotechnology Journal*, 16, 267–278, 2018.

40. Azaria, Asaph, Ekblaw, Ariel, Vieira, Thiago, & Lippman, Andrew. "Medrec: Using blockchain for medical data access and permission management." In *2016 2nd International Conference on Open and Big Data (OBD)*, pp. 25–30. IEEE, 2016.

41. Yue, Xiao, Wang, Huiju, Jin, Dawei, Li, Mingqiang, & Jiang, Wei. "Healthcare data gateways: Found healthcare intelligence on blockchain with novel privacy risk control." *Journal of Medical Systems*, 40(10), 1–8, 2016.

42. Rolim, Carlos Oberdan, Koch, Fernando Luiz, Westphall, Carlos Becker, Werner, Jorge, Fracalossi, Armando, & Salvador, Giovanni Schmitt. "A cloud computing solution for patient's data collection in healthcare institutions." In *2010 Second International Conference on eHealth, Telemedicine, and Social Medicine*, pp. 95–99. IEEE, 2010.

43. Arindam, S, Mohammad, Z. A., Moirangthem, M. S., Fattah, Abdul, Chinmay, C., & Subhendu, K. P. "Artificial neural synchronization using nature inspired whale optimization." *IEEE Access*, 1–14, 2021. doi:10.1109/ACCESS.2021.305288

44. Amit, K., Chinmay, C., Wilson, J., Kishor, A., Chakraborty, C., & Jeberson, W.. "A novel fog computing approach for minimization of latency in healthcare using machine learning." *International Journal of Interactive Multimedia and Artificial Intelligence*, 1–11, 2020, doi:10.9781/ijimai.2020.12.004

45. Anichur, R., Chinmay, C., Adnan, A., Karim, Md Razaul, Islam, Md Jahidul, Dipanjali, K., Ziaur, R., & Shahab, S. B. "SDN–IoT empowered intelligent framework for industry 4.0 applications during COVID-19 pandemic." *Cluster Computing*, 1–18, 2021, 10.1007/s10586-021-03367-4

46. Simić, Miloš, Sladić, Goran, & Milosavljević, Branko. "A case study IoT and blockchain powered healthcare." In *Proc. ICET*, 2017.

47. Saha, Himadri Nath, Supratim Auddy, Subrata Pal, Kumar, Shubham, Pandey, Shivesh, Singh, Rocky, Singh, Amrendra Kumar, Sharan, Priyanshu, Ghosh, Debmalya, & Saha, Sanhita. "Health monitoring using internet of things (IoT)." In *2017 8th Annual Industrial Automation and Electromechanical Engineering Conference (IEMECON)*, pp. 69–73. IEEE, 2017.

48. Hasan, Mahmudul, Islam, Md Milon, Zarif, Md Ishrak Islam, & Hashem, M. M. A.. "Attack and anomaly detection in IoT sensors in IoT sites using machine learning approaches." *Internet of Things*, 7, 100059, 2019.

49. Cinay, D, Brian, L. D., & Chinmay, C. Generative design methodology for Internet of MedicalThings (IoMT)-based wearable biomedical devices. *Int. Congress on Human-Computer Interaction, Optimization and Robotic Applications (HORA'21)*, 1–4, 2021. doi:10.1109/HORA52670.2021.9461370

50. Chinmay, C., Gupta, B., & Ghosh, S. K. "A review on telemedicine-based WBAN framework for patient monitoring." *International Journal of Telemedicine and e-Health, Mary Ann Libert inc*, 19(8), 619–626, 2013. ISSN: 1530-5627, doi:10.1089/tmj.2012.0215

3 Revolutionizing Healthcare by Coupling Unmanned Aerial Vehicles (UAVs) to Internet of Medical Things (IoMT)

Faris A. Almalki
Taif University, Taif, Saudi Arabia

Soufiene Ben Othman
University of Sousse, Tunisia

Hedi Sakli
EITA Consulting, Montesson, France

Marios Angelides
Brunel University London, Uxbridge, UK

CONTENTS

DOI: 10.1201/9781003247128-3

3.1   INTRODUCTION

The communications and information technology sector are witnessing rapid developments during which the roles of technology and its capabilities are increasing, as the most prominent features of the Fourth Industrial Revolution (4IR) are formed through the technologies like Internet of Things (IoT), Robotics, Drones, and Artificial Intelligence (AI). The IoT is the most important feature of this revolution, and it is widely known that IoT is the fuel for the 4IR since it consists of a network of trillions of objects and sensors that are independently capable of sensing, monitoring or interacting with the surrounding environment. In addition to the ability to collect and transmit generate real-time data. Such a technology also provides a package of smart services and options that can be used in several applications such as smart homes, smart farms, connected cars, fleet management (e.g., vehicles or robots) and many other applications (Almalki et al. [1]).

Reading the future of the IoT is possible by noting the tremendous development that is increasing daily for this technology. According to some statistics, there will be more than 40 billion smart devices connected to the Internet by 2025, and the number will soon exceed that [2]. Thus, the new rule for the future would be, 'Anything can be connected, and it will be connected.' But why do we want so many devices and things connected and in a harmonious conversation with each other? The potential value says if you are on your way to a meeting, your car will make decisions for you when traffic is heavy, and perhaps send the meeting parties a message that the meeting is postponed. Another example is that your alarm will tell the coffee maker that you will wake up at 6 am, saving you time [3].

There are many companies that have produced and are still developing this section of products and devices significantly, and when we reach a stage where these devices from different manufacturers can cooperate with each other, and communicate smoothly, we will overcome many simple and routine tasks, which these devices will perform instead for us, and they devices will be able to read their surroundings, and communicate with other devices to obtain the data they need to carry out their tasks to the fullest. We notice that the home is no longer the only place where this technology works, and we can imagine a smart city connected to the Internet, where the streets can talk to each other, and you can tell us how long it will take to get to work, and perhaps show us a better way in the event of a traffic accident smart traffic lights that will immediately give priority to ambulances and firefighters and direct you to an alternative route to your original destination. Perhaps in a world where self-driving cars are common, communication will be much easier, and perhaps we can consider this car also as part of the world of 'IoT'. Governments are expected to focus on increasing productivity, reducing costs, and improving the quality of life of their citizens [4].

Happening now is the development in things from wearable technology to technology implanted in the body, and we will witness the integration of the body and the machine together with smart chips and advanced vision and brain lenses, and informatics in learning will be a great leap in the IoT, as the curriculum will develop to be intelligent automatically according to the scientific development of the student. Further, the IoT in the health sector also helps to monitor patients and receive vital signs such as pressure, sugar, temperature and heart rate, from remote patients and store them in data centres, so that they are analyzed in order to detect diseases, and act in a timely manner, but in the long run collected at record speed, this data will help make major leaps in science and medicine, and improve health on a global level [5].

Unsurprisingly, coupling IoT with UAVs would effectively links trillions of items and sensors, which in turn leads towards hyper-connected societies, and thus more global smart connectivity. There are many advantages over which attracts researchers' attention towards UAVs. For example, UAV reliability, line of sight (LoS) connectivity, flexibility, efficiency, applicability, rapid deployment, portability and low manufacturing, launching and maintenance cost. Furthermore, UAVs could offer wide range of applications including telecommunications, multimedia communications, smart healthcare, remote sensing, empowering smart cities, smart farming, public safety, long range surveillance, border and traffic monitoring, natural/manmade disasters response, atmospheric studies, smart service delivery, high-resolution imaging, and localization and navigation [6]. Hence, great attention from both industry and academia can be seen, due to coupling IoT and UAVs along with their advantages and wide. This subsequently leading to an intelligent and hyper-connected world, where all things are sensing, and connected to the grid network [7].

In our current digital era, approximately everything on the globe will be online or ready to be connected to the Internet, which means and according to the Economist magazine: 'By 2035, the earth will become a supercomputer.' This would take the idea of connecting trillions of items and sensors into to broader horizons to include nearly everything (things, people, processing and data). Thus, many aspects have been emerged from IoT like: Internet of Medical Things (IoMT), Internet of Everything (IoE), Internet of Vehicles (IoV), Internet of Logistics (IoL), Internet of Farming (IoF), Internet of Buildings (IoB), Internet of Cities (IoC), Internet of Industrial Things (IIC) [8]. Furthermore, the merit of IoT with all its derivatives is based not only on the ability to connect people and things to the Internet, but also the merit of the functionality that can be done automatically without human intervention. The rest of this chapter is organized as an overview on wireless communication systems for UAVs case in Section 3.2. Then revolutionizing smart healthcare is presented in Section 3.3. Section 3.4 highlights trends and smart healthcare applications of IoMT-enabled UAVs. Finally, a conclusion and future perspectives in Section 3.5.

3.2   WIRELESS COMMUNICATION SYSTEMS: A UAV CASE

Since ancient times, people have realized the need to achieve remote communication with each other. Under the pressure of this necessity, research and experiments were conducted to find the means and methods that enable the human being to transcend distances and times, and to achieve the exchange and transmission of information from a distance. Wireless technologies based their development on the breakthroughs made by great pioneers in physics, mathematics and engineering sciences in the nineteenth and twentieth centuries. The most important of them is the discovery of the ability of electricity to produce magnetism, then the discovery of magnetic induction, and the discovery of radio waves (Priyanka [9]).

Guglielmo Marconi's development in the late nineteenth century of the wireless telegraph system marked the beginning of the wireless age. He was preceded by Jagdish Chandra Bose by sending a signal to remotely strike a bell and detonate a stun on millimetre frequency in 1895. This was followed by the completion of the first radio transmission in 1906, establishing the first true wireless industry (radio equipment) in the 1920s. The Second World War played an important role in the development of wireless technologies to meet the military needs in the field of radio communication systems, radar, and encryption [10]. The first civilian wireless telephone system (first generation) appeared in the seventies of the twentieth century in the United States of America. The 1990s saw an acceleration in the wireless sector, with the first commercial GSM (global system for mobile communications) networks appearing in Scandinavia in 1991. The paging service invaded Europe in the mid-nineties of the twentieth century, and at the end of the twentieth century, medium-range wireless data networks emerged in the form of wireless local networks and Bluetooth system. The beginning of the twenty-first century is the beginning of the era of the wireless Internet [11].

The idea of Wireless Communications is based on a simple idea; It is the complete dispensation of 'wires' and the provision of various communication services to users everywhere: home, car, plane, ship, institutions, universities, etc. On the other hand, providing the same services and features as wired communications [12]. Broadly, wireless communication systems can be divided into two main types: terrestrial systems and space-based systems (e.g., satellite and UAVs). This section aims to cover cutting-edge work on UAVs and compare it against other communication systems from features like capabilities, types, applications and main limitations. This section concludes with a comprehensive comparison [13].

3.3   REVOLUTIONIZING SMART HEALTHCARE

The IoT in the health sector helps to monitor patients and receive vital signs such as pressure, sugar, temperature and heart rate. This monitoring can be done remotely, and data get stored and processed on the Internet and make it available to doctors to give a consultation anytime anywhere. Such a real-time monitoring would allow medical teams and professionals to detect diseases and take actions like advising patients in a timely manner [14].

3.3.1   RATIONALE OF CONSIDERING IoMT

Network technology has huge potential in the healthcare sector. As a result, we can classify the most popular IoT healthcare applications into four categories:

3.3.1.1   Wellbeing and Early Detection

The focus of healthcare is shifting away from sickness towards health, and consequently disease prevention. Wearable smart gadgets, for example, track basic activity and use more complex technology to measure respiratory patterns, skin behaviour, ambient light and skin temperature. Currently, non-invasive measurements and monitoring vital signs can be conducted, which can be used by applications that linked to Electronic Health Record (EHR), Personal Health Record (PHR), or Electronic Medical Record (EMR), or even more linked to ResearchKit as part of a clinical trial. Therefore, physicians, hospitals, pharmacies and other authorized sources can retrieve data remotely. People with chronic diseases and or elderly can benefit from such a smart monitoring system allow the patinates to live independently via monitoring activities analyzing health signs, where automatically alerting healthcare providers and/or patinates to take rapid actions. The use of IoMT could aid in the early detection of disruptions in daily routines or unusual events, as well as alerting family members or emergency personnel. Using smart applications and wearables to track exercise levels and monitor fitness and overall wellness can also be highly useful [15].

3.3.1.2   Patient Support

The incorporation of IoT in the healthcare field is fostering a new approach known as the Internet of Medical Things (IoMT). This term refers to a connected infrastructure of devices and software applications that can communicate with various IT systems to provide health-related services [16]. Telemonitoring for patients with chronic or long-term diseases is one instance of IoMT. This sort of therapy eliminates the need for patients to visit the hospital or doctor's office every time they have a medical concern or a change in their health, as well as inpatient wearable mHealth devices that can communicate data to nurses. Another example, in the pharmaceutical sector, is drug tracking. However, it is important to note that the healthcare sector faces many challenges. The main challenge is the processing and analysis of patient records, due to the large amount of data collected. The security of this data is another challenge to consider. These systems are vulnerable to malicious assaults due of their high connection. Furthermore, due to the sharing of sensitive data, it is difficult to maintain privacy [17].

3.3.1.3   Improving Professional Medical Services

IoT is always seen to offer good quality of medical services, such as ECall call systems as can be found in the European union. The system recognizes the severity of automobile accidents, as well as informing communicate the geolocation of the accident. Where this dataset is sent to local authorities for further actions. Further, since the vehicle is coupled with smart devices, the vehicle can gain access to personal health records, which in turn leads to rapid and better response and then save more lives. Another example of medical services is led by Ontario University Institute of Technology and the Toronto SickKids Hospital via introducing Artemis project. The project aims to diagnoses small changes in hospitalized infants before any external signs appear [18].

3.3.1.4   Data Analytics

There is a direct line between IoT and Big Data in healthcare, which can be demonstrated within three dimensions quantity, velocity and type. The first dimensions indict the volume of data that get collected from wearable devices, and medical sensors. The second dimensions indict the transmission speed in real time. The third dimensions indict various types of collected data from wearable devices, and medical sensors (e.g., charts, numbers, characters and sounds). On the other hand, powerful computers such as IBM Watson should be utilized to manage and process the healthcare activities like analyzing and storing. Despite the achievements of IoT for healthcare sector, some challenges are still existed includes data integrity, data quality and security. Thus, it is vital to enhance connectivity and security aspects to enhance experiences of IoMT and thus safe lives of many people [19].

3.3.2   IoMT Overview and Architecture

The IoMT architecture includes diagnosis and monitoring of vital signs like heart rate, pulse, temperature, blood pressure, sugar level in the body and digestive system. Diagnosis of health conditions can sense data, which is collected throughout the day, and then sending them to medical personnel for appropriate analysis and medical actions. This why IoMT has emerged to take IoT to broaden aspect [20]. Applications of IoMT can have substantial impact in enhancing access and quality, as well as reducing cost of care.

IoMT system architecture contains five main layers: Application Layer, Processing Layer, Aggregator Layer, Transport Layer and Devices Layer. Where at the devices layer, smart sensors and/or devices (e.g., wearable, smart watch, smart contact lenses, smart pills) can sense and gather data of predefined parts of human body. At the transport layer, sensed and gather data can be transferred between different layer through a wireless network, such as: Bluetooth, WiFi, RFID, or NFC [21]. Thus, in our scenario, a UAV can act as an aerial rely on node to collect data and then transferee it to the following layers. At the aggregator layer, it contains of several protocols (e.g., Message Queuing Telemetry Transport (MQTT), HTTP, gateway). These protocols are considered as messaging protocols that play a big role to enable IoMT, where they optimize towards message size, for efficiency, low computing, low power, consumption capability and small storage are the main advantages of these protocols, especially MQTT. At the processing layer, sensed and gather data can be stored and analyzed for suitable actions and/or advice. Additionally, this layer employs datasets, cloud computing and bigdata processing modules. The application layer is responsible for delivering services to the users; besides, it can manage the whole IoMT system including applications interface, models, and secured data [22].

3.3.3 IoMT Wide Application

Unsurprisingly, IoMT applications can reach many areas in the body to enhance the patients experience. Here are examples of main IoMT applications include monitoring Glucose, Electrocardiogram (ECG), arrhythmias, Blood pressure, Elevated body fever, Oxygen saturation, Congestive heart failure, Asthma inhalers, Pill bottles and Digital contact lenses. In terms of integrating IoMT with artificial intelligent monitor, Apple smart watch received approval from the US Food and Drug Administration (FDA) that rival many approved medical devices. Further, the smart watch has effective recording quality systems, which can be able to record measures like heart rate, temperature and intravenous therapy. This would send alarm messages to both healthcare providers as well as patients, which in turn helps prevent early diseases such as strokes and heart attacks. Furthermore, these kinds of smart gadgets are designed to automatically call emergency services while sending the patient's location to emergency contacts [23].

According to the World Health Organization (WHO), the COVID-19 disease has struck almost every country in the world, resulting in hundreds of millions of confirmed cases, and millions of deaths. For more than a year now, with the pandemic caused by the coronavirus disease, the world has been moving towards a technological approach to cope with the spread of the disease, which finds its strength through groupings and human-to-human contact. The IoT is also interesting in terms of traceability of the drug circuit outside the hospital. Via connected drug packaging, the various players in the care pathway will be able to know whether a patient is following his prescribed treatment. The IoT then finds a major role, through its ability to manage the condition of a patient from a distance. The instructions required by the WHO are thus applied to control and limit the spread of the disease. Researchers and tech companies worldwide are striving to develop advanced technologies to combat COVID-19 outbreak. The rest of this subsection presents the major technical trends for better understanding of directions the healthcare technology industry [24].

Trend 1: IoMT with various devices and mobile applications are now playing an important part in chasing and averting chronic diseases; thanks to coupling IoT technology with wearable devices/sensors and telemedicine technologies. To illustrate, many wearable devices can take common medical measurements like ECG, skin temperature, glucose level and blood pressure readings. Another example would be a smart pill that recognized by FDA in 2017, where medical personnel can have various options for medical investigation. Efficient connectivity to multiple medical IoT devices is one of the main issues that face the IoMT system; especially regular protocols are still used between devices. This issue gets more complicated when collecting vast data. Therefore, the idea of using heterogeneous topology is becoming necessarily rapid.

Trend 2: Telemedicine COVID-19 has significantly enhanced the use of tele-health resources. Where such a technology acts an alternative of communication between patients, healthcare workers and other patients, which can be considered as pre-cautious measure of spearing COVID-19. What even more for telehealth, wearable devices enable healthcare workers to obtain real-time measurements while they are at home. It is widely expected that the growth of telehealth will continue even after the pandemic is over, especially with development of mobile apps. An example of telemedicine applications is WebRTC, the app's versatility is a useful feature such as text and video chat, screen sharing and file transfer. Besides, the ability of demonstrate the patients' medical records in the app. Additionally, Interactive Voice Response (IVR) is another beneficial application to transmit communications to patients via digital speech. These apps and different ones can provide treasured prospects to gain real-time access to health information. Furthermore, Cloud servers are vital for running all the mentioned processes with careful consideration of significant features like security, appointment, multimedia calling, secure messaging and healthcare provider reviews.

Trend 3: AI techniques have served in battling against COVID-19 from many perspectives. For instance, pandemic detection, thermal monitoring, injection progress or facial recognition. Pandemic detection like BlueDot has been major pioneers in early cautioning systems. Various AI methods help in collaborating with human efforts to understand characteristics of virus due to the collaboration accuracy, efficiency and speed. Thus, with the help of the machine, immunologists have identified more than a million parts of cell surface proteins that can be detected by T-cells. However, without the help of Machine Learning (ML) approaches, only humans would be able to know this for sure. Thanks to ML, the development of a COVID-19 vaccine continues rapidly. Moreover, AI techniques can perform mass analysis and processing (e.g., public places) to identify people with high temperatures using smart thermal cameras or might be aerial thermal cameras onboard a drone. What even more, deep learning approaches like convolutional Neural Network (CNN) can help in recognizing people who wearing masks for security purposes.

Trend 4: AI in Healthcare a tendency that has excessive opportunity to improve healthcare services, since AI with human-style information processing and decision-making opens many potentials in accuracy, speed and efficiency of diagnosis. Early treatment can be accomplished via AI analytics that help medical personnel to find the appropriate method and actions to patients in terms of diagnosis and/or treatment. Additionally, ML algorithms can analyse thousands of drug developments to enhance chemical and biological interactions to get new drugs to market faster.

Wide range of medical applications can benefit from ML such as mental health and diagnosis of cancer. Furthermore, a recent integrating between chatbot and AI technologies that can be used to aid patients with self-diagnosis and give medical advice. This integrating help in reading and answering questions in an intuitive, faster and simpler fashion, which in turn making the whole process more useful for clinicians. Smartphones, wearable devices and the growing IoMT infrastructure promise an increase in the data sets available for ML software analysis. Deep learning can yield significant returns if the process is maintained, where AI, ML and data science are key trends envisioning the forthcoming of healthcare.

Trend 5: Augmented Reality (AR), Virtual reality (VR), Mixed Reality (MR), or Extended Reality (XR) in healthcare are significant technologies with massive potential to enhance the quality of remote medical instructions to patients during the COVID-19 pandemic. Also, this technology can help in educating medical students in simulating procedures through overlays, which can change science fiction into reality. The simulation environment of the AR, VR, MR, or XR help many patients (e.g., stroke victims, those suffering dementia and/or cognitive disabilities) to overcome motor deficiencies as well as improve their emotional wellbeing via flexibility physical therapy. Furthermore, these advanced techniques can provide in 3D space in the vision of the surgeon, or doctor or even robotic surgeries; thus, better understanding and more accurate information can be given remotely.

Trend 6: Blockchain is a method that intends to significantly improve the healthcare sector rapidly. Digital ledgers are striving to enable digital transformation to reach securely transaction records to patients. Blockchain's system allows users to securely access the patient's registers, where there is no need for a foundation of trust between two parties. Portability, interoperability and security are all desirable blockchain goals that improve healthcare and IoMT. An example of this is that medical personnel can provide advice via a secure system. Alternatively, patients can choose to provide data for research purposes, so anonymity is achieved. Blockchain is, also, can help in providing clinical study information, patient records, digital health card and wearable patient data.

3.4   TRENDS AND SMART HEALTHCARE OF IOMT-ENABLED UAVS

The ground segment contains medical sensors, relay nodes, aggregator and medical server. Where patients are equipped with wearable devices, before sending sensed information to the medical server. On the other hand, the aerial segment includes any of the UAV platform type depends on the application, configuration or user preference. The UAV can be payloaded with telecommunication devices to collect sensed information from a wireless server gateway to be directly sent to the cloud for storage and further process. Therefore, healthcare providers can access the data anywhere and anytime. Clearly, the UAV considers as median between terrestrial devices such as sensors, relays, and gateways, on one side, and the cloud on the other. This integration replicates the trustworthiness and swiftness of such a technology. The IoMT-enabled UAVs structure might be suitable in remote reigns with difficult terrines where it could be economically infeasible or may be impossible to be achieved with traditional systems.

The 5G population is designing, standardizing and implementing a layered network architecture which will drive the future of telecommunications for 5G and beyond, where UAV network one of them that promise to achieve the necessary attributes of global coverage, capacity, and seamless interconnected networks [25]. Thus, such a IoMT-enabled UAVs framework would represent the connectivity fabric which reinforces the digital transformation and the provision of digital health services. What even more, IoMT-enabled UAVs enables the shift to newly distributed patient-centric digital health ecosystems, which can integrate with Big Data analytics, cloud computing and AI. Advances in IoMT have principally focused on five main functions which are: sensing, transmission, storage, analysis and visualization of data. These functions represent the workflow of the IoMT:

- The sensor collects data from a patient or doctor/nurse for data entry.
- The IoT device analyses the collected data with the help of algorithms that rely on AI such as ML approaches.
- The device decides whether to act or send information to the cloud.
- Physicians or health practitioners are empowered to make informed and actionable decisions based on data provided by an IoMT sensors and/or devices.

IoMT can be used in many applications, due to the flexibility of UAV coverage networks. Additionally, UAV has the capability to execute diverse intelligence in many applications such as monitoring and predictions. Relay on UAV is not only vital in remote reigns with difficult terrines where it could be economically infeasible or may be impossible to be achieved with traditional systems; but also, important when integrating with terrestrial and/or satellites systems. Such an integration would increase hyper-connected societies, and thus more global smart connectivity. On the other hand, away from considering a UAV as aerial rely, UAV can provide various applications in critical times like COVID-19 [26]. For instance, UAV can support carriers deliver goods, foods, medicine and clothes to disaster areas and quarantine areas during COVID-19. Other examples would be help in monitoring people, who violate curfews or stay-at-home orders, and detecting infected person of COVID-19 from long distance and absent masks [27].

3.5   CONCLUSION

Today, with technological development and the world of technology, the IoE is a cornerstone for countries looking for economic development and prosperity. Where smart city programmes place a premium on technology that increase community quality of life and efficiency while lowering expenses. IoMT is one of several smart IoT applications that involves the continuous and comprehensive monitoring of patients using cameras and/or sensors that monitor everything about the patient, which could be the difference between life and death. This chapter aims to highlight the coupling of IoMT and UAVs in healthcare along with their capabilities, advantages, applications and challenges. This contribution is a noticeable shift from exiting work in the literature, where it provides a panoramic view on the proposed integration between IoMT and UAVs.

Clearly, UAV can help IoMT to connect everything and cover everywhere, where it can extend the network coverage with and without communication infrastructure. The connected devices wirelessly transmit important and vital data on the patient's condition 24 hours a day, 7 days a week to the doctor's computer, which then takes the appropriate action for the case, such as performing or not performing an operation, writing a medication and other procedures. Additionally, such an integration would reduce human intervention and enforce the advancement of AI for remote follow-up and monitoring of the patient. Further, this chapter provides a vision for the future of digital healthcare where it emphasizes the empowering effect of connectivity. Such a transformation would help in reshaping the provision of digital healthcare services and corresponding socioeconomic impacts.

Every technology in this modern era has its pros and cons, yet as this technology has benefits in our lives, it has some damages in return. Some the positives are quick access to information, saving time and effort, improving the quality of life, ability to control and monitor with high levels of precision, and provide limitless healthcare in timely and efficient manners. However, the main drawbacks are fears of system failure, and data integrity and security; these issues could open further research work.

REFERENCES

1. F. Almalki et al., "Green IoT for Eco-Friendly and Sustainable Smart Cities: Future Directions and Opportunities," *Springer Mobile Networks and Applications*, to be published.
2. M. Elsisi, K. Mahmoud, M. Lehtonen, and M. M. F. Darwish, "Reliable Industry 4.0 Based on Machine Learning and IoT for Analyzing, Monitoring, and Securing Smart Meters," *Sensors*, vol. 21, no. 2, p. 487, January 2021, doi: 10.3390/s21020487.
3. L. Sujay Vailshery, "Global Number of Connected IoT Devices 2015–2025," *Statista*, March 08, 2021. https://www.statista.com/statistics/1101442/iot-number-of-connected-devices-worldwide/ (accessed Jun. 24, 2021).
4. W. Li et al., "A Comprehensive Survey on Machine Learning-Based Big Data Analytics for IoT-Enabled Smart Healthcare System," *Mobile Networks and Applications*, Jan. 2021, doi: 10.1007/s11036-020-01700-6.

5. K. Hazarika, G. Katiyar, and N. Islam, "IoT-Based Transformer Health Monitoring System: A Survey," *2021 International Conference on Advance Computing and Innovative Technologies in Engineering (ICACITE)*, 2021, pp. 1065–1067, doi: 10.1109/ICACITE51222.2021.9404657.

6. Faris A. Almalki, and Ben Othman Soufiene, "EPPDA: An Efficient and Privacy-Preserving Data Aggregation Scheme with Authentication and Authorization for IoT-Based Healthcare Applications," *Wireless Communications and Mobile Computing*, vol. 2021, p. 18, 2021, Article ID 5594159. doi: 10.1155/2021/5594159.

7. F. A. Almalki, B. O. Soufiene, S. H. Alsamhi, and H. Sakli, "A Low-Cost Platform for Environmental Smart Farming Monitoring System Based on IoT and UAVs," *Sustainability*, vol. 13, no. 11, p. 5908, May 2021, doi:10.3390/su13115908.

8. C. Chinmay, and N. A. Arij, "Intelligent Internet of Things and Advanced Machine Learning Techniques for COVID-19," *EAI Endorsed Transactions on Pervasive Health and Technology*, pp. 1–14, 2021, doi: 10.4108/eai.28-1-2021.168505.

9. D. Priyanka, and C. Chinmay, Application of AI on Post Pandemic Situation and Lesson Learn for Future Prospects, *Journal of Experimental & Theoretical Artificial Intelligence*, pp. 1–24, 2021, doi: 10.1080/0952813X.2021.1958063.

10. C. Chinmay, "Performance Analysis of Compression Techniques for Chronic Wound Image Transmission under Smartphone-Enabled Tele-wound Network," *International Journal of E-Health and Medical Communications (IJEHMC), IGI Global*, vol. 10, no. (2), pp. 1–20, April. 2019.

11. F. A. Almalki, "Developing an Adaptive Channel Modelling using a Genetic Algorithm Technique to Enhance Aerial Vehicle-to-Everything Wireless Communications," *International Journal of Computer Networks & Communications*, vol. 13, no. 2, pp. 37–56, 2021. Available: doi: 10.5121/ijcnc.2021.13203.

12. S. H. Alsamhi, M. S. Ansari, O. Ma, F. Almalki, and S. K. Gupta, "Tethered Balloon Technology in Design Solutions for Rescue and Relief Team Emergency Communication Services," *Disaster Medicine and Public Health Preparedness*, vol. 13, pp. 1–8, May 2018, doi: 10.1017/dmp.2018.19.

13. F. A. Almalki, "Optimisation of a Propagation Model for Last Mile Connectivity with Low Altitude Platforms using Machine Learning," Ph.D. dissertation, Dept. Elect. Eng., Brunel Univ., London, UK, 2018.

14. F. A. Almalki, and M. C. Angelides, "Empirical evolution of a propagation model for low altitude platforms," *2017 Computing Conference*, London, 2017, pp. 1297–1304, doi: 10.1109/SAI.2017.8252258.

15. F. A. Almalki, and M. C. Angelides, "Propagation modelling and performance assessment of aerial platforms deployed during emergencies," *12th International Conference for Internet Technology and Secured Transactions (ICITST)*, Cambridge, UK, 2017, pp. 238–243, doi: 10.23919/ICITST.2017.8356391.

16. F. A. Almalki, "Comparative and QoS Performance Analysis of Terrestrial-Aerial Platforms-satellites Systems for Temporary Events," *International Journal of Computer Networks & Communications*, vol. 11, no. 6, pp. 111–133, 2019, doi:10.5121/ijcnc.2019.11607.

17. D. Sachin, C. Chinmay, F. Jaroslav, G. Rashmi, K. R. Arun, and K. P. Subhendu, "SSII: Secured and High-Quality Steganography Using Intelligent Hybrid Optimization Algorithms for IoT," *IEEE Access*, vol. 9, pp. 1–16, 2021.

18. C. Chinmay, "Joel JPC Rodrigues, A Comprehensive Review on Device-to-Device Communication Paradigm: Trends, Challenges and Applications, Springer," *International Journal of Wireless Personal Communications*, vol. 114, pp. 185–207, 2020.

19. D. Sachin, C. Chinmay, F. Jaroslav, G. Rashmi, K. R. Arun, and K. P. Subhendu, "SSII: Secured and High-Quality Steganography Using Intelligent Hybrid Optimization Algorithms for IoT," *IEEE Access*, vol. 9, pp. 1–16, 2021.

20. F. Almalki, and M. Angelides, "Deployment of An Aerial Platform System for Rapid Restoration of Communications Links After a Disaster: A Machine Learning Approach," *Computing*, vol. 102, pp. 829–864, November 2019.

21. S. Alsamhi, F. A. Almalki, S. Gapta, M. Ansari O. Ma, and M. Angelides, "Tethered Balloon Technology for Emergency Communication and Disaster Relief Deployment," *Springer Telecommunication Systems*, vol. 75, pp. 235–244, 2019, doi: 10.1007/s11235-019-00580-w

22. F. A. Almalki, and M. C. Angelides, "An Enhanced Design of a 5G MIMO Antenna for Fixed Wireless Aerial Access," *Cluster Computing*, July 2021, doi: 10.1007/s10586-021-03318-z.

23. F. A. Almalki, and M. C. Angelides, "Considering near space platforms to close the coverage gap in wireless communications; the case of the Kingdom of Saudi Arabia," *FTC 2016 San Francisco – Future Technologies Conference*, 2016, pp. 224–230.

24. F. A. Almalki, and M. C. Angelides, "Evolution of an Optimal Propagation Model for the Last Mile with Low Altitude Platforms using Machine Learning," *Elsevier Computer Communications Journal*, vol. 142–143, pp. 9–33, May 2019, DOI: org/10.1016/j.comcom.2019.04.001.

25. R. K. Usman, U. Ubaid, K. Shehzad, R. Umar, C. Chinmay, and A. T. Fadi, "Path Loss Modelling at 60 GHz mm Wave Based on Cognitive 3D Ray Tracing Algorithm in 5G," *Peer-to-Peer Networking and Applications*, pp. 1–17, 2021, doi:10.1007/s12083-021-01101-w.

26. Faris A. Almalki, Soufiene Ben Othman, Fahad A. Almalki, and Hedi Sakli, "EERP-DPM: Energy Efficient Routing Protocol Using Dual Prediction Model for Healthcare Using IoT," *Journal of Healthcare Engineering*, vol. 2021, p. 15, 2021, Article ID 9988038. doi: 10.1155/2021/9988038.

27. F. A. Almalki, "Implementation of 5G IoT-Based Smart Buildings using VLAN Configuration via Cisco Packet Tracer," *International Journal of Electronics Communication and Computer Engineering*, vol. 11, no. 4, pp. 56–67, 2020.

4 Public Perception toward AI-Driven Healthcare and the Way Forward in the Post-Pandemic Era

Spandan Datta, Nilesh Tejrao Kate, and Abhishek Srivastava
Pune Institute of Business Management, Pune, Maharastra

CONTENTS

4.1 INTRODUCTION

Now, there should arise one fundamental question: what is Artificial Intelligence? According to IBM, AI uses computers, machines and robust datasets that can impersonate the different capabilities of the human mind. It (AI) has the capabilities to augment human intelligence in its present form.

In machine learning, algorithm models are used to attain AI concepts; as the algorithms are exposed to fresh data, they adapt and adjust themselves independently over time to perform better in the future. As they process data, the machines are learning. AI systems can use this method to select activities that have the best chance of succeeding.

The deep learning method discovers patterns in data by utilizing numerous layers of the network, including abstract layers not built by human engineers. This technique aids in the organization of unstructured data and allows machines to learn to classify data on their own.

Now, as fascinating as it may sound today, AI was not always there from the start. It was surely with us through science fiction stories but in reality, it was gradually evolved. The concept of AI, as a machine that thinks is credited to British mathematician Alan Turing. Starting as a concept, AI has come a long way, where we are today talking about self-driving cars to the potential use of AI in the healthcare system. Can AI augment human intelligence in the healthcare system? if yes, then in which spheres it can contribute? AI can help in medical diagnostics, drug discovery, clinical trials, pain management, improving patient outcomes, etc. These are just a few examples. The use of AI can be wider and deeper as we progress in time. It can also help in clinical data management, clinical decision support system, personalized treatments, etc. In May–June this year, when the COVID-19 second wave hit the nation hard, a critical conversation was going on among the peers. The discussion point was that in some hospitals where there was sufficient oxygen availability, and some healthcare touchpoints were facing a severe scarcity of oxygen. 'Can AI solve the issue?' Some may ask. One can argue that is there no instance of AI saving lives in India? A full-scale searching yielded a very interesting case.

Strokes have always been one of the major causes of human demise in the state of Assam. A local hospital conducted a study in 2018 which concluded that the cases of strokes were around 150 per day. There is a scarcity of trained radiologists in Assam, as well as India as a whole. It is projected that there are around 15,000 radiologists in India and they are based mainly on Tier-I and II cities, far from interiors.

In the case of stroke, minutes of delay can be fatal, so a Baptist hospital of Tezpur found a solution to this problem after partnering with a technology start-up. The hospital, integrated AI to interpret brain CT scans in seconds. The hospital has had the technology since March 2021 and now it is diagnosing hundreds of patients every month.

Now the question is, how effective can these AI systems be? They can surely augment healthcare professionals in some way. But can they replace them?

Professor Alastair Denniston and his team from England researched in 2019 to try to understand if AI can determine illnesses as successfully as medical workers.

The research inferred suchlike AI accurately identifies illnesses in 87% of the occurrences, whereas observations by medical professionals shown an 86% accuracy rate [1].

According to research published in 'International Journal of Interactive Multimedia & Artificial Intelligence', as our present lifestyle is heavily dependent on technology and associated devices (smartwatch, etc.), these IoT devices are providing huge multimedia information about patient health in the form of data which is being stored in the cloud. Analysis on a real-time basis can revolutionize the healthcare system for the better. The authors suggested that by adopting 5G as greater network access, in the future the reliability of e-healthcare solutions and latency for high-risk data may be enhanced. The fog model may be used to create a smart medical system [2].

In the case of India, where there is a huge gap in terms of health services available to the common people, AI can surely bridge the gap; i.e., sustainability. Managerial decision to patient data harvesting and predicting the likelihood of next outbreak, AI is effective and successful in every aspect. India is in its infancy in terms of adoption of AI. It ranked 19th on the AI adoption list. Not an impressive score, however, leaving plenty of opportunity to improve. Bangalore-based NetApp, one of prominent cloud storage providers, has come up with the indigenous plan to provide various citizenship services. With the help of the Government of India, NetApp is planning to implement a project named Ayushman Bharat Mission. It is an auspicious plan to provide health insurance to the needy persons. 10 crores Indian families will benefit from health insurance of ₹5 lakhs each, from the Government, at a highly affordable price. The massive operational and technological infrastructural services will be provided by the NetApp. Ayushman Bharat Mission can be exemplified as one of the biggest spending by the Indian Government on health insurance and at the same time it also signifies investment in terms of AI in order to maintain record and seamless updating of record with minimal human intervention [3]. The data used in this project can help future generation for the predicting and finding cure for the diseases. Finding patterns for disease, remedy strategies and early detection of chronical and fatal diseases can become substantially easy to understand. Insurance providers can benefit by joining hand with the Government and providing various innovative services.

Whether people will accept these services and trust them as they trust conventional modes of diagnoses and treatment that needs to be found out. A new technology before adoption generates some fundamental issues that need to be addressed. One of them being data privacy concerns as medical data contains very personal and specific health-related information of a patient which he/she may or may not want to reveal in the public. So, there should be a system that will guarantee data safety.

Another concern can be that there should be proper government guidelines to regulate these kinds of services. In absence of proper guidelines, the technology can be misused for business purposes.

Besides that, accuracy, ease of use, pricing, etc. can also be of concern for the potential users.

In this chapter, we analyse the general public understanding and perception towards AI-driven smart healthcare systems. Recent and extensive literature based on public perception towards AI awareness and its enabled smart healthcare system covered and through research gap research problems were identified. We study if there is any relation between income, age, education, technical literacy, regulatory concerns, COVID-19 and perceived usefulness, perceived trust towards Smart AI-driven Healthcare System. Analysis section of this chapter consist of detailed (figures and tables) analysis of research variables and their outcomes. In discussion and conclusion section, we established that most of the significance and relevant factors to be useful for AI-based healthcare system for socio-economic development.

4.2   LITERATURE REVIEW

The paper 'Perception of Artificial Intelligence in Spain' was reviewed. It was published in *Telematics & Informatics Journal* in 2021. The variables found in the research paper are attitude, perception, scientific discoveries and technological development, AI, and robots. The research methodology used was survey-based descriptive research. Target respondents were 6,308 Spanish Individuals. After analyzing with the binary logit regression model, individuals have a dismissive view if they are not engaged in scientific findings and technological breakthroughs and if AI and robots are ineffective at work, according to the research. The study's limitations include the fact that it is a country-specific study [4].

The paper 'Understanding user perception toward artificial intelligence (AI) enabled e-learning' was reviewed. It was published in *International Journal of Information and Learning Technology* in 2020. The constructs identified are being perceived ease of use, perceived usefulness, personal learning environment (PLE), artificial intelligence (AI), personal learning profile (PLP), personal learning network (PLN), attitude and satisfaction. Online survey-based descriptive research was done among students and professionals who have used e-learning. After smart partial least square-structural equation modelling it was observed that the PLE is impacting both perceived ease of use and perceived usefulness. The study has shown that perceived ease of use showed a moderating effect between PLE and perspective and fulfilment. Limitations being the details are collected from students and professionals who have ever used the e-learning module and wholly based on their understanding, directing to self-awareness bias [5].

The paper 'Public Perception of Artificial Intelligence in Medical Care: Content Analysis of Social Media' was reviewed. It was published in *Journal of Medical Internet Research* in 2020. The variables identified are being technology and application, trade growth, impact on society, people attitudes. Online survey-based descriptive research has been done. The researchers gathered a data set from China's Weibo platform consisting of above 16 million users throughout China by crawling all individual posts from January to December 2017. Rooting on this data set, they have pointed out 2,315 broadcasts related to Artificial Intelligence in medical care and assorted them through content scanning. After analyzing this content of social media data, it was discovered that 59.4% (568), 34.4% (329), and 6.2% (59) of all the postings indicated favourable, impartial and dismissive attitudes, respectively, out of 956 posts where public attitudes were expressed. The two main explanations for the negative sentiments were the infantility of AI-driven technology (27/59, 46%) and mistrust of connected organizations (15, 25%). The majority of respondents had positive sentiments of AI doctors and believed that they would eventually replace human doctors totally or partially. Limitations include China's social media analysis [6].

The paper "Intelligent Conversational Agents in Mental Healthcare Services: A Thematic Analysis of User Perceptions" was reviewed. It was published in *Pacific Asia Journal of the Association for Information Systems* in 2020. The constructs found are perceived risk, perceived benefits, trust and perceived anthropomorphism, user's adoption, use of mental healthcare. Qualitative research was done based on netnography. After doing Thematic analysis of publicly available user reviews in an iterative process the authors created a complete thematic map that includes four primary themes: perceived danger, perceived advantages, trust and perceived anthropomorphism, as well as 12 subthemes that visualize the aspects that influence an end user's acceptance and application of mental healthcare CA [7].

The paper 'Use of AI-based tools for healthcare purposes: a survey study from consumers' perspectives' was reviewed. It was published in *BMC Medical Informatics and Decision-Making* in 2020. The variables/constructs identified are technological, ethical, regulatory concerns, Perceived Risk, Perceived Benefit. Online survey-based descriptive research was done on 307 US individuals. After doing hypothesis testing a model was developed. In the development of AI-based gadgets, the suggested model recognizes the sources of motivation and pressure for patients. The findings reveal that technological, ethical factors, as well as regulatory concerns all, have a role in people's perceptions of the hazards of utilizing AI in healthcare. Technological considerations (i.e., execution and transmission features) are found in all three groups to be the most powerful indicators of risk attitudes. The limitations being it was a US-based study [8].

The paper 'E-health and wellbeing monitoring using smart healthcare devices: An empirical investigation' was reviewed. It was published in *Technological Forecasting & Social Change* in 2020. The variables identified are intrusiveness (INTR), Comfort (C), perceived usefulness (PU), perceived ease of use (EOU), attitude, intention. Exploratory research was done with 273 respondents, age group between 25 and 40 years. As analysis, Partial Least Square Structured Equation Modelling was done and it was found out that officiousness and easiness have no direct influence upon the intent to use BI (Behaviour Intention) BI SWH devices; nevertheless, intrusiveness has a substantial influence upon the PU of SWH devices, and comfort has a significant influence upon the perceived usability and perceived ease of intelligent wearable devices. The limitation of the research is that research in this area is still at a very rudimentary stage. Exploratory research design and detailed descriptive research are needed [9].

The paper 'Smart healthcare: Challenges and potential solutions using the internet of things (IoT) and Big Data analytics' was reviewed. It was published in *PSU Research Review* in 2019. The variables identified are healthcare, IoT, Big Data, smart health, Connected Health, and Digital Health [10–12]. A detailed literature review was done by the author, and he talked about how IoT and Big Data technology can be used in conjunction with smart health to address some of the issues around healthcare availability, access and prices. The paper's limitation is that it is a review of research [13].

The paper 'Future Trends of the Primary Healthcare System in Iran: A Qualitative Study' was analyzed. It was published in *International Journal of Preventive Medicine* in 2019. The variables identified are social/value, Technological, economic, environmental and political inclinations, demographic transition, epidemiological transition, internet and cyberspace, budgeting limitations, resource management, Pollution of the environment, natural catastrophes and health governance. Exploratory research was done. Data were collected through the interview from 25 experts in primary healthcare. After analyzing by The STEEP model revealed that demographic transition, epidemiological transition, sociocultural changes, the rise of new of comprehensive and innovative technology solutions, internet and cyberspace, budgetary restrictions, strategic planning and shifting the framework from volume to providing valuable primary healthcare were among the most effective social, technological, and social/cultural changes. Natural catastrophes, health leadership, the intellectual worldview of a top official, regional stability, global development and other internal healthcare system challenges are all factors to consider. The limitation of the research is it is an exploratory research work and further research work is needed in this space [14].

The paper 'Engagement in Healthcare Systems: Adopting Digital Tools for a Sustainable Approach' was reviewed and analyzed. It was published in *Sustainability* in 2019. The variables identified from the paper are satisfaction, social sustainability, online engagement, physician loyalty. Descriptive research was done after collecting data from 293 doctors. After doing multiple regression analyses it was found out that online involvement had a direct impact on the digital health's social sustainability platform, this has a positive impact on physician loyalty. For the platform's re-use, the human component of social sustainability, in particular, proved to be crucial. The study's limitation was that it was limited to medical practitioners [15].

The paper 'Patients' Adoption of WSN-Based Smart Home Healthcare Systems: An Integrated Model of Facilitators and Barriers' was reviewed and analyzed. The paper was published in *IEEE Transactions on Professional Communication* in 2017. The variables identified from the paper are facilitators, barriers, wireless-sensor-network-based smart home healthcare systems (WSN-SHHS), sociotechnical, cognitive, affective and contextual factors. They have used both quantitative and qualitative research. Data were collected from 15 patients and healthcare experts who get home healthcare, online and paper-based surveys facts from 140 respondents. Qualitative data was analyzed through Kvale's approach and quantitative data was analyzed by partial least square analysis. Several new constructs about WSN-SHHS adoption have been identified, concerns about human separation, privacy and life expectancy are among them, even financial concerns. Additionally, the structures from the generic adoption model were confirmed. The researchers developed a research model based on the outcomes of the qualitative study. The quantitative investigation backed up the model, which has a high level of prediction accuracy, accounting for more than 50% of the contrast in WSN-SHHS adoption. Human detachment issues, rather than performance expectations, were found to be the most important factor influencing patients' willingness to use WSN-SHHS. The limitation of the paper is a small sample size [16].

The paper 'The potential for artificial intelligence in healthcare' was reviewed and analyzed. The paper was published in *Future Healthcare Journal* in 2019. The constructs identified are being types of AI, patients' involvement and compliance, administrative duties, screening and therapeutic recommendations. After doing a thorough analysis of various articles the authors deduce, although in many situations, AI can do medical tasks as well as or greater than humans, implementation problems may cause large-scale digitization of health professional jobs to take a long time. Ethical issues about AI usage in healthcare are also raised. The limitation of the paper is that it is a literature review [17].

The paper 'Explainability for artificial intelligence in healthcare: a multidisciplinary perspective' was reviewed and analyzed. The paper was printed in *BMC Medical Informatics and Decision-Making* in 2020. The constructs identified are explainability in medical AI, technological, legal, ethical, societal perspective, use of AI-powered technologies in medical care. The authors have taken as a case study and looked into AI-based CDSS (Clinical Decision Support System) and thematically analyzed the literature on the subject. They drew many significant factors and then compared them to ethical consequences. After conducting research, the authors discovered that explainability is a critical factor for various stakeholder groups. Explainability is a requirement for success. The limitation of the study is that the paper is a literature review work [18].

The paper 'Methodologic Guide for Evaluating Clinical Performance and Effect of Artificial Intelligence Technology for Medical Diagnosis and Prediction' was reviewed and analyzed. The paper was published in the *Radiological Society of North America* in 2018. The constructs identified are high-dimensional or over parameterized diagnosis or prediction algorithms, medical assessment of AI technologies for application in medicine, discrimination and calibration performances of a framework for diagnosis or prediction, effects of the impact of illness presentation range, and incidence on productivity. After analysis, the authors deduced that discrimination, calibration, external validation and effect on patient outcomes are the major validation and testing techniques for AI-based predictive models for medical diagnosis [19].

The paper 'Machine learning for medical diagnosis: history, state-of-the-art and perspective' was reviewed and analyzed. The paper was published in *Artificial Intelligence in Medicine* in 2001. The study gives a machine learning-based overview of the evolution of medicine, advanced analytical analysis is crucial, including a historical perspective, a state-of-the-art perspective and a forecast of possible future developments in this subject of applied AI. The study's goal is not to present a thorough overview, but rather to describe specific subareas and future objectives [20].

The paper 'Artificial Intelligence in Medicine and Cardiac Imaging: Harnessing Big Data and Advanced Computing to Provide Personalized Medical Diagnosis and Treatment' was reviewed and analyzed. The paper was published in *Nuclear Cardiology* in 2013. The constructs identified are AI, Big Data, on-demand healthcare database, personalized medicine. The author deduced in addition to in silico research, Big Data mining and advanced analysis in healthcare based on empirical data, give authentic diagnosis and (possibly) curative recommendations The ability to create customized medicine will be supported and sustained by on-demand access to quality systems and large healthcare datasets [21].

The paper 'Artificial neural networks in medical diagnosis' was reviewed and analyzed. The paper was published in *Journal of Applied Biomedicine* in 2013. The constructs identified are artificial neural networks' philosophy, skills and limits in clinical diagnosis. After analyzing the cases chosen, the authors concluded that clinical specialists now have access to a variety of data, which includes everything from clinical symptom descriptions to biochemical data and imaging gadget outputs. Each piece of data collected throughout the diagnostic procedure offers data that must be analyzed and assigned to a specific aberration. Machine learning and AI techniques (particularly computer-assisted examinations and neural networks i.e., ANNs) must be utilized to speed up and avoid misdiagnosis in everyday life. These adaptive learning algorithms can incorporate a wide range of medical data into classified outputs [22].

The paper 'Overview of artificial intelligence in medicine' was reviewed and analyzed. The paper was published in *Journal of Family Medicine & Primary Care* in 2019. The constructs identified are Artificial Intelligence, medicine, terms, concepts, current and future application of AI. The key phrase 'artificial intelligence' was searched for in PubMed and Google. Cross-referencing the major papers yielded new recommendations. After analysis, the authors concluded Although AI has the potential to alter medicine in previously unthinkable ways, many of its practical applications are still in their early stages and require extensive research and development. To give better healthcare to the general people, medical practitioners must also understand and adapt to these innovations [23].

The paper 'Advocating for Safe, Quality and Just Care: What Nursing Leaders Need to Know about Artificial Intelligence in Healthcare Delivery' was reviewed and analyzed. The paper was published in *Nursing Leadership* in 2019. The constructs identified are nurses' influence on the development, deployment and evaluation of AI technologies. The research was based on an upgraded Arskey and O'Malley framework which was presented following the important nursing management positions as defined by the Canadian Nurses Association. Throughout this investigation on the use of artificial intelligence in healthcare, the use and potential ramifications of AI integration were not discussed with nurses. As noted in the review of current AI-based capabilities and concerns, nurses are ideally positioned to assist in the moral and successful deployment of AI [24].

The paper 'Artificial Intelligence-enabled Healthcare Delivery and Digital Epidemiological Surveillance in the Remote Treatment of Patients during the COVID-19 Pandemic' was reviewed and analyzed. The paper was published in

American Journal of Medical Research in 2021. The constructs identified are in the distant care of patients during the COVID-19 pandemic, Artificial Intelligence-enabled medical service and electronic epidemiological monitoring are important. The study was descriptive research with collected data from 4,200 respondents. The author conducted research and generated projections about how smart healthcare might reduce COVID-19 spread using data from Accenture, Amwell, Brookings, Deloitte, Gartner, Kyruus and Sykes, etc. [25].

The paper 'Developing a delivery science for artificial intelligence in healthcare' was reviewed and analyzed. The paper was published in *npj Digital Medicine* in 2020. The constructs identified are the characteristics of the total AI-enabled structures (what are the constructions, trends, and procedures of the workflows, groups, and technologies that make up the new AI-enabled system for providing advance treatment) and the adjustments that lead to the desired healthcare outcomes (how did the ML model's fatality projection functions mediate the improved performance in advance care planning) are both facilitated by AI and machine learning. SEIPS14 (Systems Engineering Initiative for Patient Safety) is a sociotechnical systems model that may be used to investigate the complicated relationships between people and technology in the workplace. RE-AIM13 (range, efficiency, acceptance, deployment, and preservation) is a framework that can help define the aspects to assess implementation and continuing distribution activities. To enhance clinical care, the authors concluded that AI research should go beyond in silico model creation and into real-world architecture, implementation and assessment. Machine learning models will almost definitely be required, but not adequate, components of larger AI-assisted solutions. How such systems are created, deployed, and assessed will be tackled in AI delivery [26].

The book chapter 'Application of Artificial Intelligence in Modern Healthcare System' was reviewed and analyzed. It was published in a book called *Alginates – Recent Uses of This Natural Polymer* in 2020. AI, machine learning, Natural Language Process (NLP), medical imaging and SVM are the variables that have been identified. After careful consideration, the authors concluded that AI, machine learning and other similar technologies are significantly altering the healthcare scene. There is a lot of excitement about AI-based healthcare's potential applications, but there are several constraints, such as data storage and security [27].

The research paper 'Applications of Artificial Intelligence and Big Data Analytics in m-Health: A Healthcare System Perspective' was reviewed and analyzed. It was published in *Journal of Healthcare Engineering* in 2020. The constructs identified are AI, Big Data analytics, m-health. The researchers have presented a solution based on the use of AI and Big Data analytics, a complete analysis of the healthcare system. Several m-health benefits are offered as a result of this combination. All key technological domains and building blocks related to mobile health are covered in detail, including communications, sensors and computation. While there are many advantages to the suggested m-health architecture based on AI and Big Data analytics, there are also some disadvantages to consider:

a large percentage of the population, the process can never be too accurate, the need to rely only on technology, and various confidentiality issues [28].

The research paper 'Application of Artificial Intelligence-Based Technologies in the Healthcare Industry: Opportunities and Challenges' was reviewed and analyzed. It was published in *International Journal of Environmental Research & Public Health* in 2020. The variables identified are AI-based innovation, its advantages and disadvantages, as well as legislative and managerial support, the healthcare industry. After research, the authors have identified several important aspects like necessity to establish a legal framework, social consensus, collaborations or multidisciplinary approach, value creation, awareness, participation and data security. The recommendations in this study are based on existing AI-based technology use, which may limit the comprehension of future technology's full potential [29].

The research paper 'Societal Issues Concerning the Application of Artificial Intelligence in Medicine' was reviewed and analyzed. The paper was published in the journal *Kidney Diseases* in 2019. The constructs identified are AI, machine learning, fairness, privacy and anonymity, explainability, interpretability, ethics and legislation. The authors have concluded that to fulfil the goal of increasing adoption of AI and machine learning-based technologies, as well as to comply with growing legislation regarding the influence of digital technologies on ethical and privacy-related concerns, the social factors should be taken into account [30].

The research paper 'Artificial Intelligence Transforms the Future of Healthcare' was reviewed and analyzed. The paper was published in *The American Journal of Medicine* in 2019. The constructs identified are medical informatics, precision medicine, Artificial Intelligence (AI), integrated healthcare systems, machine learning, medical informatics. The authors explored machine learning applications in medical services, focusing on therapeutic, experimental and healthcare applications, as well as the important importance of confidentiality, information sharing, and genetic data [31].

The article 'Artificial intelligence approach fighting COVID-19 with repurposing drugs' was reviewed and analyzed. The article was published in *Biomedical Journal* in 2020. The constructs identified are AI, DNN, COVID-19, SARS-CoV-2, Feline coronavirus, Drug repurposing. Using two separate learning databases, an AI platform was created to find probable old medications having anti-coronavirus activities; In an in vitro cell-based experiment, all AI projected substances were evaluated for activity against a feline coronavirus. The AI system used the test findings as input, allowing it to retrain and create a novel AI model to hunt for old medicines. Using AI, the researchers were able to find earlier medicines that have anti-FIP coronavirus activity. More research is being done to establish that they are efficacious in vitro and in vivo against SARS-CoV-2 at clinically significant doses and dosages [32].

The article 'Artificial Intelligence and Internet of Things Enabled Disease Diagnosis Model for Smart Healthcare Systems' was reviewed and analyzed. The article was published in *IEEE* in 2021. The construct identified is the Internet of Things (IoT), cloud computing, and Artificial Intelligence (AI), disease diagnosis model for heart disease and diabetes. The proposed technique uses a Crow Search

Optimization algorithm-based Cascaded Long Short-Term Memory (CSO-CLSTM) model for illness detection. CSO is used to fine-tune the CLSTM model's weights and bias factors to enhance medical data categorization. This study also uses the isolation Forest (iForest) approach to remove outliers. During the trials, the reported CSO-LSTM model had the highest levels of accuracy of 96.16% and 97.26% in detecting diabetes and heart disease, correspondingly. As a result, the suggested CSO-LSTM model can be used in smart healthcare systems as a disease diagnosis tool as suggested by the authors [33].

The article 'An artificial intelligence-based referral application to optimize orthodontic referrals in a public oral healthcare system' was reviewed and analyzed. The article was published in *Seminars in Orthodontics* in 2021. The constructs identified are Computational Formulation of Orthodontic referral Decisions (CFOD), orthodontic diagnosis. Following validation by 15 experienced orthodontist experts, the CFOD method was adopted, and clinical dentists were educated. Orthodontic referral trends were compared before and after the CFOD system was implemented. The authors after analyzing concluded a major public oral healthcare system could benefit from an AI expert system for orthodontic patient referral [34].

The article 'The rise of artificial intelligence in healthcare applications' was reviewed and analyzed. The article was published in *Artificial Intelligence in Healthcare* in 2020. The constructs identified are AI, healthcare applications, machine learning, precision medicine, environmental assisted living, natural language programming and machine vision. It is commonly anticipated, according to the authors, that AI technologies would help, and augment human labour rather than fully substitute the job of doctors and other medical staff. AI can help healthcare personnel with a variety of activities, such as admin work, patient records and patient engagement, as well as specialized assistance in areas like image processing, medical device control, and monitoring patients [35].

The article '5G and intelligence medicine-how the next generation of wireless technology will reconstruct healthcare?' was reviewed and analyzed. The article was published in *Precision Clinical Medicine* in 2019. The variables identified are the IoT, Big Data, AI, and 5G wireless transmission technology, patient experience, healthcare service quality, healthcare cost. According to the authors despite its limitations and challenges, 5G has begun to demonstrate considerable advantages in boosting hospital intelligence services, automated patient tracking, accurate remote surgical procedures, rationally allocating high-quality healthcare resources, and managing enormous wearable devices and monitoring equipment carried by patients. The limitation of the paper is that it is a research review work and proper quantitative or qualitative research work is needed [36].

The article 'Artificial Neural Synchronization using Nature Inspired Whale Optimization' was reviewed and analyzed. The article was published in *IEEE Access* in 2021. The constructs identified are whale optimization-based DLTPM (Double Layer Tree Parity Machine), authentication, confidentiality and integrity, neural network, neural synchronization. The authors concluded that this paper suggests utilizing nature-inspired whale optimization to synchronize Double Hidden Layer Neural Networks for the cryptographic public-key exchange protocol. The weight vector of two DLTPMs is optimized utilizing whale optimization techniques for quicker synchronization in this article. The security and synchronization time of DLTPM are also investigated. Geometric assaults have been proven to have a reduced success rate. DLTPM security is proven to be greater than existing TPM security with identical settings. Future studies can conduct more detailed risk assessment studies, according to the authors [37].

The article 'A Novel Fog Computing Approach for Minimization of Latency in Healthcare using Machine Learning' was reviewed and analyzed. The article was published in *International Journal of Interactive Multimedia and Artificial Intelligence* in 2020. The constructs identified cloud computing, data segregation scheme, fog computing, latency, machine learning, multimedia healthcare data analytics, multimedia transmission, and quality of service. Following an investigation, the authors developed a unique intelligent multimedia data segregation (IMDS) method in the fog computing environment utilizing machine learning (k-fold random forest). The latency characteristics, such as transmission delay, network delay, and calculation delay, are assessed, and the high latency is reduced. The suggested paradigm improves the e-healthcare customer experience and is adaptable to diverse networks. Latency and network use are also factors in QoS. As a result, reducing latency and network utilization enhances QoS [2].

The paper 'Application of AI on Post Pandemic Situation and Lesson Learn for Future Prospects' was reviewed and analyzed. The article was published in the *Journal of Experimental and Theoretical Artificial Intelligence* in 2021. The constructs identified are Gaussian mixture model-universal background model GMM-ubm, deep neural network (DNN), bottleneck feature, voice signal, COVID-19 detection. The authors presented methods based on a supervised/unsupervised approach and continuous physiological variable tracking. Finally, utilizing the speech signal, the effectiveness of COVID-19 identification with the Gaussian mixture model-universal background model (GMM-UBM) approach was proven. In terms of areas under receiver operating characteristic (ROC) curves, the proposed system achieves COVID-19 detection accuracy in the region of 60%–67%. Furthermore, suggestions for the future are offered based on the many lessons learned from the current COVID-19 problem [38].

A literature review has helped to identify the correct variables. Without finding proper variables or the construct of the research it is impossible to move further. After analyzing these quality research papers carefully, exact variables have been determined for our research topic. PU, perceived EOU, perceived risk, benefits, etc. was decided as variables. Most of the papers had followed exploratory research design as Artificial Intelligence-related perception research is a relatively new field of study. This field has a lot of room for more study and analysis.

4.2.1 RESEARCH GAP

The research papers reviewed are mostly talks about the application of AI and its effectiveness in the healthcare system. The public perception towards AI-based healthcare has not been properly understood. For a smooth delivery of AI-based health services, it is necessary to do specific targeted research to understand the factors affecting the peoples' trust towards Smart AI-based healthcare systems. Also, the research there is a necessity to do the research using quantitative methods and proper analysis in the Indian context. If successfully done, it could provide direction towards further studies in this context.

4.2.1.1 Research Variables

Independent variables will be (as found out from the literature review): Income, Age, Education, Technical literacy, regulatory concerns, COVID-19.

The dependent variable will be (as found out from the literature review): perceived usefulness, perceived trust.

4.2.2 RESEARCH OBJECTIVES

To find out if there is any relation between income, age, education, technical literacy, regulatory concerns, COVID-19 and PU, perceived trust towards Smart AI-driven Healthcare System.

4.2.3 METHODOLOGY

A descriptive research design was used in the study. The target population was every individual who experienced the healthcare system. Data collection was primarily done by a self-administered structured questionnaire. Sampling is a very important part of quantitative research.

4.2.3.1 Sampling

Sampling is an essential part of quantitative research. Sample should reflect the overall essence of the population. In this particular study, non-probability convenience sampling was selected as the sampling procedure due to the constraints of the pandemic. 105 respondent data have been collected through an online survey (Figures 4.1–4.2).

The age group is being considered as an independent variable in this study. So, here is an analysis of the sample's age group to have a clearer perspective. It is visible that most of the respondents are in the 20–30 age group. The second-largest age group being 31–40 years.

Education qualification is also an important variable as identified from the literature review. From the pie chart, it is deduced that most of the respondents are graduates, the second-largest qualification group is the master's group and lowest number of respondents are doctorates.

4.2.4 DATA ANALYSIS

The significance testing method, the chi-square test was chosen as the analysis method for determining whether or not there is a strong association between the independent and dependent variables (Tables 4.1–4.4).

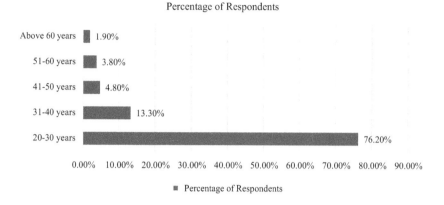

FIGURE 4.1   Age group of respondents.

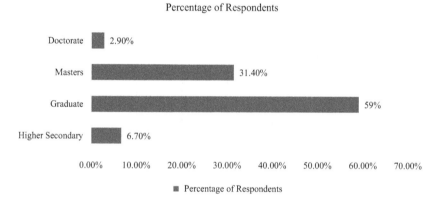

FIGURE 4.2   Educational qualification of respondents.

TABLE 4.1
Income vs. Perceived Trust Analysis

Chi-square Tests	Value	df	Asymp. Sig. (2-Sided)
Pearson chi-square	6.023[a]	4	0.197
Likelihood ratio	6.395	4	0.172
Linear-by-linear association	0.716	1	0.397
N of valid cases	105		

[a] 1 cell (10.0%) has expected count less than 5. The minimum expected count is 4.86.

TABLE 4.2
Age Group vs. Perceived Trust Analysis

Chi-square Tests	Value	df	Asymp. Sig. (2-Sided)
Pearson chi-square	7.663[a]	4	0.105
Likelihood ratio	9.347	4	0.053
Linear-by-linear association	1.503	1	0.220
N of valid cases	105		

[a] 6 cells (60.0%) have expected count less than 5. The minimum expected count is 97.

TABLE 4.3
Income vs. Perceived Usefulness Analysis

Chi-square Tests	Value	df	Asymp. Sig. (2-Sided)
Pearson chi-square	2.493[a]	4	0.646
Likelihood ratio	4.023	4	0.403
Linear-by-linear association	1.244	1	0.265
N of valid cases	105		

[a] 5 cells (50.0%) have expected count less than 5. The minimum expected count is 76.

TABLE 4.4
COVID-19 vs. Perceived Usefulness Analysis

Chi-square Tests	Value	df	Asymp. Sig. (2-Sided)	Exact Sig. (2-Sided)	Exact Sig. (1-Sided)
Pearson chi-square	18.966[a]	1	0.000		
Continuity correction	13.675	1	0.000		
Likelihood ratio	10.946	1	0.001		
Fisher's exact test				0.002	0.002
Linear-by-linear association	18.785	1	0.000		
N of valid cases	105				

[a] 1 cell (25.0%) has expected count less than 5. The minimum expected count is 69.
[b] Computed only for a 2 × 2 table

Hypothesis 1: Income vs. Perceived Trust

H_0: There is no noteworthy effect of income on perceived trust towards AI-driven smart healthcare systems.[1]

---

[1] '*' refers to vs (versus).

H_1: There is a notable effect of income on perceived trust towards AI-driven smart healthcare systems.

The p-value calculated in SPSS is.197 which is greater than 0.05. So, it can be suggested that the null hypothesis is accepted, and the alternate hypothesis rejected.

So, it can be clearly said that income has no significant impact on perceived trust towards AI-driven smart healthcare systems.

Hypothesis 2: Age Group vs. Perceived Trust

H_0: There is no table effect of age on perceived trust towards AI—driven smart healthcare system.

H_1: There is no table effect of age on perceived trust towards AI—driven smart healthcare system.

The p-value calculated in SPSS is 105, which is greater than 0.05. So, it can be suggested that the null hypothesis is accepted, and the alternate hypothesis rejected.

It can therefore be clearly said that age has no significant impact on perceived trust towards AI-driven smart healthcare systems.

Hypothesis 3: Income vs. Perceived Usefulness

H_0: There is no notable effect of income on perceived usefulness of AI—driven smart healthcare system.

H_1: There is notable effect of income on perceived usefulness of AI—driven smart healthcare system.

The p-value calculated in SPSS is 646 which is greater than 0.05. So, it can be suggested that the null hypothesis is accepted, and the alternate hypothesis rejected.

Therefore, it can be clearly said that income has no significant impact on the PU of the AI-driven smart healthcare system.

Hypothesis 4: COVID-19 vs. Perceived Usefulness

H_0: There is no noteworthy effect of COVID-19 on perceived usefulness of AI-driven smart healthcare system.

H_1: There is noteworthy effect of COVID-19 on perceived usefulness of AI-driven smart healthcare system.

The p-value calculated in SPSS is 0.002 which is less than 0.05. So, it can be suggested that the null hypothesis is declined, and the alternate hypothesis is accepted.

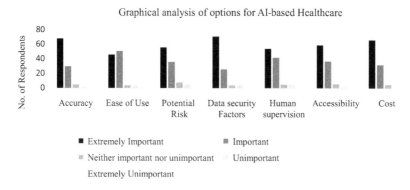

FIGURE 4.3 Graphical analysis of options for AI-based healthcare.

Therefore, it can be clearly said that COVID-19 has a significant impact on the PU of AI-driven smart healthcare systems.

After analyzing every dependent and independent variable through the chi-square test by the above method it is found out that independent variable age group, income, education, technical literacy, regulatory concerns and covid-19 do not have any significant impact on the dependent variable, perceived trust. The same is the case with the dependent variable PU except for COVID-19, which has a significant impact upon the PU of AI-based healthcare techniques.

If we analyse the Likert scale-based questions graphically, we can see a pattern. Most of the respondents think that parameters like accuracy, potential risk, data security, human supervision, accessibility, cost are extremely important while opting for AI-based healthcare. The ease-of-use parameter is considered as important by most of them. If we benchmark 60 respondents count, then we will see clearly that three of the seven parameters being most important. Those parameters are accuracy, data security and cost. Accessibility is one of their closest parameters.

4.3 DISCUSSION

From the above analysis, it has been found out that earnings, educational background, technical literacy, regulatory concerns, etc. are not impacting the perceived trust in the AI-based healthcare system. In the Indian context, it shows us the way to develop a proper AI-based healthcare system that can create a balance. In Tier-I, Tier-II cities and rural areas where government-provided health service is the only way out for the people, AI can bring revolution and increase the quality of service and ensure that health services can be provided to everyone out there. By augmenting human services, AI can give relief to the burdened healthcare professionals thereby improving the quality of human-given care as well. It can be suggested from the analysis that people may or may not trust AI-based smart

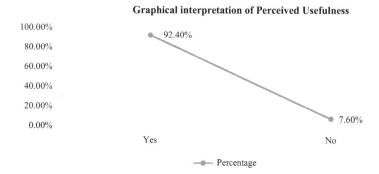

FIGURE 4.4   Graphical interpretation of perceived usefulness.

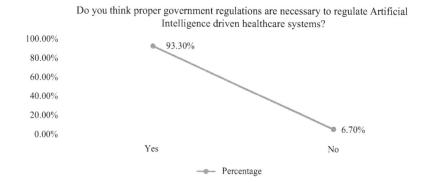

FIGURE 4.5   Graphical representation of regulatory concern responses.

healthcare systems despite being in any social class, having any income range, educational background. Technical literacy, regulations and COVID-19 have minimal impact on perceived trust.

In the case of PU, the situation is kind of identical except for COVID-19. According to the analysis, earnings, educational background, technical literacy, regulatory concerns, etc. have no impact on the PU of AI-based healthcare, but COVID-19 has a notable effect on the PU of AI-based smart healthcare systems. The impact of these variables on PU is very important as it is reflective of public opinion.

If we analyse the specific responses of usefulness, we can see that most of the respondents i.e., 92.4% perceive AI-driven healthcare as useful irrespective of their income, age, educational qualification. It shows that there is a basic awareness in the people about the AI and they might accept technological advances in the form of AI-driven care as well.

Another important aspect is Govt. regulation (as many of the reviewed articles are focussed on regulatory concerns specifically).

If we analyze the regulatory concerns of the people, the responses are indicating that the majority of the respondents are in favour of a clear government guidelines that can regulate any kind of AI intervention in the healthcare system.

From the Likert scale-based questions' graphical interpretation, we can infer that majority of the respondents think that these seven factors will be important while opting for an AI-based smart healthcare system. The degree of importance may vary from person to person but accuracy, EOU, potential risk, data security, human supervision, accessibility, costs are major factors. The importance of these factors cannot be undermined.

Accuracy is a major factor as healthcare sometimes life and death situation and for trusting a technology for your life is not an easy choice to make. So, AI should be accurate while delivering health services. Ease of use is important because we are discussing people from every stratum of the society can be benefitted from the system, so the system should be all-inclusive. Ease of use ensures that people from any walk of our society will be able to use or take benefit of AI.

If we want a successful implementation of any health services (be it human-driven or AI) we must ensure to minimize risk. Lower the risk factor, there will be more participation of the people.

Today, in this age of technical advancement, data security is one of the key concerns of the users. From financial information to personal ones, there is always a threat to data security. Health information is a very personal kind of information and most of the patients do not want to share those with all. Ensuring the data security of the concerned will be one of the key challenges to any AI-based healthcare provider. Human supervision is a key component to deliver proper health services to people as AI is there to only augment or help health workers in their work. The purpose is not replacing humans and it is not going to happen in near future as well. Accessibility and proper costing will also be two major factors while implementing AI in healthcare. Though AI-based healthcare research incur huge costs, the prices of the services must stay within the very limit of common people. The lower costing will help the masses to use it as well it will be helpful to the government to use these services in government setup as well.

This paper depicts and indicate one critical understanding about the AI and its relevance on healthcare system. It is the future of every aspect of healthcare economy. Starting from the business to next outbreak of a disease can be effectively measured by using AI. The adoption process might be slow especially in healthcare system, however, it is inevitable for developing economies across the globe, be it a large one or small, to adopt and rip the benefits of AI. The future holds promising aspects for us. There might be fear over losing job and replacing human race from its apex position in the intelligence pyramid, but the key to success will always remain in the hand of innovation. According to [39], Global Innovation Index; India's rank jumps from 81 in 2015 to 46 in 2021. AI is the innovation which will bring the transformation in smart healthcare system.

4.4   CONCLUSION

In this research, it is established that most of the important hierarchies of our social being are not related to the perceived trust towards AI-based healthcare and they also do not affect the PU. But will people accept AI-based healthcare with ease, and will they trust it, which creates the space for further discussion among peers. There are innumerable possibilities of achieving a 'smart' healthcare future where AI can augment (if not replace) human-based healthcare and it will bridge the healthcare gaps.

There are two directions of this discussion, one is that if we can provide access to an AI-based smart healthcare system to every citizen of this country or for that anyone opting for it? The second question is will they adopt it or trust it? Which factors are important for their trust? In this research paper, we have focussed our discussion on the second question more. But there is ample scope of discussion about this question, and further research can surely pinpoint the right answers.

4.5   FUTURE SCOPE

In this research, higher secondary has been taken as the lowest educational qualification, whereas uneducated people also use (and are entitled to) basic healthcare facilities. So, to make it more comprehensive and cohesive, further studies should try to be more inclusive in terms of respondents. Due to COVID-19 and current unforeseen conditions, the survey was floated online, so it can be clearly stated that whoever has filled out the survey has basic technical literacy. Further research can be done with physical responses.

The lowest income group taken in this research is 'less than Rs. 20,000', which can easily be subdivided further at least in the Indian context. This research can further be elaborated with more sample size and a bigger context. The sample size is 105 in this research work, and it can be increased further to understand the bigger Indian context. The effect of the aforementioned elements (accuracy, EOU, potential risk, data security, human supervision, accessibility, costs) can be calculated by peers. It has been determined that the factors have impacts, but the degrees of these could be determined in further research.

REFERENCES

1. Bhalla Kritti. *A small Hospital in a Remote Corner of Assam is Using AI to Detect Strokes in Tea Planters*, 2021. Tezpur: Businessinsider.in.
2. Amit K, Chinmay C, Wilson J, Kishor A, Chakraborty C, and Jeberson W. "A Novel Fog Computing Approach for Minimization of Latency in Healthcare using Machine Learning." *International Journal of Interactive Multimedia & Artificial Intelligence* 6, 1–11, 2020.
3. Pramanik A. "Ayushman Bharat can Open Up Opportunities for AI-Based Services: NetApp–The Economic Times." *The Economic Times*, 2019.https://economictimes. indiatimes.com/tech/ites/artificial-intelligence-can-help-improve-citizen-services-locally-anil-valluri-netapp-president/articleshow/71966499.cms?from=mdr

4. Albarrán, Irene, Lozano José, Manuel Molina, and Covadonga Gijón. "Perception of Artificial Intelligence in Spain." *Telematics and Informatics63*, 2021.
5. Kashive, Neerja, Leena Powale, and Kshitij Kashive. "Understanding User Perception Toward Artificial Intelligence (AI) Enabled e-Learning." *International Journal of Information and Learning Technology 38*, 1–19, 2020.
6. Gao, Shuqing, Lingnan He, Yue Chen, Dan Li, and Kaisheng Lai. "Public Perception of Artificial Intelligence in Medical Care: Content Analysis of Social Media." *Journal of Medical Internet Research 22*, 2020.
7. Prakash, Ashish Viswanath, and Saini Das. "Intelligent Conversational Agents in Mental Healthcare Services: A Thematic Analysis of User Perceptions." *Pacific Asia Journal of the Association for Information Systems 12*, 2020.
8. Esmaeilzadeh, and Pouyan. "Use of AI-Based Tools for Healthcare Purposes: a Survey Study from Consumers' Perspectives." *BMC Medical Informatics and Decision-Making 20*, 2020.
9. Papa, Armando, Monika Mital, Paola Pisano, and Manlio Del Giudice. "E-Health and Wellbeing Monitoring Using Smart Healthcare Devices: An Empirical Investigation." *Technological Forecasting & Social Change 153*, 2020.
10. Sujata D, Chinmay C, Sourav KG, Subhendu KP, and Jaroslav F. "BIFM: Big-data Driven Intelligent Forecasting Model for COVID-19." *IEEE Access*, 1–13, 2021, 10.1109/ACCESS.2021.3094658
11. Anichur R, Chinmay C, Adnan A, Razaul Karim MD, Jahidul Islam MD, Dipanjali K, Ziaur R, and Shahab SB. "SDN-IoT Empowered Intelligent Framework for Industry 4.0Applications during COVID-19 Pandemic." *Cluster Computing*, 1–18, 2021, doi:10.1007/s10586-021-03367-4
12. Hemanta KB, Chinmay C, Yogesh S, and Suvendu KP. "COVID-19 Diagnosis System by Deep Learning Approaches." *Expert Systems*, 1–18, e12776. "https://www.google.com/url?q=https%3A%2F%2Fdoi.org%2F10.1111%2Fexsy.12776&sa=D&sntz=1&usg=AFQjCNGgsanW5cLFl2YY-QWRX_4zSwBFUg", "https://www.google.com/url?q=https%3A%2F%2Fdoi.org%2F10.1111%2Fexsy.12776&sa=D&sntz=1&usg=AFQjCNGgsanW5cLFl2YY-QWRX_4zSwBFUg" doi: 10.1111/exsy.12776
13. Zeadally, Sherali, Farhan Siddiqui, Zubair Baig, and Ahmed Ibrahim. "Smart Healthcare: Challenges and Potential Solutions Using Internet of Things (IoT) and Big Data Analytics." *PSU Research Review 4(2)*, 2019.
14. Dehnavieh Reza, Sajad Khosravi, Mohammad Hossein Mehrolhassani, AliAkbar Haghdoost, and Saeed Amini. "Future Trends of the Primary Healthcare System in Iran: A Qualitative Study." *International Journal of Preventive Medicine 10(1)*, 2019
15. Presti, Letizia Lo, Mario Testa, Vittoria Marino, and Pierpaolo Singer. "Engagement in Healthcare Systems: Adopting Digital Tools for a Sustainable Approach." *Sustainability 11(1)*, 2019.
16. Alaiad, Ahmad, and Lina Zhou. "Patients' Adoption of WSN-Based Smart Home Healthcare Systems: An Integrated Model of Facilitators and Barriers." *IEEE Transactions on Professional Communication (IEEE Transactions on Professional Communication) 60*(1), 1–20, 2017.
17. Davenport, Thomas, and Ravi Kalakota. "The Potential for Artificial Intelligence in Healthcare." *Future Healthcare Journal (Future Healthcare Journal) 6(2)*, 94–98, 2019.
18. Amann, Julia, Alessandro Blasimme, Effy Vayena, Dietmar Frey, and Vince I Madai. "Explainability for Artificial Intelligence in Healthcare: A Multidisciplinary Perspective." *BMC Medical Informatics and Decision-Making (BMC Medical Informatics and Decision-Making) 20(1)*, 2020.

19. Park, Seong Ho, and Kyunghwa Han. "Methodologic Guide for Evaluating Clinical Performance and Effect of Artificial Intelligence Technology for Medical Diagnosis and Prediction." *Radiological Society of North America 286(3)*, 800–809, 2018.

20. Kononenko, Igor. "Machine Learning for Medical Diagnosis: History, State of the Art and Perspective." *Artificial Intelligence in Medicine 23*(1), 89–109, 2001.

21. Dilsizian, Steven E., and Eliot L Siegel. "Artificial Intelligence in Medicine and Cardiac Imaging: Harnessing Big Data and Advanced Computing to Provide Personalized Medical Diagnosis and Treatment." *Nuclear Cardiology 16(1)*, 2013.

22. Amato, Filippo, Alberto López, Eladia María et al. "Artificial Neural Networks in Medical Diagnosis." *Journal of Applied Biomedicine 11(2)*, 47–58, 2013.

23. Amisha, Paras Malik, Monika Pathania, and Vyas Kumar Rathaur. "Overview of Artificial Intelligence in Medicine." *Journal of Family Medicine & Primary Care 8(7)*, 2328–2331, 2019.

24. Risling, Tracie L., and Cydney Low. "Advocating for Safe, Quality and Just Care: What Nursing Leaders Need to Know About Artificial Intelligence in Healthcare Delivery." *Nursing Leadership 32(2)*, 31–45, 2019.

25. Phillips, Angela. "Artificial Intelligence-Enabled Healthcare Delivery and Digital Epidemiological Surveillance in the Remote Treatment of Patients During the COVID-19 Pandemic." *American Journal of Medical Research 8(1)*, 40–49, 2021.

26. Li, Ron C, Steven M Asch, and Nigam H Shah. "Developing a Delivery Science for Artificial Intelligence in Healthcare." *NPJ Digital Medicine 3(1)*, 2020.

27. Datta, Sudipto, Ranjit Barua, and Jonali Das. "Application of Artificial Intelligence in Modern Healthcare System." In *Alginates–Recent Uses of This Natural Polymer*, by Leonel Pereira, 121–138. London: Intech Open, 2020.

28. Faizal Khan, Z., and Sultan Refa Alotaibi. "Applications of Artificial Intelligence and Big Data Analytics in m-Health: A Healthcare System Perspective." *Journal of Healthcare Engineering 10*, 1–15, 2020.

29. Lee, DonHee, and Seong No Yoon. "Application of Artificial Intelligence-Based Technologies in the Healthcare Industry: Opportunities and Challenges." *International Journal of Environmental Research & Public Health 18*(1), 2021.

30. Vellido, Alfredo. "Societal Issues Concerning the Application of Artificial Intelligence in Medicine." *Kidney Diseases 5*(1), 11–17, 2019.

31. Noorbakhsh-Sabet, Nariman, Ramin Zand, Yanfei Zhang, and Vida Abedi. "Artificial Intelligence Transforms the Future of Health Care." *The American Journal of Medicine 132*(7), 795–801, 2019.

32. Ke, Yi-Yu, Tzu-Ting Peng, Teng-Kuang Yeh et al. "Artificial Intelligence Approach Fighting COVID-19 with Repurposing Drugs." *Biomedical Journal 43*(4), 355–362, 2020.

33. Mansour, Romany Fouad, and Adnen El Amraoui et al. "Artificial Intelligence and Internet of Things Enabled Disease Diagnosis Model for Smart Healthcare Systems." *IEEE*, 45137–45146, 2021.

34. Mohameda, Mariam, Donald J Fergusona, Adith Venugopal, Mohammad Khursheed Alam, Laith Makki, and Nikhilesh R Vaida. "An Artificial Intelligence Based Referral Application to Optimize Orthodontic Referrals in a Public Oral Healthcare System." *Seminars in Orthodontics*, 157–163, 2021.

35. Bohr, Adam, and Kaveh Memarzadeh. "The Rise of Artificial Intelligence in Healthcare Applications." *Artificial intelligence in Healthcare*, 25–60, 2020.

36. Li, Dong. "5G and Intelligence Medicine—How the Next Generation of Wireless Technology will Reconstruct Healthcare?" *Precision Clinical Medicine 2*(4), 205–208, 2019.

37. Arindam S, Mohammad ZA, Moirangthem MS, Chinmay C Abdulfattah, and Subhendu KP. "Artificial Neural Synchronization Using Nature Inspired Whale Optimization." *IEEE Access*, 1–14, 2021.

38. Dwivedi, Priyanka, Achintya Kumar Sarkar, Chinmay Chakraborty, Monoj Singha, and Vineet Rojwal. "Application of Artificial Intelligence on Post Pandemic Situation and Lesson Learn for Future Prospects." *Journal of Experimental & Theoretical Artificial Intelligence*, 1–24, 2021.

39. Sharma, Yogima Seth. "India jumps 2 places to rank 46 on Global Innovation Index." *The Economic Times*. 2021. https://economictimes.indiatimes.com/news/economy/indicators/india-jumps-2-places-to-rank-46-on-global-innovation-index/articleshow/86371513.cms.

5 Security, Privacy Issues, and Challenges in Adoption of Smart Digital Healthcare

Aditee Swain
Utkal University, Bhubaneswar, India

Bhabendu Kumar Mohanta
Koneru Lakshmaiah Education Foundation, Green Fields,
Vaddeswaram, Andhra Pradesh, India

Debasish Jena
IIIT Bhubaneswar, Odisha, India

CONTENTS

5.1 INTRODUCTION

Conventional healthcare is not able to house everyone's wishes due to the huge growth in population. Despite having strong infrastructure and cutting-edge technologies, clinical offerings aren't approachable or economical to everybody.

DOI: 10.1201/9781003247128-5

The current generation is the only computerized generation. With the development of intergenerational and clinical concepts, traditional medicines based on genetic engineering continue to digitize and integrate information. Smart health management originated from the concept of Smart Earth presented by IBM (Armonk, New York, USA) in 2009. Smart healthcare represents a new timeline of information. One of the purposes of smart healthcare is to assist customers through instructing them about their medical records along with preserving their health. Smart healthcare authorizes customers to restrain some circumstances. It offers a better experience for the buyer. Smart medicine enables you to reach your full potential. It supports remote patient observation, and assists in reducing maintenance cost for the consumer. Furthermore, it facilitates clinical professionals to increase their utilities lacking any geographical limitations. With the developing trend of smart cities, an effective smart health system provides a healthy home for natives. The major contributions of this chapter are as follows:

- Initially this paper identified the associate protocols and technologies used in smart healthcare system.
- An extensive survey was conducted regarding the existing work in healthcare system.
- The security and privacy challenges are identified and discussed in detail.
- The problem statement is formulated from the literature survey outcome, and the need to address the security challenges in healthcare system.
- The blockchain-based solution model proposed to address the security and privacy issues in smart healthcare system.
- The smart contracts are mentioned with implementation details at the end of this paper.

5.1.1 Smart Healthcare System Associate Technologies

The smart healthcare system concept has various users associated with it, such as doctors, patients, hospital staff and research institutions. Hospitals deal with several functionalities, including diagnosis of disease, maintenance and monitoring, prognosis and treatment, facility management, fitness decision-making and medical research. The Internet of Things [1], mobile internet, cloud computing, Big Data, 5G, microelectronics, artificial intelligence and other information technologies and modern biotechnology together form the cornerstone of smart health. These technologies are widely utilized in all factors of smart healthcare.

5.1.2 Smart Healthcare Planning: Essentials, Elements and Features

Necessities of health could be extensively categorized in the functional and non-functional necessities, as manifested in Figure 5.1. Functional necessities labels particular necessities of a smart healthcare structure. However, non-functional necessities aren't very specific. Non-functional necessities talk over with attributes primarily based on which the fine of the healthcare gadget may be decided.

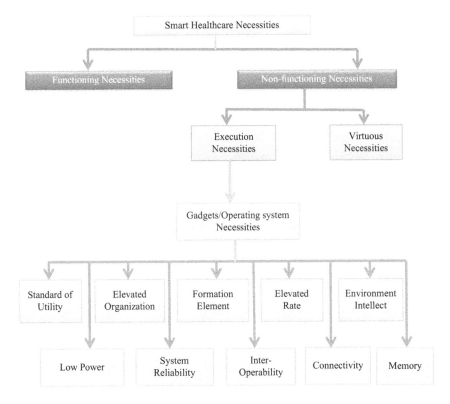

FIGURE 5.1 Requirements in smart healthcare.

Important prerequisites for an effective smart medical care are little strength, portable from issue, machine accuracy, excellent of carrier, rich user experience, high throughput, capability to engage throughout one-of-a-kind structures, ease of deployment, recognition of the smart healthcare machine to provide non-stop support, scalability of the system to upgrade to newer versions and technology, and ample connectivity since the very high cause of designing a smart healthcare is to make certain clinical service directly.

5.1.3 IoT Enables Smart Healthcare System

IoT is a smart topic, involving interconnectivity as well as processing of collected information in real time. The computerized model is mentioned every day in which all the actual-global elements could live related. With maximized profit and traits consisting of identity and place, connection to the Internet of Things is essential for smart Medicare, as illustrated in Figure 5.2. Imposing a smart healthcare machine, the IoT could carry out a wide variety of tasks, beginning with measuring medical devices every day with a customized tracking machine.

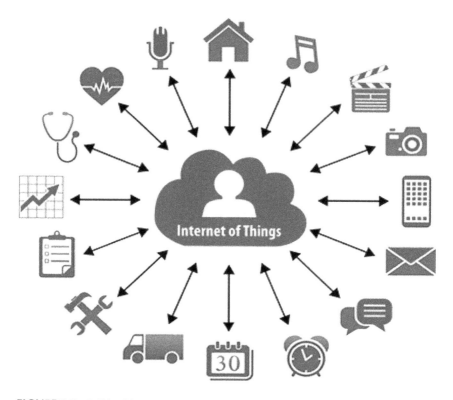

FIGURE 5.2   IoT healthcare components.

The Internet of Things plays a considerable part in healthcare implementation, from treating chronic diseases by blocking the spectrum of chronic diseases to monitoring the daily activities of the body everyday which helps achieve health goals. The IoT may be used every day to display the system of manufacturing.

IoT features as a crossover between the everyday as well as affected persons by means of presenting remote access that can assist the day-to-day monitoring of the patient and provide remote sessions. A combination of sensors, actuators, micro-controllers and processors, together with cloud computing, the IoT enables obtaining of exact effects and putting together healthcare that is workable day-to-day for anybody. The use of the IoT in healthcare has guided analysts globally with a layout encouraging structure and technology that can offer clinical help every day to everyone.

Privacy and security are the main concerns of the Internet of Things. The presence of malicious devices, loss of effective and reliable security protocols, people's ignorance, and daily active monitoring are different challenges facing the Internet of Things. We checked the remaining the issues of IoT security systems and functions, and determined (a) various security and privacy issues, (b) daily use strategies weaken the daily environment and IoT systems, (c) protection measures must be provided, and (d) important and appropriate high-quality data protection models must be applicable to all layers of the IoT application.

The rest of the chapter is organized thus: The literature survey regarding the previous work done in the field of security and privacy issue in healthcare systems is in Section 5.2. Section 5.3 addresses security and privacy issues. In Section 5.4, in-depth analysis of security and privacy of digital healthcare systems are discussed. The problem statement is identified in Section 5.5. The proposed method has been presented in Section 5.6. The implementation details and conclusion are presented in Section 5.7.

5.2   LITERATURE SURVEY

Tawalbeh et al. proposed new hierarchical IoT models, and these models appear regularly and are extended to include data protection and security as well as the identity of the layers [2], created by Amazon Web Service as a virtual machine host. Under the guidance of the inexperienced green grass environment on AWS, the middle layer is implemented as a Raspberry Pi 4 hardware package. The top layer, the cloud, is the IoT environment. There are security logs and critical control periods between each layer to ensure the confidentiality of customer events. We use security certification to ensure the exchange of information between quotation levels. Cloud/Edge-ready IoT version. We study the benefits and risks of the Internet of Things. With all these advantages, risk can harm the end user by allowing unauthorized access to sensitive private data, allowing attacks on structures and increasing data protection risks. With the emergence of IoT devices on the market, we hope to equip them with appropriate security features to improve their availability, performance and integration with existing systems. We hope to build a dynamic security framework to reduce security and privacy risks with the help of researchers, rather than eliminate them now, and be smart enough to adapt to new communication technology changes and exclusive software implementations.

Abdullah Algarni critically reviewed studies articles that addressed safety and privacy in SHS [3]. Doing so has shown the distribution of labour on security and privacy. Distributions and categorizations have been provided based on book venue, eBook year, objective, application area, and protection method. Further maximum commonplace security attacks in SHS are summarized, at the side of their countermeasures. Furthermore, an evaluation of the approaches modern-day research handles SHS security and privateness is furnished. Open research challenges are mentioned, as well as instructions for future studies. Alam et al. have drafted a survey on most probable security in addition to privacy troubles related to healthcare which needs to seize the eye for permitting the healthcare device extra dependable, more powerful in phrases of advancement of scientific technology and curing extra sufferers at a time predicting the viable illness [4]. Sachin et al. endorses an agile software infrastructure for flexible, price effective, secure and privacy preserving deployment of IoT for smart healthcare applications and services [5]. It integrates state-of-the-art networking and virtualization techniques throughout IoT, fog and cloud domains, using Block chain, Tor and message agents to offer security and privacy for patients and healthcare carriers. We recommend a novel platform for the usage of Machine-to-Machine (M2M) messaging and rule-primarily based beacons for seamless information control, and play a modern role in information and selection fusion within the cloud and the fog, respectively, for smart healthcare programmes and offerings. Gupta et al. propose a widespread version for software in density IoT healthcare structures [6]. This survey then presents the state-of-the-art research relating to each location of the model, evaluating their strengths, weaknesses, and general suitability for a wearable IoT healthcare device. Challenges that healthcare IoT faces inclusive of security, privacy, wear ability, and low-power operation are offered, and pointers are made for future research directions. It was found that access control rules and encryption can appreciably improve security, however no preferences were expressed for immediate application into a wearable, IoT-based healthcare system. Daojing He et al., after giving a top stage view of security threats of healthcare IoT, studies safety vulnerabilities of password constructing and offers a password strength evaluation approach that takes under consideration users' personal facts. In this article, we have targeted password-guessing assaults [7]. We have proposed a password strength meter that takes into account customers' personal records. It permits clients to select passwords with a higher degree of security. Shreshth Tuli et al. throw light on some of the critical traumatic situations in providing low-value, green, secure and reliable healthcare from the viewpoint of laptop and clinical sciences [8]. We deliver a reason for a conceptual version which could offer whole answer for those growing desires. In our model, we elucidate the components and their interaction at top notch degrees, leveraging state-of-the-art technologies in IoT, fog computing, AI, ML and blockchain. Many efforts have been made to improve company operation in fog environments, with a goal to provide extra accurate sickness prediction and automated prescription. Eight studies also design new techniques to increase the security and reliability of such systems. In addition, architecture-degree optimizations were proposed in wireless body sensor nodes (WBSNs) that make the most rising technology, so one can lessen the electricity intake and enhance performance. Tariq et al. and Manpreet et al. provide up-to-date surveys on unique demanding situations and open problems faced in smart healthcare due to the updated conventional security measures, along with the safety necessities of such domains [9, 10]. These also amalgamate the potentials of blockchain generation as a promising protection measure, highlights potential challenges in the healthcare domain, and provides an analysis of different blockchain-based security solutions. In this study, we addressed the safety necessities of IoT-enabled smart healthcare systems to update the utility of blockchain with protection solutions. It also mentioned how blockchain up-to-date answers can conquer one of kind security problems in a green, distributive, and scalable manner. Similarly, the challenges of blockchain deployment in the infrastructure are also mentioned. In the future, we propose an intense evaluation of the authentication mechanism design and blockchain-based identification authentication mechanisms.

5.3   SECURITY AND PRIVACY CHALLENGES IN SMART HEALTHCARE

Recently, information privacy has grown to be an important subject for corporations in each industry, particularly healthcare. Healthcare agencies should properly manage patient data, not only to satisfy strict records privacy regulations and legal guidelines, but also to build a culture of honesty and transparency with patients.

Data privacy in healthcare is ever evolving, with laws and regulations being constantly updated, so that patients acquire the privacy they assume and deserve. Protecting the security of information in health studies is vital due to the fact health research calls for the gathering, storage and use of big amounts of in my view identifiable health data, a lot of which can be sensitive and doubtlessly embarrassing. If security is breached, the people whose health data was inappropriately accessed face a number of capacity harms. Artificial intelligence [11] and machine learning [12] techniques are used to address some of the security issue in smart healthcare system. Despite the fact that smart healthcare allows in providing better healthcare worldwide, it additionally will face further risks. Due to its dynamics and small dimensions the safety requirements for smart sanitation range from the conventional safety strategies. Figure 5.3 suggests the important protection necessities in preserving a procured smart fitness-control machine. To reduce costs, the mainframes utilized in smart healthcare structures are slow, and have features that cannot fit in with extra safety procedures because of the growth inside the amount of IoT gadgets within the healthcare community, it is miles of extremely demanding project work for designers to supply protection and refurbishment or a valid answer for computing records. Smart health-maintenance organizations are vulnerable for safety assaults at diverse tiers of the machine. To continue statistics originality within the fitness-supervision community, the password and clue should need to be updated regularly. Assaults targeting data forwarding within the community could involve obtrusion of the provider accessibility, amendment of initial statistics and fraud

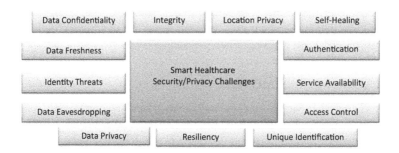

FIGURE 5.3   Security requirements of smart healthcare.

news. Assaults can also meddle with the gadgets, i.e., the interrelated bodily gadgets or the freeware; i.e., the working structures and implementations. Confidentiality is a key safety condition in smart healthcare information, that encompasses personal data and preferences. Consequently, at least a two-stage substantiation procedure should be carried out to ensure recognition of the user. Data integrity or data probity means that every actual value compiles with connation quality lacking uncertified or unofficial changes. It includes precision along with trust.

It can be divided into four categories, namely: object integrity, domain integrity, referential integrity and customer elucidated integrity, and can be supported by foreign keys, restrictions, rules and enkindle. Integrity wishes to be continued inside the medical management community, guaranteeing the customers that the facts that are conveyed and accepted aren't amended or compromised. If the facts of the interrelated tool are ruptured, then the safety machine should guarantee that there may be no access to data or functions within the healthcare system. The interconnected tools must have easy-recuperation to various diploma, to make certain that if a tool fails, it has minimal effect on the health community. Access control or restriction of access is a method of statistical equipment to determine the specification of consumers and a predetermined strategy to avert unsanctioned customers from retrieving assets. Many enciphering procedures or techniques have been implemented to gain controlled access, including Symmetric Key Encryption (SKE) or regularity solution cipher, Asymmetric Key Encryption (AKE) or lopsided solution cipher and Attribute Based Encryption (ABE) or quality established cipher. According to popular understanding, cryptanalysis is based on solutions. The key size and age implementation will influence the security of the cryptanalysis structure without hesitation. Therefore, the cue conducting mechanism controls the security lifecycle of the cryptographic system. Due to the extensible pointer control and flexible approach operation guideline ABE has become a step-by-step method. In Health Information Exchange (HIE) or medical knowledge swapping, the patient's medical records can be transmitted digitally with direct permission for controlled transactions. Nevertheless, current processes for endorsing health data structures show off specific disadvantages in assembling the requirements of HIE, with non-cryptographic strategies missing a secure and dependable apparatus to get entry to coverage enforcement, even as cryptographic tactics being too high-priced, complex, and constrained in specifying regulations. Anichur et al. described the use of software defined network, for IoT application [13].

5.4   PROBLEM STATEMENT

Hospital therapy has been a fundamental a part of our lives, and so the scientific facts – for example, prescriptions and preceding medical statistics – have additionally become essential elements for patient analysis, and likewise for treatments. The healthcare enterprise has unique data control preferences as it offers patient information that is sensitive, non-public, and private; however, this information is often saved and distributed across large facilities and companies, which can result in tedious and inefficient methods, which is not desirable if records need to be accessed during an emergency. Traditionally, clinical information was recorded on paper, which has been at risk of being damaged or altered. Therefore, it became necessary to hold information electronically. But the scientific database could still be tampered with or deleted entirely. Usually, patients may additionally have a lot of carrier providers in phrases of clinical healthcare that include general physicians or professionals and therapists. When you consider that an ailment may be resultant of a previous ailment, they may want to share health documents securely without manipulation. Patient information is critical for various purpose, such as treatment and further research to learn more about diseases. If a health facility desires to share a patient's records for research, there should be consent from that patient. Once more, if consent is delayed then the transfer of information is time consuming. Moreover, if the statistics which might be transferred are on paper or email, there are time, speed, storage, and security issues. Storing data in a database has many limitations, including storage and vulnerability to cyber-attacks. Attackers may intrude into the system and obtain patient data. One can also no longer rely upon a centralized database, because with the development of emerging technology, existing architectures are converted into a decentralized architecture (see Figures 5.4–5.7).

5.5   PROPOSED METHODOLOGY

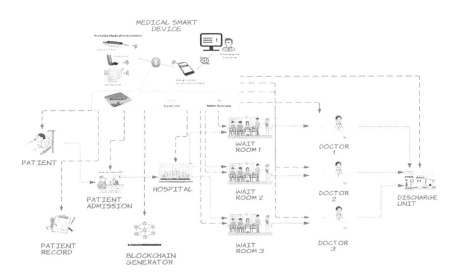

FIGURE 5.4   Hospital system with blockchain technology and medical smart device.

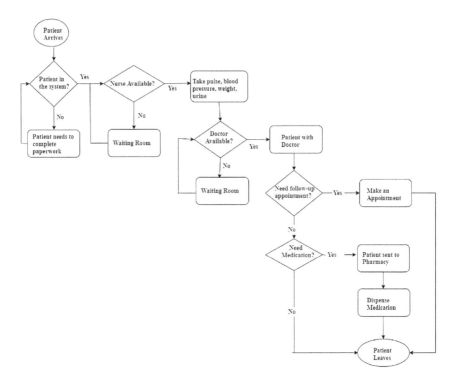

FIGURE 5.5   Patient process flow cycle in the smart healthcare system.

5.6   IMPLEMENTATION

It's inconvenient and insufficient to exchange scientific paper files with distinct infirmity by patient. Handing out health-maintenance information is reckoned to be an important attitude to improve the best of health protection provider and decrease medicinal expenses. Although ongoing EHR (Electronic Patient Record) methodology carries plenty of comfort, numerous hurdles nonetheless prevail in the medical management statistics structures during the exercise. Other than that, victims are incapable of maintaining position in their own nonpublic statistics. This may lead to unaccredited use of personal data by unknown companies.

In view of this particular example, it is necessary to ensure production together with seclusion for the proper management of data returned to customers so that it will inspire information sharing. It's fairly simple to address protection and privacy issues whilst the record resides in a single company, but it will be challenging in the case of secure health statistics passed through different domains. This mechanism includes accessing coverage normally such as access control list (ACL) related to statistics owner. ACL is a list of users who can get admission to records, and have associated authorization (read, write, update) to precise statistics. Concurrence is

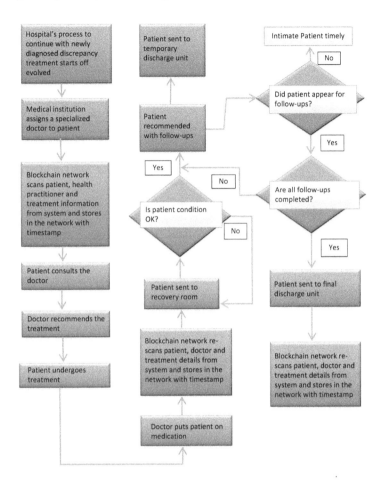

FIGURE 5.6 Working process flow in integration with blockchain technology in health-care system.

the purpose of allowing authentication authority to customers so as to achieve the covered assets backing presumed get entry to strategies. Customers constantly anticipate the mediator (e.g., cloud servers) carry out corroboration and have access to information requirements. Although, in reality, the host is sincere yet peculiar. It's encouraging that merging blockchain with access to check devices enables a sincere device. Buyers can feel reassured that their data is safe. In this new model, patients can predetermine access rights (authorize, deny, revoke) operations (check, write, update, delete) and provide statistical data duration through smart contracts on the blockchain without lost correct access. After all prerequisites are met, a smart contract can be generated on the blockchain, and an audit mechanism can also be provided for each request recorded in the ledger.

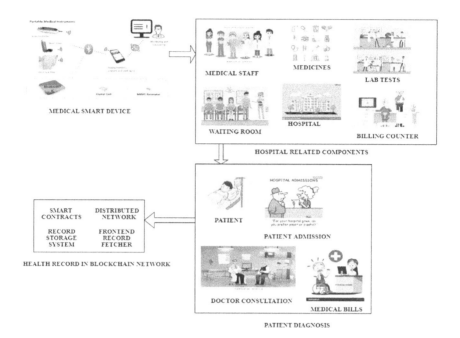

FIGURE 5.7   Blockchain enables smart healthcare network.

5.6.1   RECOMMENDATIONS FOR THE DEVELOPMENT OF SMART CONTRACT AND THEIR COOPERATION WITH SMART MEDICAL SYSTEM

Figure 5.8 shows all owners or smart contracts proposed by six smart contracts (person, medical centre, wounded, department, doctor or practitioner and nurse) for smart healthcare machine contracts both are directly and indirectly linked (using the concept of the "is-a" relationship, as per the entity relationship (ER) diagram) with the clinic, as shown in Figure 5.9. The list and explanations of all smart contracts shown in Figure 5.8 looks like this: people's settlement stores data about all people who are directly connected to health. List of people – it is a memorized list that contains a permanent and unchanging record of men and women related to the healthcare institutions, even if they are fired or given up from work. First call, call centre, remaining calls, registration date, treatment by gender and phone number in the facility are also stored correctly. The smart contracts are used to implemented different non-financial application in blockchain environment [14]. The secure communication is one of the essential requirements in the smart healthcare network because all the collection data needs to be transmitted in secure channel [15].

5.7   CONCLUSION

The healthcare system is facing global challenges to provide healthcare facilities to patients. Recently, due to the pandemic of COVID-19, the worldwide healthcare system has become so important to provide patient treatment. The numbers

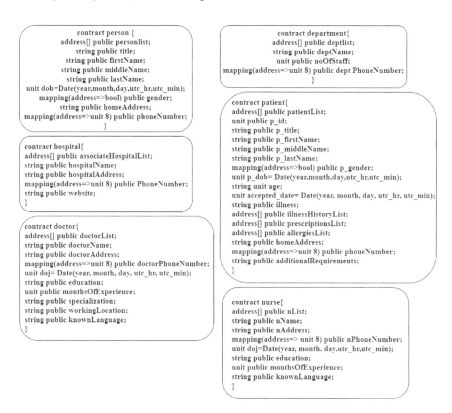

FIGURE 5.8   In smart healthcare system having list of smart contracts with list.

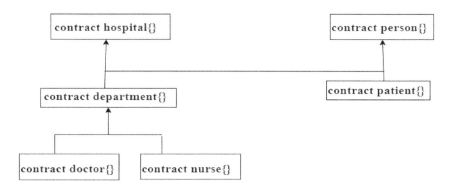

FIGURE 5.9   Smart contracts proposed for smart healthcare system.

of patients are very high, whereas that of doctors, nurses and hospitals are less. Here come the uses of technology into the smart healthcare system to introduce system automation. Using emerging technologies like IoT, machine learning, artificial intelligence and blockchain, the system becomes easy to access for both patients and doctors. Every application comes with implementation challenges, and in this smart healthcare system it is essential to address security and privacy issues. In this chapter, the details of security and privacy challenges have been explained. The blockchain-based solution was proposed to address security issues. Smart contracts are written to automate the system. In the future, proposed model scalability issues will need to be addressed. In blockchain there is requirement for high computational power to execute different transactions.

REFERENCES

1. Jaiswal, Kavita, et al. "An IoT-Cloud Based Smart Healthcare Monitoring System Using Container Based Virtual Environment in Edge Device," *2018 International Conference on Emerging Trends and Innovations In Engineering And Technological Research (ICETIETR)*, Ernakulam, India 2018, pp. 1–7, doi: 10.1109/ICETIETR.2018.8529141.
2. Tawalbeh, Lo'ai A, Fadi Muheidat, Mais Tawalbeh, and Muhannad Quwaider. "IoT privacy and security: Challenges and solutions." *Applied Sciences* 10, no. 12 (2020): 4102.
3. Algarni, Abdullah. "A survey and classification of security and privacy research in smart healthcare systems." *IEEE Access* 7 (2019): 101879–101894.
4. Alam, Zahid, and Hiral Patel. "Security and privacy issues of big data in IoT based healthcare system using cloud computing." *International Journal on Recent and Innovation Trends in Computing and Communication* 5, no. 6 (2017): 26–30.
5. Sachin, D., C Chinmay, F Jaroslav, G Rashmi, KR Arun, and KP Subhendu, "SSII: Secured and high-quality steganography using intelligent hybrid optimization algorithms for IoT." *IEEE Access* 9, (2021): 1–16, 10.1109/ACCESS.2021.3089357.
6. Gupta A, C Chakraborty, and B Gupta. "Secure transmission of EEG data using watermarking algorithm for the detection of epileptical seizures." *Traitement du Signal, IIETA* 38, no. 2 (2021): 473–479, doi:10.18280/ts.380227.
7. He, Daojing, Ran Ye, Sammy Chan, Mohsen Guizani, and Yanping Xu. "Privacy in the Internet of Things for smart healthcare." *IEEE Communications Magazine* 56, no. 4 (2018): 38–44.
8. Tuli, Shreshth, Shikhar Tuli, Gurleen Wander, Praneet Wander, Sukhpal Singh Gill, Schahram Dustdar, Rizos Sakellariou, and Omer Rana. "Next generation technologies for smart healthcare: Challenges, vision, model, trends and future directions." *Internet Technology Letters* 3, no. 2 (2020): e145.
9. Tariq, Noshina, Ayesha Qamar, Muhammad Asim, and Farrukh Aslam Khan. "Blockchain and smart healthcare security: A survey." *Procedia Computer Science* 175 (2020): 615–620.
10. Manpreet K, ZK Mohammad, G Shikha, N Abdulfattah, C Chinmay, and KP Subhendu. "MBCP: Performance analysis of large scale mainstream blockchain consensus protocols." *IEEE Access* 9 (2021) 1–14, doi. 10.1109/ACCESS.2021.3085187.
11. Arindam, S, ZA Mohammad, MS Moirangthem, Chinmay C Abdulfattah, and KP Subhendu. "Artificial neural synchronization using nature inspired whale optimization." *IEEE Access* (2021): 1–14, doi: 10.1109/ACCESS.2021.305288.
12. Amit, K, C Chinmay, J Wilson, A Kishor, C Chakraborty, and W Jeberson. "A novel fog computing approach for minimization of latency in healthcare using machine learning." *International Journal of Interactive Multimedia and Artificial Intelligence*, (2020): 1–11, doi:10.9781/ijimai.2020.12.004.

13. Anichur, R, C Chinmay, A, Adnan, Md Razaul Karim, Md Jahidul Islam, K Dipanjali, R Ziaur, and SB Shahab. "SDN-IoT empowered intelligent framework for industry 4.0 applications during COVID-19 pandemic." *Cluster Computing*, 1–18, 2021, doi: 10.1007/s10586-021-03367-4.
14. Mohanta, BK, SS Panda, and D Jena. An overview of smart contract and use cases in blockchain technology. In *2018 9th International Conference on Computing, Communication and Networking Technologies (ICCCNT)* (pp. 1–4). IEEE, 2018, July.
15. Satapathy, U, BK Mohanta, SS Panda, S Sobhanayak, and D Jena. A secure framework for communication in Internet of Things application using hyperledger based blockchain. In *2019 10th international conference on computing, communication and networking technologies (ICCCNT)* (pp. 1–7). IEEE, 2019, July.

6 Tapping the Big Data Analytics and IoT in the Pandemic Era

Yashikha Dhiman
TCS, Ahmedabad, India

Ashish Joshi and Isha Pant
THDC Institute of Hydropower Engineering and
Technology, Uttarakhand, India

CONTENTS

DOI: 10.1201/9781003247128-6

6.1 INTRODUCTION

For a long time, the technology and healthcare sectors have been inextricably linked. The volume of patient and customer health statistics has risen enormously in the healthcare domain; this has happened because of contemporary computer-based information systems. The extensive and complicated requirements of medical record keeping, combined with rigorous patient privacy regulations, resulted in an immensely cumbersome maze of health data demands. Empowering healthcare with Big Data and IoT investigates the convergence of these two areas and forecasts the future of utilizing modern technology and building data ecosystems in the healthcare industry. However, the prompt growth of IoT and Big Data has stemmed in the embryonic new opportunities in the field of the medical and healthcare sectors. The emergence of wearable equipment, biosensors, and m-health in recent years has increased the amount of biological records and data congregated [3]. Additionally, when folks all over the sphere began to embrace wearable biosensors, innovative applications for tailored eHealth and m-health devices appeared. The merits of these technologies and devices are evident: they are widely accessible, solely available, and guileless to familiarize; they equally make it guileless for suppliers to deliver custom-made economically and at scale devices. The manifestation of 'Big Data' was thought up during the last span of around ten years as an outcome of the enormous bulk of information flowing into our modern digital environs. Big Data is usually considered as immense collections of data that, owing to their absolute bulk, can only be observed by computers to picture patterns, fashions and associations, mainly with reference to human manners [1].

Big Data is frequently divided into three categories:

Transactional data – Data from bills, payment briefings, storage registers, distribution archives, claim activities and expense data are samples of transactional data. These are beneficial to both clients and benefactors in the healthcare domain and medical sector.

Machine or clinical data – This might contain statistics attained from industrialized tools, instantaneous data from measuring device and wearable machinery (for instance, the sensors on your smartphone or a heart rate observer), and web records that trail consumer activities online.

Social data – Facts and information descended from social media facilities like Facebook Likes, LinkedIn Reactions, Twitter Tweets, Instagram Activities or YouTube views that deliver visions on patient conduct and emotion statistics.

In the perspective of healthcare, the term 'Big Data' indicates the convergence of arithmetic, figures, statistics, facts, data science, machine learning and healthcare.

Acceptance of this technology is vigorous not just for providing higher quality treatment to patients, but also for the overall sustainability of healthcare systems. Big Data is actually drilling into the details that make a difference in quality outcomes and profitability in industries other than healthcare across the globe. The rapid expansion of COVID-19 has revealed and worsened several fundamental flaws in countries' health-response systems. All of these trepidations subsidize to an incompetence to balance the remedy in reaction to the epidemic's spread. Locating the origin of an epidemic, isolating most likely diseased patients, handling censoriously sick patients and avoiding cross-spread of infection among medical workforces and patients all need a huge human resource; a faster epidemic will put even more burden on the system. Through the speedy expansion of technology in the medical domain, officialdoms all over the sphere are awaking to the need to use the massive amounts of data being generated to serve their patients and providers. Big Data analytics is rapidly expanding in IoT for better judgement building. MIoT is a crucial facet of healthcare's digital transformation since it enables new business models to evolve and changes in work processes, efficiencies, cost containment, and enhanced customer experiences [1]. Big Data analysis in IoT demands the treating of a huge volume of statistics and its room in various packing systems. Combinations of sensing and actuating devices can exchange material on sites from side-to-side cohesive manner and establish a single functional system to allow novel solicitations. In all-purpose, IoT expands the quantity and variety of data. As a result, it facilitates the application and development of Big Data analytics. Furthermore, IoT fundamental and applied models are accelerated by the usage of Big Data technology. The first approach is to maintain IoT databases, which are used by linked sensors to interact with one another. For instance, communiqué strategies such as smart home apparatuses, insolent traffic lights and CCTV cameras produce massive volumes of data in a variety of forms. This information will be reserved on the bank of cloud at a minimal cost. The subsequent stage involves the generation of data, which is referred to as Big Data due to its size, rapidity and diversity. This massive quantity of information will be reserved in Communal disseminated fault manager data stations. The last stage employs analytics technologies such as Map Reduce, Spark, Splunk and Skytree to examine massive IoT data volumes. Starting with training data, the four stages of analysis go through analysis tools, queries and reports. It is commonly accepted in healthcare that the efficacy of Big Data analytics (BDA) tools is dictated by the value of the information used to train them. Algorithms trained on faulty, low-quality data will produce incorrect findings, resulting in insufficient care delivery. Obtaining excellent training data, on the other hand, is a tough and time-consuming endeavour, leaving many businesses without the resources to devise models. As healthcare establishments depend on analytics algorithms to support them create maintenance selections, it is essential that these apparatuses be barren of inherent or overt preference that might intensify health discrepancies. With the current inequities in the healthcare business, creating defects is a hazard [4]. The apprehension of data privacy and security is great on the grade of problems in algorithm improvement. Right of entry into huge, varied data sets required to train analytics tools might be hampered by legal, privacy and cultural barriers.

The remainder of the article is structured as follows. Section 6.2 discusses connection of IoT and Big Data for digital health, the BDA support. Section 6.3 contains the resilience building in pandemic conditions. Section 6.4 depicts how to fight pandemic using Big Data modules. Section 6.5 shows role of BDA during pandemic times. Section 6.6 demonstrates the exploratory study. Section 6.7 contains notion of IoT to IoMT. Finally, Section 6.8 concludes with the idea of future considerations.

6.2   CONNECTING BIG DATA AND IOT TO DIGITAL HEALTH

It's no secret that healthcare is plagued by a deficiency of continuous, across-the-board health records interoperability. Over the last decade, the healthcare sector has made gigantic achievements in the gathering of health-related information and the use of knowledge to assess and produce actionable stuffs from it. Conversely, the factual influence of medical-related Big Data is not just in the statistics composed, but also in how statistics and figures are smeared and what that data demands in relations of its effect on the efficacy and output of our healthcare and medical arrangement. Positive as well as life-saving results are the key factors that have made a significant and effective dent in the world of Big Data. In recent times, the impact of digital health seems to have become crucially influential for both care practitioners and patients. Today's healthcare breakthroughs have had a significant influence on the whole healthcare business, prompting us to embrace vital digital health trends. The taking on of allied healthcare equipment such as smart devices, wearable health devices, and smart health one-to-one care arrangements is one of these advances [5]. These technologies are intended to improve patient care and provide accurate and efficient health tracking for patients and clinicians alike. The rising popularity of IoT in healthcare and medical areas has also fuelled the rise of the Internet of Medical Things (IoMT), which is well-defined as an assemblage of medical devices and apps that can access to healthcare information technology systems via networking technologies. The fact that networks are always evolving in terms of speed, reliability, and availability, and that connected devices are benefitting on that speed and throughput, is a massive boon to companies seeking to implement connected solutions, obtain valuable data and respond. Sensors can obtain data, and cloud-based services can use that data to help automate the labour-intensive operations that keep the economy moving as much as feasible. This can span from rapidly assessing the body temperatures of visiting consumers to monitoring the cargo temperature of food and medications in transit to sending work tickets when actions are desired. Two primary growth forces are influencing demand for IoT-based healthcare solutions: affordability and widespread use of IoT tools and linked devices. By lowering hospital readmissions and simplifying operations, IoT healthcare solutions can dramatically reduce healthcare expenditures.

6.2.1 THE BIG DATA ANALYTICS BDA SUPPORT

Big Data enables long-term methods that actively manage healthcare value by lowering costs while maintaining or improving excellence. It also emboldens invention to impulse the borders of medicine and elevate R&D throughput in innovation, growth and protection. Healthcare is a multi-layered system planned with the rapid agenda of averting, identifying and handling health-related ailments or damages in humans. Big Data is being brought together in healthcare to predict surge, treat illness, improve value of life and decrease needless deaths. It is often used to edify consumers on life adoptions that improve welfare and dynamic customer contribution in their own carefulness. Big Data is utilized in healthcare settings to provide evidence-based treatment that has been shown to provide desired results aimed at each individual while maintaining wellbeing. It also permits a care specialist to choose the utmost suitable location for conveying the specified healing impact. They might together support the subdivision in addressing issues such as unpredictability in healthcare quality and increasing healthcare costs. A physician can hire statistics from varied bases (such as medicinal and assurance cover data, wearable devices, genomic data, and even social media usage) to develop a completed eviction of the patient as a being in order to yield a personalized healthcare package from a patient-centred viewpoint. Big Data can also be used to spot diseases prior to their growth, when they can be cured more solely and efficiently; to cope specific individual and people fitness; and to identify fitness care scam more rapidly and proficiently [6]. Data analytics can answer a diverse variety of queries.

Specified the massive possibility for Big Data uses in the upcoming times, healthcare corporations can consume the Big Data collected in the multiple segments:

- **Enact solid digital health platform**: To get the most out of the linked digital health environment for Big Data analytics, you need a stage on which to construct and accomplish apps, conduct analytics, and collect, stock and guard your records. A stage or platform, similar to operating system software for a desktop, executes a number of things in the background to make the lives of developers, users, stakeholders and ourselves simpler and less expensive.
- **Enabled system and stakeholder integration and interoperability**: Big Data's assurance in medical sector depends upon gathering and distributing data from numerous bases, organizations and shareholders. The statistic that numerous health records bases have remain desolated is a limitation to Big Data growth. Incorporation and interoperability are precarious when numerous databases and software systems hoard dissimilar subgroups of information.
- **Spur innovation and openness**: Medical Sector industries are assigning financial encouragements to data dimension and study; presenting noble and associate data on patient gratification and value methods; and leveraging consoles, all in a determination to bind cooperation and enhance clinician performance.

BDA is reported to help hospital management enhance their efficacy in providing healthcare programmes that offer customized maintenance to the patients [7]. Continuous investigation is requested to examine the role of BDA in enlightening service quality in hospitals. Academics and Researchers are required to overcome new methods of giving more refined personal support to persons, particularly older peoples and patients suffering from prolonged illnesses.

6.2.2 IoT Support: Sensing Systems That Collect Data

The cornerstone of IoT is perception and identification technology. Sensors are machines and gadgets that incorporate various fluctuations in their environments, like radio frequency identification (RFID), cameras, infrared devices, GPS, health devices and smart device instruments. These devices provide a comprehensive insight through object recognition, location recognition, and topography recognition, and can adjust this information to digital signals for an easy network transmission. Sensor machineries allow real-time observing of treatments and the assembly of an overabundance of physical constraints about a patient, permitting diagnoses and high-quality treatment to be accelerated. During the last two decades, science, particularly biosciences and manufacturing, have seen extraordinary rates of technical improvement. The enlargement of molecular biology gears, visual and imaging gears such as tomography, additive and subtractive engineering, robotics, new production technologies, diminishment of semiconductor chips and energy rooms, upsurge in computational supremacy and parallel processing, data storage on semiconductor chips, network enlargement and sensor technologies have made momentous progress [6].

- **Research assistance**: IoT provides real-world information to medical researchers via real-time data from IoT devices, which can then be analyzed and evaluated to provide further accurate results.
- **Moodables**: According to researchers, this will be humans' biggest supporter in the coming years. These tools will aid in the relaxation of persons suffering from stress problems and ADD. Moodables can scan brain waves and transmit low-intensity currents to the brain as needed. This gadget can help both healthy and stressed brains. These gadgets are intended to enhance or modify a person's mood; these devices are primarily conceived and developed through neuroscience research driven by IoT.
- **Emergency Medical Assistance**: Using IoT-based applications and devices, medical-aid providers are informed before any disaster occurs, allowing them to take proper steps to improve healthcare service.
- **Tracking and alerts**: Continuous surveillance may be done manually or automatically, since IoT-based devices gather and exchange data in real time, allowing notifications to be sent based on a person's fluctuating health.

- **Ingestible sensors**: Swallowable sensors or ingestible sensors are one of the most intriguing aspects of the IoT in the medical business. They open up whole new avenues for monitoring patients remotely. These sensors are used to more accurately clock medications as well as to reflect lifestyle choices and overall medication-taking behaviours. The programme will have an impact on precision during dose assurance on patients and will reduce adverse effects caused by incorrect prescription. Ingestible sensors, for example, may use stomach fluids as a source of energy to treat schizophrenia, depressive disorders and bipolar illness. They will assess diet adherence, which is useful in the treatment of depressive disorders [8]. These are the most unusual IoT-powered innovations that may assist to monitor and identify any anomalies in the body because they are pill-sized and can remain within the body without causing any harm while also benefitting healthcare.

6.3 BUILDING RESILIENCE USING BIG DATA ANALYTICS AND IOT IN PANDEMIC CONDITIONS

Few events in our lives will have the same far-reaching influence as the COVID epidemic. Nations, corporations and individuals all around the world have seen many aspects of their life flipped upside down. The growing need for data insights and remote access in every commercial, industrial, and government environment has created the circumstances for the rapid adoption of technologies and systems that rely on the IoT.

There are several explanations for this occurrence. We require the capacity to interact, meet and collaborate with people without physically being present. We can practise algorithms to examine health records and trace patients' interaction past to assist detected forms of viral range by uniting data from several bases. With the aid of movement and interaction finding, these apps can be used to determine not only current areas with a great number of cases, but also help in predicting upcoming occurrences. Businesses, medical professionals and governments want crucial information supplied quickly via linked devices and high-speed networks. To create resistance against the COVID-19 pandemic, it has become imperative to even provide precise and timely data on the outbreak. The IoT and Big Data can become unconditionally vital to medical sector (IoT). In the case of medical research, any device that generates data on a patient's wellbeing and transfers that information to the cloud would be considered IoT. Wearables are unquestionably the most famous sample of such a device. To get the maximum from the connected digital health situation, or IoT, you need a platform to build and manage apps, perform analytics, and collect, stock and guard data. In the digital health corporate, the manifestation 'connected health' is referred to designate how healthcare is associating [7]. In the digital health sector, a connected health scheme will make the most of healthcare sources and provide suppler replacements for customers to appoint with clinicians and vice versa to better self-manage their treatment. For the digital healthcare sector, a stage is vital in an associated health scheme. Health data systems have giant potential for increasing care provision efficacy, depressing entire healthcare prices, and meaning fully enlightening patient consequences. With the adoption of this rule and the related know-hows, it is precarious to correctly establish and précis the ever-increasing amount of data that is numerically collected and deposited inside medical organizations. The use of leading-edge know-hows to defend info altercation during a pandemic like COVID-19 can be hugely obliging. Suitable calibration procedures for new-fangled communication and network protocols are crucial in this respect to confirm their continuous and unbroken assimilation in medical sector organizations. Because IoT use delivers wide access to system observing statistics, new data-driven safe keeping methods for constructing predictive machine learning algorithms to classify IoT fears may be generated. Distributed record technology and blockchain may promise data reliability without engaging an intermediary party for reliable information exchange across different stakeholders in the healthcare sector, allowing privacy-preserving solutions for smart healthcare systems [9]. The technological growth and IoT features that can be used to help a medical system deal with disease outbreaks already exist; however, they are fragmented and not yet integrated. As a necessity, the system must be able to rapidly construct its infrastructure in order to connect the components of data collecting, processing and storage, allowing the system to grow and extend for disease surveillance, preventive quarantine and inpatient treatment of the afflicted.

6.4   FIGHTING PANDEMIC USING BIG DATA ANALYTICS

With a noteworthy number of active cases around the sphere, the novel coronavirus creates a serious community wellbeing challenge. Due to the extreme pandemic's eruption, travel restrictions have been enacted, creating information gathering a hard job for the improvement investigation community. During these times, customary information gathering approaches that need field official visit can be dangerous. In this situation, Big Data is more pertinent and valuable than ever before if suitable confidentiality and moral protections are in place. Global Positioning System (GPS) coordinates collected from mobile phone histories, for example, may be valuable in chasing individual's actions. During an epidemic, this information has massive possibility for forecasting hotspots and faltering virus spread. As another example, sentiment analysis grounded on data mining of social media repositories can be used to deliver useful understandings to help in the expansion of suitable health messaging for the common people. It has generated a new CEDIL-sustained methodical map that collects an exclusive and wide-ranging gathering of educations that use Big Data to ration or assess improvement consequences [9]. The map comprises influence assessments that use Big Data to assess improvement consequences, methodical appraisals of Big Data influence assessments, and other dimension readings that used Big Data in unique conducts to ration improvement consequences.

Of the studies, 63 out of 437 comprised in the map observed at health-related improvement consequences. Twenty-eight researches observed at intermediations intended at depressing death, and a further 28 observed at intermediation intended at placing an end to a transmissible disease widespread. Conversely, there is an absence of influence assessments that measure the influence of an epidemic outburst, both in minor areas like districts and bigger parts such as a state or country. Satellite statistic was used in 29 researches and was over and over again used basis of Big Data. Among one of those researches, for instance, observed at the obtainability of measles outburst vaccines in Niger. The study joined satellite-observed inhabitant's dissemination sizes with high resolution measles cases stated in the country [11]. This was carefully tracked by the mobile phone call detail record (CDR), which was used in 27 dissimilar researches. The aim of a research in Haiti was to understand if CDR could forecast the prompt spatial growth of the cholera widespread. Additionally, this map displays that Sub-Saharan Africa has had the largest statistics researches associated to disease widespread, with the Middle East and North Africa containing the least. When it comes to researches on disease widespread in delicate circumstances, this map discloses a noteworthy evidence gap. In terms of global evidence gaps in further wellbeing results, road traffic demises, material misuse and sexual and reproductive medical facilities have hardly been studied.

With the rapid growth in coronavirus infections, Big Data keeps the ability to assist in epidemic prediction. By integrating data from multiple sources, we may utilize algorithms to evaluate health records and trace patients' contact histories to assist discover viral transmission trends. Natural Language Processing (NLP) is an AI technique worth mentioning here. By studying normal human interactions in the form of text and speech, NLP may help trait with more meaning to human communication. It may be used to examine social media links and online news stories, possibly triggering an alert when new COVID-19-related events occur throughout the world. In the future, NLP and other Big Data approaches might be used to detect incidents, ensuring that such health problems are handled with as quickly as feasible [12]. Despite recent advances, these technologies are still relatively new, and numerous implementation problems, such as data ambiguity and information overload, continue. Many nations are seeking to halt the spread of the epidemic with the aid of smartphone apps. These apps monitor people's travels to see if they're in high-risk regions or have come into contact with high-risk individuals.

However, the increasing use of Big Data has generated ethical and legal problems. These mobile phone apps have access to a lot of personal data. Privacy compromises, a loss of personal liberty, and public desire for openness and justice in the use of Big Data are all ethical issues. It is important to properly evaluate and execute data privacy regulations when working with large data. Despite privacy issues, Big Data in medicine has a promising future. As long as travel limitations exist in many nations, there may be more chances to use Big Data to compensate for the absence of in-person data collecting. This will, however, necessitate financial investments. When it comes to Big Data, healthcare businesses must invest in the appropriate technology, infrastructure and personnel training. Employees would need to be trained in data analysis techniques first and foremost. The research community needs to perform a more systematic review of the current techniques in order to fully exploit the promise of Big Data in healthcare. Given the present public health crisis, it will be fascinating to see if Big Data can be used to forecast future disease outbreaks.

6.5 COLLECTING BIG DATA ANALYTICS IN HEALTHCARE DURING A PANDEMIC

Many sectors have been impacted by Big Data, and many have been forced to embrace technology that allows for better analytical capabilities. This isn't only a trend in the healthcare business. So according to the market research, the worldwide Big Data in healthcare market will reach $34.27 billion by 2022, with a compound annual growth rate (CAGR) of 22.07% throughout the projected period [14]. The healthcare business is being affected by Big Data in the following ways:

- With over 30 billion healthcare transactions performed each year, the healthcare sector is overwhelmed with data. In healthcare, Big Data analytics has the potential to become a promising sector, tackling some of the industry's most pressing challenges, such as cost inefficiencies and prescription mistakes. Advantages of Big Data have sparked the interest of the healthcare industry, which is seeking for more effective business strategies to increase production and service quality. While Big Data has the potential to assist the healthcare business, it must overcome several challenges.
- Big Data refers to enormous volumes of complicated, raw data that may give significant insight when processed by clever analytics tools. Regrettably, conventional equipment has still not expanded to match the volumes of data that we now have exposure to, and typical data-processing equipment is inefficient of handling large amounts of data [13]. Modern technology is necessary to gather, store and disseminate large data. The value of large data is established by what can be done with it, not by the amount of data it contains. By appropriately analyzing Big Data, industry leaders have lowered costs, saved time and initiated the creation of new products.
- The healthcare business stands to gain a lot by digitizing, integrating and efficiently utilizing Big Data. Big Data can help healthcare companies develop holistic, customized and comprehensive patient profiles, as well as diagnose and cure diseases at an earlier stage. Individual and population health information is now readily available to medical professionals. Healthcare businesses can also expect to enhance security by more simply and efficiently detecting healthcare fraud. Data integration helps not just healthcare practitioners, but it also has the potential to dramatically improve customer product quality. Consumer healthcare services will be provided through mobile health applications such as telehealth and wearables such as the Fit Bit.
- However, the advantages and potential of Big Data in healthcare look to be bright, Big Data and healthcare face significant fundamental obstacles. The technical skills necessary and the capacity to assure compliance

with all security procedures around Big Data are the two primary hurdles to its use in healthcare. Big Data demands a particular skill set due to the complexity of the files [15]. Hospitals will need to seek the help of data scientists to manipulate information in a Big Data environment since IT specialists who are acquainted with SQL programming and conventional databases are not equipped for the learning curve. Security is another key obstacle to Big Data and healthcare. Hackers and sophisticated persistent threats are known to target Big Data storage (APTs). Although the security measures in most businesses are acceptable, policies such as HIPAA compliance must be protected.

• Big Data analytics has the ability to enhance medicine, technology, and finance in the healthcare business, and as it gains traction, more healthcare companies will use it. Healthcare providers may create thorough patient profiles, enhancing client loyalty, and consumers can anticipate greater quality treatment both within and outside of healthcare facilities. Big Data enables us to transform previously acquired and stored data into practical solutions for enhancing healthcare infrastructure.

Big Data, IoT and AI have all shown their usefulness when they were most needed [16]. This is discussed in further detail as follows:

I. As a way of fighting the fast spread of COVID-19, Big Data has become a buzzword recently. The World Health Organization (WHO) been advocating for extensive testing and tracking to battle the infection since mid-March. The best approach to ensure that this information has the greatest impact is to collect it on a national level. Although some nations, such as Germany, South Korea, Hong Kong, New Zealand and Canada, were fast to establish integrated logistics laws, others trailed behind.

Many nations have encountered challenges in adopting countrywide testing. To identify probable cases of the virus in this region, companies have created unique Artificial Intelligence and IoT smart solutions. Fever and potential breathing abnormalities, both of which are frequent signs of the virus, can be detected by smart cameras integrated with facial recognition technology and temperature detection software.

II. DeepMind, a part of Google, revealed the findings in order to create therapies utilizing AI algorithms and computer capacity. Benevolent AI uses AI systems to discover medicines for severe illness treatments, and they are aiding in coronavirus therapy. It utilized its predictive powers to propose current medications that may be beneficial within weeks of the epidemic.

III. Screening hospitals and clinics is a time-consuming and important operation. Hospitals around the world are turning to smart robots to fill empty beds as a result of personnel shortages and rising admissions. Robots were used to transport medicine across the hospital, clean and conduct admission processes in China. Because robots cannot become infected with the virus, they pose no risk while dealing with patients.

IV. Physicians are attempting to reinvent their services as a result of the issue. Since consumers cannot be seen in reality, other methods must be used to contact them, and this is where healthcare has had to develop [10]. Due to tight rules, the healthcare sector has frequently trailed behind other industries in terms of digitization. People may now get remote treatment in many clinics for the first time, due to video conferencing and apps. These applications utilize Artificial Intelligence-powered chat bots and diagnosis tools to get to the bottom of your ailments. Artificial Intelligence does not pose a danger to the medical profession; rather, it is the finest assistance a doctor can have.

6.6 EXPLORATORY STUDY

Experimental research was conducted in the present situation of COVID-19 pandemic. The pandemic has presented a lot of problems to the medical industry [17]. These problems can be handled utilizing techniques like as IoT, ML and AI. The next section describes the additional research.

6.6.1 INTRODUCTION

On December 31, 2019, the Wuhan Municipal Health Commission in China stated a cluster of pneumonia cases in Wuhan, Hubei Province, which was later recognized as a different virus called SARS-COV-2, foremost in the illness known as Coronavirus Disease 2019, also known as COVID-19. Officials verified the first known COVID-19 case outside of China on January 13, 2020. After the sickness began dispersal throughout the world, the WHO professed it an epidemic on March 11, 2020. As of August 24, 2020, COVID-19 has reached 213 countries and the world, resulting in unevenly 23,586,023 verified cases of infection and 812,527 mortalities. The healthcare sector has made considerable expenditures in COVID-19 diagnosis, screening and treatment of infected people in order to combat this epidemic. Governments and international organizations are collaborating to ensure that enough healthcare is available to battle the disease. There has yet to be found a medicine or vaccine that can totally remove the chance of getting this disease. As a result, a variety of therapeutic techniques and medicines are utilized to treat this disease as needed. To avoid the virus from spreading, administrators are implementing measures such as social segregation, area lockdown and adequate sterilization. Additionally, combining future technologies with effective healthcare administration and strong governance will enhance society's ability to fight itself against COVID-19 infection. Improved AI methods assure extensive application in a large area of organizations with the introduction of intelligent technology in this information era from a broader perspective. While social quarantining and the practice of wearing masks/gloves have been demonstrated to inhibit the growth of the epidemic, effective interventions and defensive positioning must be developed to achieve pandemic resistance through better management and surveillance. AI and machine learning, which have been efficaciously utilized in an extensive range of study fields, might offer a number of possible applications for achieving brilliance. AI can be used at the cellular scale to estimate the structure of SARS-COV-2 associated proteins, classify current treatment drugs that may be used to treat the sickness, propose new composites that may underwrite to medicine improvement, design probable vaccine objectives and create documentation procedures as well as an improved understanding of the infection expand. AI may help improve COVID-19 detection by analyzing computed tomography, provide various strategies for tracking illness development using appropriate tools, and create prognostications on communicable diseases based on compound numerical responses, including digital health information [15]. AI may be utilized in epidemiological exploratory modelling, experience statistics and projecting the number of cases based on various public policy alternatives from a social standpoint. Generating and publishing research ideas, as well as gathering insights from numbers and simulations, are all necessary components in expediting the epidemic responses.

6.6.2 APPLICATIONS OF ARTIFICIAL INTELLIGENCE AND MACHINE LEARNING IN THE MEDICAL SECTOR

The application of AI in identifying infectious illnesses is very significant in the medical business and has the potential to revolutionize healthcare procedures. Integrating AI into imaging procedures has increased a ration of interest in the healthcare and medical industry. Machine learning prototypes can look at medical images in the early stages of a disease and diagnose it. Big Data and deep learning techniques are used to power these prototypes to fulfil the objective. Microbiology, optometry, radiology and skincare are among the fields where image-based learning could be used. The avoidance of diseases like COVID-19 is highly relied on patients being screened by pathogenic diagnostics, which is a much time-consuming procedure, therefore precision is critical. By assessing and organizing large volumes of patient data stored in digitized medical records, machine learning may assist healthcare professionals [18]. Machine learning is also utilized in a number of therapeutic diagnostics, such as recognizing patients with severe illnesses that require immediate intensive care unit (ICU) services, classifying initial indications of the disease, analyzing chest X-rays to understand the patient's respiratory status, and so on. As a consequence, AI and machine learning improve the performance of identification and prediction procedures in the medical sector, as well as the way administrative choices are made.

Computed tomography and X-rays are common diagnostic and therapeutic tools in diagnostic imaging. CT scans and X-ray imaging were essential for determining the SARS-COV-2 infection during the COVID-19 epidemic. Disease type classification enabled by AI will aid in the automated processes of the screening procedure, lowering the period of time clinicians and patients must engage. As a consequence, it safeguards medical imaging professionals while also aiding in viral transmission. To assess the concentration of any type of RNA, the Reverse

Transcription-Polymerase Chain Reaction (RT-PCR) assay is widely employed. COVID-19 infection is diagnosed with this RT-PCR. The RT-PCR test, on the other hand, has certain flaws. The most sophisticated Artificial Intelligence-powered technologies and techniques will undoubtedly aid in the establishment of resilience against the COVID-19 pandemic. The identification technique was utilized on CT scans of the abdomen in a study that showed rapid recognition of COVID-19 using machine learning approaches. Qualified radiologists found that COVID-19 was different from other viral pneumonias based on CT scans. As a consequence, medical practitioners will be able to diagnose COVD-19 infection early on.

6.6.3 IMPLICATIONS OF AI AND ML IN SOCIAL AND INFORMATION SCIENCE

The proposed machine learning approach utilizes a bunching method to modify a three-dimensional picture of COVID-19 activity throughout China, as well as a data augmentation methodology to deal with the paucity of previously available disease activity reports and developing epidemic trends. SIRNET combines machine learning, theoretical physics and outbreak modelling into a single system. From a physical standpoint, the epidemic modelling creates important factors, which provides a spontaneous knowledge of how the prototype may be utilized for anticipating illness patterns. It is critical to categories data and assess how it is disseminated on social media in order to implement appropriate data-sharing rules. Different techniques should be utilized when releasing various sorts of circumstantial news or information. In the public sector, the use of computerized decision-making systems has particular benefits and requirements. In the current COVID-19 epidemic, this type of computerized system is important, since authorities are developing applications or technology to track human mobility in an effort to reduce the risk of transmission.

6.6.4 THE POSSIBLE USES OF IOT

IoT technologies have the potential to improve the COVID-19 diagnostic and treatment method by speeding it up, increasing its accuracy and making it more efficient. Research demonstrates how the COVID-19 Intelligent Diagnosis and Treatment Assistant Program could be coupled with cloud-based software. [19]. Electronic medical records and machine learning techniques are used in the program for automated diagnosis. It can assist the health department by collecting data from patients, organizing coordination and allowing patients to self-diagnose. Chabot is being developed by a number of health agencies for automated disease screening and follow-up planning. Autonomous ophthalmology carts (such as the Vici InTouch) can be used to support individuals under quarantine without the requirement for medical staff to be there. The proliferation of IoT-enabled devices has generated a plethora of smartphone apps for tracking physiological data like heart rate, temperature and sleeping habits. These devices or detectors can be combined with machine learning technologies to predict COVID-19 infection phases. Alarms generated by computerized temperature and blood oxygen monitoring can be utilized to direct medical personnel's attention. Data from Fitbit or Apple Watch has been utilized in a variety of studies, such as Digital Engagement and Tracking for Early Treatment and Control, to connect heart rate and activity pattern with that reported by COVID-infected people.

6.6.5 THE RISKS THAT CAN ARISE WHILE USING THESE INTELLIGENT EQUIPMENT AND TECHNIQUES

Because of all the erroneous input, policy choices, as well as patient monitoring and diagnosis, may be skewed or incorrectly conducted. GAN may produce new pictures or datasets with the same characteristics as the training dataset, based on a deep learning and machine learning class. As a result, GAN is capable of producing pictures that have never existed before. As a result, a hacker might use this learning model to create false CT scan data or other diagnostic imaging data and pictures. Cyber-attacks on healthcare organizations can have a significant influence on the primary treatment and patient health, and have become a severe issue in contemporary healthcare organizations as hacking assaults have become more common [18]. Because they rely on data gathered from linked networks, IoT-based apps can exacerbate this vulnerability. According to a poll of older/senior individuals, not every age group in society will have the same level of technological readiness, which creates additional hurdles in the adoption of IoT-based applications in healthcare. Distributed ledger technology like blockchain can assure information integrity across various organizations in the healthcare industry without requiring a third party, allowing privacy-preserving system for sustainable healthcare services.

6.7 DRIVE THROUGH THE FUTURE: IOT TO IOMT

Contemplate your last latest clinical encounter; it was most probably a medical gadget or piece of equipment, such as a blood pressure cuff, a glucose levels monitor, or perhaps an MRI scanner. Contemporary Internet-connected gadgets are intended to enhance efficiency, decrease treatment costs and improve overall healthcare results. With rise of IoT and Big Data analytics in medical, information can still be acquired in areas where it was formerly done manually or not at all. Smart thermometer, for instance, sends real-time data to global health facilities; bench-top testers quickly examine sample data and share data in near real alongside disease monitoring instruments placed kilometres away. Presently, a variety of influences monitor every type of patient behaviour, from glucose screens to prenatal screening to electrocardiograms or circulatory strain. A substantial majority of these estimates necessitate a follow-up consultation with a physician [12]. IoMT solutions are quickly altering clinical practice due to their capacity to gather, analyze and communicate healthcare information. These apps are playing an essential part in assessing and avoiding chronic diseases for both doctors and patients, and they have been set to usher in a new era of care. The IoMT is a networked backbone of medical equipment, software products, health services. And, while an expanding pool of IoT applications as well as widespread adoption affects several more firms, it is a surge of sensor-based equipment, such as wearable tech or even stand-alone gadgets for remote health monitoring, as well as the cohabitation of Internet operable medical products with patient records, that is most promising.

6.7.1 MEDICAL IoT

Evidently, there are numerous prospects for additional IoMT evolution. It already has been expanded for use in emergency treatment, insurance offices and pharmacies. The IoT has significantly decreased emergency room waiting times. The very same analysis is valuable to Emergency Health Technicians, who transfer patient to the hospital. If EMTs learn that one hospital is out of patient beds, they might divert to another. Infrared sensors track the stockpile of blood supplies and kinds accessible at the hospitals, in addition to aiding with bed occupancy. The IoMT has made pharmaceutical inventory operations easier. IoT sensors in manufacturing and production centres, like RFID tags and barcode, give real-time insight into medicine supply and trace its travel from a site to another. This has enhanced replenishing and drug fulfilment while also saving the pharmaceuticals supply network a considerable amount of money. Since this pharmaceutical sector is tightly controlled, the IoT aids in the documentation of manufacturing processes by continually giving factual information on quality assurance compliance. This in itself reduces the quantity of documentation, but also assures correctness. Furthermore, the connection of medical equipment & sensors is improving evolving healthcare management thus contributing to an incremental increase inpatient care, both within and outside of care facility doors. IoMT's strengths have included accurate diagnoses, fewer errors, and lower healthcare expenditures. When combined with smart devices, the technology enables people to submit their medical information to specialists in order to effectively monitor ailments and detect and avoid illnesses. This sort of development not only improves the clinical practice by removing a need for more in-person medical visits, but that also helps to decrease expenses. As in systems is incorporated into network devices and proves capable of real-time, remote measurement techniques of patient records, this aspect of IoMT is set for yet more growth [19]. Despite of a patient's area or ailment, the IoMT ecological development will have a greater influence. As linked medical equipment carry on making their way into the hands among both physicians and patients, even with the most distant locales will benefit from enhanced access to services.

6.7.2 IoT TO DISSECT AN OUTBREAK

As we all realize, the Advent of the Internet things has given us hopes for a great future of the Internet via machine–machine connection. The ongoing worldwide COVID-19 epidemic had already crossed provincial, radical, intellectual, moral, social, & educational borders. By utilizing an integrated system, an AI (IoT) powered healthcare system is beneficial for efficient evaluation of COVID-19 victims. This approach evolves patient satisfaction and lowers hospital readmissions. IoT seems to have the capacity to induce COVID-19 through rising attention and constant monitoring. Drones have already been used in a variety of locations to assess the response of certain specific groups [18]. It is also used by IoT nodes to improve the condition of quarantine patients. Gadgets too can aid in the detection of potential breakout hotspots. The system offers enormous potential for communication via linked gadgets. The gadgets would be used to pinpoint the precise site of origin. You may also obtain GIS data on the afflicted people. Epidemiologists can assist in the quest for patient zero. The IoT can indeed be utilized to deduce the source of a dangerous illness. IoT could confirm and ensure patient conformity as long as severely irritated individuals enter quarantine. Healthcare professionals can determine which patients remain detained and which patients have violated the quarantine. Those IoT information will even aid them in determining why anyone may have been exposed as a result of the incident. The versatility of IoT is also viable for tracing all patients who are high-risk enough even to necessitate quarantine but not serious enough as to require in-hospital treatment [11]. Currently, patients' daily check-ups are conducted manually by medical professionals who go directly.

6.7.3 Protocols for Preventive Containment

When an epidemic is identified, IoT technologies aid in the supervision of containment & response [13]. The Delta variant is a 'hyper-transmissible' strain of COVID-19 that is thought to be responsible for almost half of new infections worldwide. The sooner and more accurately variant data is disseminated, the higher the chances of assimilation. Leveraging IoT to deconstruct an epidemic given the numerous and diverse statistics gathered by communication phones, IoT would have many additional uses at certain point during a pandemic. When reaction time is important, IoT allows new technologies and apps that can aid in the quick identification of new epidemics. The apps may also help with crisis management by rolling out quick notifications to a location to enforce travel restrictions or lockdowns.

6.7.4 Upgrades in Connectivity Eternity

Rapid diagnostic sensors, data exchange, and telehealth for consultation & diagnosis have all been technical advances that can aid in the suppression of future epidemics. Furthermore, far more will be done to protect the world from future viral dangers. Individually, specific volatile organic component sensors may be mass-produced in the billions at a cheap unit cost. IoT, encompassing embedded technology, actuators, or devices, as well as data-driven apps, might assist prospective smart connected community to enhance nations' health and social postures in order to effectively combat the prevailing COVID-19 crisis and potential future disease outbreaks [13]. At an era when the entire globe is battling a certain threat, we have indeed got to accept new technology and find their virtues, even if there is still much work to be done. As a corollary, COVID-19 may even be considered the personification of the IoT.

6.7.5 CONSULTATIONS IN M-HEALTH

Due to the extremely infectious nature of this coronavirus, professionals have resorted to talking to patients through video chat in order to determine if anybody has been a target of the spreading without actually meeting in person [15]. Using technology to interact and keeping patients at home is a fantastic alternative to a chaotic rush to the hospitals for severe cases of the disease.

6.7.6 THE ADVENT OF THE ROBOTICS

Meeting social distance on an assembly line is a problem for industrial maintenance managers. Many firms will now have to redesign their layouts in order to fulfil all building codes; some will have to work with smaller teams. Several enterprises would have to rely on IoT to thrive and digitize operations in order to avoid a production collapse. Clever robots can still be employed to carry supplies and meals (just as is happening in certain hospitals), as well as to disperse medicines or goods (as is the case in some pharmacies). Although they're not solely with us while we're unwell! Drones are being used by certain businesses to make secure home shipments. This minimizes the danger of contaminating healthcare professionals while also saving protective material for everyday activities. Quite certainly, just after the 'fiery test' of COVID-19, this sort of system will become more prevalent. Production is indeed one of the leading pillars of IoT deployment [19] that has aided pandemic response. Medicinal manufacturing facilities now have their hands full, with several generating millions of items for testing, treatments and personal protective equipment (PPE) every month. Retaining these levels of production in the face of widespread disruptions is a daunting problem, but IoT devices can assist.

6.8 CONCLUSION

The proposed chapter discusses numerous applications of Big Data analytics using IoT to combat the COVID-19 outbreak. Methods and approaches were also explored in order to demonstrate the importance of Big Data analytics in fixing the issues and their contribution to the state of science. Wearable's and Smartphone applications are now being used to aid with wellbeing, wellness education, side-effect tracking, and group infection management and care coordination. Each of these stages of research has the ability to boost informational returns' relevance. The connection between IoT and Big Data analytics in regard to m-health was emphasized, as well as other analytics methodologies. Conversely, the use of Big Data in smart healthcare and pandemic conditions is investigated, as is the use of IoT to track down an outbreak. In interacting with the healthcare sector, there are still numerous obstacles to overcome. Emerging novel variations, vaccine effectiveness and adverse effects, health protocol relaxation and new normal adaption, and medical waste management are all challenges that will need to be addressed in the future. A broad range of Big Data technological solutions are available to address these issues. As a result, for COVID-19, insights into current stages of knowledge on Big Data technology are presented, as well as references for further research. New enhancements are entirely feasible with the combination of Big Data and promising applications such as machine learning, Data Science, IoT and AI, which can maximize the efficiency of the healthcare and medical sectors.

CONFLICT OF INTEREST

There is no conflict of interests.

FUNDING

There is no funding support.

DATA AVAILABILITY

Not applicable.

REFERENCES

1. Sachin D, Chinmay C, Jaroslav F, Rashmi G, Arun KR, Subhendu KP, SSII: Secured and High-Quality Steganography Using Intelligent Hybrid Optimization Algorithms for IoT, *IEEE Access*, 9, 1–16, 2021, 10.1109/ACCESS.2021.3089357
2. Gupta A, Chinmay C, Gupta B, Secure Transmission of EEG Data Using Watermarking Algorithm for the Detection of Epileptic Seizures, *Traitement du Signal*, 38, 2, 473–479, 2021, doi:10.18280/ts.380227
3. Ghubaish, A, Salman, T, Zolanvari, M, Unal, D, Al-Ali, A, Jain, R, Recent Advances in the Internet-of-Medical-Things (IoMT) Systems Security, *IEEE Internet of Things Journal*, 8, 11, 8707–8718, 1 June, 2021, doi:10.1109/JIOT.2020.3045653.
4. Manpreet K, Mohammad ZK, Shikha G, Abdulfattah N, Chinmay C, Subhendu KP, MBCP: Performance Analysis of Large Scale Mainstream Blockchain Consensus Protocols, *IEEE Access*, 9, 1–14, 2021, doi:10.1109/ACCESS.2021.3085187
5. Sarkar A, Khan MZ, Singh MM, Noorwali A, Chakraborty C, Pani SK, Artificial Neural Synchronization Using Nature Inspired Whale Optimization, *IEEE Access*, 9, 16435–16447, 2021, doi:10.1109/ACCESS.2021.305288.
6. Rahman A, Chakraborty C, Anwar A, Karim M, Islam M, Kundu D, Rahman Z, Band SS, SDN-IoT Empowered Intelligent Framework for Industry 4.0Applications during COVID-19 Pandemic, *Cluster Computing*, 1–18, 2021, doi:10.1007/s10586-021-03367-4
7. Maritz J, Eybers S, Hattingh M, Implementation Considerations for (BDA): A Benefit Dependency N/w Approach, In: Hattingh M, Matthe M, Smuts H, Pappas I, Dwivedi Y, Mäntymäki M, eds., *Responsible Design, Implementation and Use of Info and Communication Technology I3E 2020. Lecture Notes in Computer Science*, vol. 12066, Springer, Cham, 2020

8. Abir SMA, Islam SN, Anwar A, Mahmood AN, Oo AMT Building Resilience Against COVID-19 Pandemic Using AI, Machine Learning, IoT: A Survey of Recent Progress, *IoT*, 1, 506–528, 2020

9. Nasajpour M, Pouriyeh S, Parizi RM, IoT for Current COVID-19 and Future Pandemic: An Exploratory Study, *Journal of Healthcare Informatics Research*, 4, 325, 2020.

10. The Big Data and IoT Applications Fighting Coronavirus, Telefonica, 5 June, 2020, https://business.blogthinkbig.com/the-big-data-and-iot-applications-fighting-coronavirus/

11. Vishnu S, Ramson SJ, Jegan R, Internet of Medical Things – An Overview, in *5th International Conference on Devices, Circuits and Systems (ICDCS)*, p. 101, 2020, doi:10.1109/ICDCS48716.2020.243558

12. Koutras D, Stergiopoulos G, Dasaklis T, Kotzanikolaou P, Glynos D, Douligeris C. Security in IoMT Communications: A Survey. *Sensor*, 20, 4828, 2020

13. Jagadeeswari V, Subramaniyaswamy V, Logesh R, et al., A Study on Medical Internet of Things and Big Data in Personalized Healthcare System, *Health Information Science and Systems*, 6, 14, 2018, doi:10.1007/s13755-018-0049-x

14. Kishor A, Chakraborty C, Jeberson W, A Novel Fog Computing Approach for Minimization of Latency in Healthcare using Machine Learning, *International Journal of Interactive Multimedia and Artificial Intelligence*, 1, 1–11, 2020, doi:10.9781/ijimai.2020.12.004

15. Duplaga M, Tubek A, mHealth – Areas of Application and the Effectiveness of Interventions, *Zdrowie Publiczne i Zarządzanie*, 16, 155–166, 2018, doi:10.4467/20 842627OZ.18.018.10431.

16. Joyia G, Liaqat R, Farooq A, Rehman S, Internet of Medical Things (IOMT): Applications, Benefits and Future Challenges in Healthcare Domain, *Journal of Communications*, 12, 240–247, 2017, doi:10.12720/jcm.12.4.240-247

17. Dimitrov V, Medical IoT and Big Data in Healthcare, *Healthcare Informatics Research*, 22, 3, 156–163, 2016

18. Internet of things (IoT), Techtarget, https://internetofthingsagenda.techtarget.com/definition/Internet-of-Things-IoT

19. Big Data in the Time of a Pandemic, reliefweb, 7 January, 2012, https://reliefweb.int/report/world/big-data-time-pandemic

7 The Clinical Challenges for Digital Health Revolution

Ramkrishna Mondal and Siddharth Mishra
All India Institute of Medical Sciences, Bhubaneswar, India

CONTENTS

7.1 INTRODUCTION

The healthcare profession has become immensely challenging in the twenty-first century with increase in chronic disease load due to increased life expectancy, inadequate manpower and the rising cost of providing healthcare. This is further aggravated by the ever-increasing administrative paperwork as described by Mesko et al. [1]. This has led to the advent of digital technologies which are redefining the doctor–patient relationship and healthcare in general. The doctor today is tech savvy and is trained to use technology to their advantage in treating patients. More and more new digital health technologies are becoming acceptable under the law and the modern-day patient is also empower with the latest information for treatment options as well as outcomes. Nowadays, both the e-physician and the e-patient are digitally literate and know where to find information and data for insights into treatment. However, economic, legal and administrative issues are holding back the physicians today to make maximum utilization of these upcoming digital technologies in healthcare. Miller et al. [2] rightly said that the digital revolution has changed the product and service development in almost all aspects of human life, including human health. Digital health bears risks of dehumanizing care, but made an array of know-hows from genome sequencing to smartphone linked ECG gladly accessible. Digital health is a swiftly growing therapeutic ground with a significant impact on improving the excellence of healthcare, its effectiveness, lowering healthcare costs for patients, and clinical research as mentioned by WHO [3], Fischell et al. [4], Serbanati et al. [5], and Swan et al. [6]. However, despite rapid growth of digital technologies, involvement of the various stakeholders, including patients, clinicians, the insurance industry and regulators in medicine, remains relatively low as cited by Birnbaum et al. [7]. This article aims to deliver the outline of the present position of digital health, forthcoming viewpoints, and the challenges want imminent solution.

7.2 HISTORY OF DIGITAL HEALTH

Greaves et al. [8] stated that digital health is a multidisciplinary domain that aims to enhance the efficiency of monitoring of the patients, diagnosis, management, prevention, rehabilitation and long-term care delivery. Digital health is not an instant overnight phenomenon. The history of digital health dates to the 1970s when health telematics came into existence as cited in WHO report [9]. Telecommunications give the healthcare systems a great opportunity to improve health, health education and follow-ups using health telematics. Meister et al. [10] and Stanberry [11] opined that Health telematics which initially focused only on techniques of improving diagnosis and treatment has now evolved into telemedicine, which is now the dominant area of digital health. The concept of personal data which include health and medical data, social data, financial data, behavioural data as shown in Figure 7.1 schematically and it shows the contribution of health data in perspective of personal data.

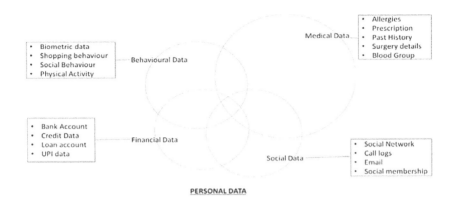

Medical Data
- Allergies
- Prescription
- Past History
- Surgery details
- Blood Group

Behavioural Data
- Biometric data
- Shopping behaviour
- Social Behaviour
- Physical Activity

Financial Data
- Bank Account
- Credit Data
- Loan account
- UPI data

Social Data
- Social Network
- Call logs
- Email
- Social membership

PERSONAL DATA

FIGURE 7.1   Health and medical data in perspective of personal data.

As we entered the twenty-first century, the desktop PC and use of internet grew to be integral parts of every household. These were great tools to reach out on a mass scale to promote health. Thus 'e-health' emerged, and it focused primarily on promoting health rather than on treatment of disease conditions as stated by Meister et al. [10]. In the 2010s, emergence of the mobile phone technology and the smartphone took the internet to every individual's hand. Thus arrived 'm-health', which promised greater adherence than 'e-health'. WHO [12] describe m-health as having a device that always is with people gives the community an ability to use healthcare services at any time, anywhere. Finally, in 2015, with the widespread use of smartphones, tablets and improvement in other technologies like robotics, a broader term than e-health and m-health emerged, and McAuley [13] and Meister et al. [10] called it 'digital health'. Bhavnani et al. [14] says that today digital health has a broad scope and encompasses telemedicine, m-health, wearable devices and biosensors, electronic health records (EHRs) and Big Data, artificial intelligence (AI), and machine learning (ML). Augmented reality (AR), Blockchain and virtual reality (VR) are other domains of digital health.

Healthcare has adopted these digital solutions with great enthusiasm, yet there is limited evidence about the usefulness and benefits of these technologies. With the popping up of innumerable digital solutions it has become imperative to identify genuinely evidence-based solutions for adoption into the real-world scenario. After a critical analysis of the available resources, WHO (2019) has released a guidance document on the same. Evaluation of digital applications are also being promoted in various clinical studies as done by Al-Durra et al. [15] and WHO [16]. The USFDA [17] has released regulatory guidelines for medical device software's. As digital health technologies continue to develop rapidly; these guidelines are proving to be extremely useful is setting standards. Nowadays, WHO is also recommending adoption of digital means for the training of healthcare professionals. However, one of the recent studies by George et al. [18] has shown that adopting online training methods for doctors does not actually show any benefit of cost reduction against the standard methods of face-to-face teaching. According to Tim Kelsey [19], electronic medical records are another important offering of digital health technology and accurate medical recorded are critical to providing quality healthcare. In AXA PPP Health Tech & You Forum [20], it is concluded that the rising burden of chronic disease conditions demands earlier diagnosis, better treatment and reduced hospital stay to contain the costs of healthcare and digital health brings immense possibilities to achieve this.

7.3   DIGITAL HEALTH AND THE HEALTHCARE PROFESSIONALS

It is proven by numerous studies that the extreme demands of the healthcare profession results in frequent burnouts, and almost half of all healthcare professionals are affected by it at some time in their career, as stated by Lee et al. [21] and Mulero A [22]. In the current scenario, recent advances in the medical profession are increasing at a phenomenal pace. Medical professions not only have to keep pace with these, but also learn how to integrate digital technologies into their daily work. Unfortunately, developments in digital health technologies are sometime not up to the mark and doctors have to deal with inefficient software's and technologies which further adds to their frustration and deprives them of spending time with their patients as agreed by Mesko [23].

The era of digital healthcare will usher in affordability and many under bridges sections of the society and those in remote places will be access healthcare easily as mentioned by many like Goodrige et al. [24], Balatsoukas et al. [25], Maher et al. [26], Laranio et al. [27], and Ranney et al. [28]. It was shown in one of the studies by Rollin et al. [29] that when digital health is used to access cases of melanoma for post treatment follow up then it helped in reducing the urban and rural divide with regards to incidence, mortality and compliance. Similarly, social media platforms can also help immensely in healthcare. Online social support and information-sharing through live interaction, has an impact on individual's health and behaviour. As described by de Bronkart et al. [30] a popular terminology 'e-Patient', who used technology to support the treatment of his cancer illustrations the contribution individuals will play in the intricacies of treatment. Unfortunately, disruptive technologies that have been brought in by digital health have so far been more helpful to the patent than the healthcare provider. Infect the pressure on the healthcare provider has increased as they have to keep abreast with these new technologies that are evolving too quickly. This is often resulting in some healthcare providers being reluctant in adapting digital health as described by Gagnon et al. [31]. However, as per Engel GL [32], with healthcare systems all over, and the work gradually becoming economically unviable, a shift to the digital medium is inescapable. With patients now having quick access to information, the doctor–patient relationship has also changed. Digital health has helped in shared decision-making, open and frequent communication. It has also made it possible for the healthcare provider to adapt a team approach when treating a patient by enabling simultaneous communication to multiple colleagues by the click of a button, as described by Mesko B [33], Dassau et al. [34] and in Digital Health Strategy in 2018 [35]. Digital health has made it possible for healthcare to shift from the hospital to the patient's home. Wearable sensors, portable equipment and telemedicine have made this possible. Wallace et al. [36] says that, at the same time, it compels the healthcare provide to acquire a new set of skills to deal with telemedicine.

In summary, digital health technologies are inescapable while practicing medicine today and the empowered patient of today has much different expectations. However, our medical education system has to adapt to enable the modern healthcare provider to accept and skill up to digital health technologies keeping in mid the expectation of the new age patients.

7.4   DIGITAL HEALTH REVOLUTION

It is evident that the digital health revolution has commenced. The digital health industry was already worth $25 billion globally in 2017 and it had the capability to reduce healthcare cost by at least $7 billion in the United States alone. Digital health products are being released into the market in an exponential pace. 2015 witness the launch of 153,000 products in the United Sates while this figure was 320,000 globally in the same year as cited by Fischell et al. [4]. Unfortunately, since there is lack of robust regulatory framework to monitor the quality of these digital products, it has led to the development of mistrust among the consumers. This phenomenon is often causing valuable technology to be ignored or abandons by the patients and healthcare providers. The environment for innovation in digital technology has thus become further challenging.

Some observers, however, worry that digital health will depersonalize healthcare [5]. In contrast, a review on telemedicine studies reports that 80% of the medical studies have shown that telemedicine has been rated favourably in relation to provider–patient interactions. According to Mesko et al. [1] patients have a multitude of new ways to communicate with medical providers and access health information. This is allowing patients not only to have more information about their disease condition but also enabling them to exercise some degree of control over their treatment. Gagnon et al. [31] says, although the advantages of digital health solutions are many, yet some sections of the population are still not fully comfortable with this option.

7.5   CHALLENGES IN DIGITAL HEALTH

As per the description of We forum Digital Health (2018) [37], there is a phenomenal chance to transmute the healthcare segment and allow citizens to take control of individuals' health [37]. Though, for the fruitful expansion, implementation and integration of novel knowhow requires a fresh approach to science and health research.

7.5.1   MULTIDISCIPLINARY COLLABORATION

Many disciplines like computer learning, manufacturing, data science, broadcasting, budget, quantifiable medicine, community wellbeing, epidemiology, and so many together contribute to the field of digital health. New frameworks and algorithms are contributed by computer science and technology. However, these may be theoretical. To successfully implement digital solutions to solve real word clinical and public health problems there must be multidisciplinary collaboration between medical science and other technologies. Along with a closer collaboration between the industry and scientific academia, the policy makers must also be included. More research needs to be carried out to identify quantitatively the positive outcomes from the new developments in digital health technologies as cited by Lewis et al. [38].

7.5.2 DISSOCIATED TECHNOLOGICAL, INSTITUTIONAL AND REGULATORY FRAMEWORKS

At present the regulations governing digital health technologies by Mcaskill [39] is not evolving rapidly enough to keep pace with the technologies which are being launched at an exponential rate. Even today, FDA as described by Hamel et al. [40] requires takes 3–4 years to grant commercial approval to any digital product. Due to such delay there is risk of new digital technologies becoming obsolete after 2 or 3 years of waiting.

7.5.3 DATA GOVERNANCE

Availability of health data is no longer limited to the government establishments or to providers of amenities only. By gathering a large quantity information from numerous industrial players, ensuring transparent data governance is a challenge. The sensitive nature of the data and vulnerability to manipulation, can give these players great power over information. This tendency certainly leads to a data imbalance amongst business and the authorities. There needs to be proper laws regarding the safety, accountability, time and place of storage, traceability, possessions and marketplace cost of health information of the population.

7.5.4 ECONOMIC AND FINANCIAL CONSIDERATIONS

As per Rosenberg L [41], digital technologies are on the identical gauge of distraction as the detection of antibiotics. Digital applications could substitute approximately current models of care with regard to the reimbursement of healthcare services. It is thus essential to establish systems to evaluate the value of new digital health technologies with esteem to enduring results Goodrich K [42] added. World report on ageing and health [43] says digital health in bringing in new ways to deliver healthcare. Hamel et al. [40] says, many mobile applications have come up that can function as a microscope, stethoscope, electrocardiogram or camera which can be used for clinical examination and diagnosis with quality no less than the traditional devices. Any person with a smartphone and basic digital literacy can use these devices easily. This will enable patients to be involved in theory own treatment and thereby increasing compliance in monitoring or follow up.

7.5.5 CULTURAL, SOCIAL AND LOCAL INFRASTRUCTURE ISSUES

The cultural, religious and moral backgrounds of users should be kept in mind in order to increase acceptability of digital technologies during the current emergency with focus on the immediate local benefit, as described by Pan X [44]. As agreed by Mackerte et al. [45], Sim I [46], and Gamble et al. [47] that due to the economic and education imbalance, a digital divide may exist in the population which can cause vulnerable communities to be overlooked while implementing of digital approaches. Nguyen et al. [48] added that this may specifically affect certain subclasses such as minorities, senior citizens or rural or low-income communities with low health literacy levels. Due to all these reasons, as per Ferretti et al. [49], digital interventions may not be uniformly effective when they are useful in high, medium or low-income zones or when they are organized in different types of nations.

Keesara et al. [50] opine the feasibility of implementing successful billing systems for telehealth lies with the government authorities. Patient data protection is of prime importance in telemedicine consultations and for this, it is essential that the various stakeholders work in close collaboration. Lack of basic infrastructure or inefficient digital infrastructure as well as remotely located populations are challenges often faced by some developing countries. These countries may also face problem in funding the establishment of digital infrastructure as mentioned by Muinga et al. [51] and Kruse et al. [52].

7.5.6 HUMAN RIGHTS, ETHICAL AND POLICY CHALLENGES

It is believed that digital health technologies will fill in the gaps to enable to deliver quality healthcare and in order to achieve the United Nations' projected Sustainable Development Goals 2030. Threats to data privacy, patient confidentiality if not attended to in time will widen the "digital divide" that will undermine the effect of these efficient technologies. In a study by Davis et al. [53] mentioned that, till now the efforts to overcome the negative aspects of digital health technologies has revolved around the adoption of legal framework for implementing international human rights obligations. Various experts of IEEE Global [54] have established possessions associated to morals and digital know-hows. The United Nations Board for Coordination [55] has also developed recommendations on the ethics related to AI. All these ethical guidelines from various organizations emphasize on principles like beneficence, autonomy, consent, privacy, participation, transparency, non-discrimination, equity and accountability. In short, the consensus is that digital health technologies should not harm in any way, and they should maximize benefits for humanity as mentioned in US Belmont Report (1979) [56]. However, it may be noted that moral values can lack specificity and sometimes application systems can be feeble. Thus, it is important that adequate steps should be taken for enforceability and accountability. Some of the main moral and strategy contests in digital health are:

7.5.6.1   Security and Confidentiality of Data

Maximum of the discussion on digital health and Big Data has focused on privacy. As the science progresses and more and more gets available, high-end analytics can be applied to these data for obtaining various results. In such a situation managing data privacy becomes herculean task. In the study by Vayena et al. [57] says a simple consent obtained by the click of a virtual button may not provide adequate safeguard against misuse. Similarly, with cyber-attacks, databases hacking and theft of bigdata being reported frequently, data security has also been a challenge as described by Gayle et al. [58]. In the United Kingdom Commissioner's office [59], the health sector reports the most incidents data security breech. Growing concerns about data privacy and security among public are creating a negative impression among public regarding the future of this sector.

7.5.6.2   Trust

Tsioulas et al. [60] stated that all stakeholders of digital health must create a culture of trust in the ecosystem of Big Data so that all can benefit from the developments. The future of digital health needs much more than just data privacy. It has to ensure transparency, accountability, share all benefit and certainly show more clarity about ownership and control of data. Mere innovative consent models cannot achieve this trustworthiness. There must be clearness on how people and societies will be helped after digital health progresses.

7.5.6.3   Accountability

As the possibility of automated decisions for clinical or public health interventions becomes a near reality, the issue of accountability is of critical importance. It is anticipated in the study of Kawamoto et al. [61] and Hsu et al. [62] that there will be tremendous use of AI in the judgement, treatment decisions and surgical procedures in near future [61, 62]. However, as more AI-guided digital health tools become autonomous, human operators will have little independence to override machine decision and this has the potential to compromise the present rules of professional accountability in clinical practice.

7.5.7   COVID-19 Challenges and Digital Health

Coronavirus caused by SARS-CoV2 is our newest guest. This epidemic affects people's lifestyles in all ways, as described by Wen et al. [63]. According to Fagherazzi et al. [64] due the lack of enough medical resources many countries faced problems and it has compelled them to put 'digital health' into more consideration. Digital health helps the healthcare system to fight against COVID-19 in many different ways starting from prevention and primary care, screening, monitoring to finally remote surveillance.

7.5.7.1   Digital Health and COVID-19, Community Health Reactions

COVID-19 epidemic has crippled both financial prudence and wellbeing structures and consider as the global pandemic of such a dimension in this digital era. S mentioned by WHO [65] and Mahmood et al. [66]. Barsa et al. [67] cited that conventional modelling has indicated that few health systems are predominantly susceptible, together with numerous emerging nations in Asia and Africa. Telehealth, AI, Big Data, predictive analytics, proposition considerable potential to alleviate the possessions of COVID-19 as mentioned by Rasmussen et al. [68] Leung et al. [69] stated that digital health technologies did not highlight glaringly in earlier major disease epidemics like, severe acute respiratory distress syndrome (SARS) and middle east respiratory syndrome (MERS). Still, secluded reports of real-world expansion and authentication of these solutions, current works of Murray et al. [70] has emphasized noteworthy encounters in disposition, and confines of diverse excellence and strategy. Consequently, as described by Li et al. [71], the flood of distortion during this pandemic has go down out certified information, coined as 'infodemic' by WHO. As per Mesko et al. [1] here persist substantial encounters and breaches in implementation, scale-up and incorporation of digital health into healthcare even in developed nations.

7.5.7.2 Digital Communication During the Pandemic

Wetsman et al. [72] rightly said that it is important that the political leaders and the scientific community work in sync during the pandemic. From the beginning of this pandemic, fake news and misinformation has been present not only on social media and the Internet, but also in government communications. This has propagated fear in the community. It is extremely important to have a good communication plan to effectively influence health behaviours of the society. Digital health technologies provide an efficient and effective communication platform. The WHO [73] and other health agencies have been using this medium for quick communication of correct information on a mass scale. Various apps and websites as described by Liu et al. [74] can also be used by governments and official agencies for communication as well as contacting health workers remotely. According to Zhou et al. [75], Torous et al. [76], and Signorini et al. [77], Telemedicine and digital health play important roles in the present crisis not only to fight this disease, but also to attend to psychological issues related to isolation or quarantine.

7.5.7.3 Digital Data to Classical COVID-19 Blowout, Progression and Awareness

Digital epidemiology, or monitoring of online or social media behaviours of people for capturing health-related trends and modelling disease outbreaks, has existed since 2010, most of the models were developed to gain insight into the trends of disease for H1N1 [78], measles [79], the Zika virus [80] and Ebola virus [81, 82]. However, though these internet surveillance systems are very helpful for public health, yet they lacked proper methodology and standardization as mentioned by Ayyoubzadeh et al. [83] This also raises question on their reliability, and thereby depending on them to implement public health interventions. However, moving beyond the initial mistakes and building more complain technologies in the background of a more open data mentality has allowed to use social media like

TABLE 7.1
Challenges of Digital Health Revolution Cited in Different Studies

Behavioural	Administrative	Procedural
1. Resistance to change	1. Absence of regulations	1. Inadequate Internet
2. Meagre real knowledge	2. ICT infrastructure criteria	2. Time-consuming
3. Data secrecy concern	3. Less government support	3. Lack of security
4. Deficiency of awareness	4. Poor privacy	4. Lacks interoperability
5. Cost concern	5. Reimbursement glitches	5. Software inadequacies
6. Legalities concern	6. Poor e-health resources	6. Electricity dependence
7. Inadequate relationship	7. Technical support deficit	7. Dependence on Internet
8. Poor patient input	8. Lack of guidelines	8. Problematic treatment
9. Apparent time-consuming	9. Poor provider training	9. Hardware restrictions
10. Suitability concern	10. Unclear accountability	10. Insufficient structure
11. Usefulness concern	11. Difficult implementation	11. Artificial intelligence limit
12. Proficiency concern	12. Lack of studies	12. Unclear display
13. Worried about consent	13. Time-consuming process	13. Expensive
14. Safety concern	14. Environment constraints	14. Poor empathy
15. Sustainability concern	15. Deficiency of equipment	15. Lacks contextualization
16. Lack of satisfaction	16. Poor community policy	16. Poor correlation with
17. Paper culture	17. Scarce validated tools	direct assessment
18. Poor communication skills		17. Licensed software

Twitter, Google Trends, Wikipedia, Baidu Index and Weibo Index in China for effectively studying the COVID-19 virus and its trends, as described by Li et al. [84]. In China, using these technologies, Alessa et al. [85] made it possible to predict peaks and daily incidences in the real world much in advance so that preventive public health interventions could be planned. Viboud et al. [86] opined that this method also provides a very economic method for gathering data on public health. However, using data from online activities has never been used on a large scale to predict public health interventions and disease trends. COVID-19 may be the primary outburst where so many forthcoming studies like Luo et al. [87] is being done successfully. Abd-Alrazaq et al. [88] and Coiera et al. [89]. Social media data analysis is also relevant in understanding how people are responding to interventions the evolution of the pandemic over time. Table 7.1 shows the different challenges of digital health revolution cited in different studies.

There are lots of benefits of digital health usage. But there are challenges or barriers too. Below a summary of different benefits, barriers and possible solutions given in the perspective of digital health revolution in medical practice in Table 7.2.

7.6   FUTURE RESEARCH

Digital literacy is quickly growing universally specially among the human resources field of healthcare industry, which denotes to an individual's capability to discovery, appraise and constitute vibrant information over writing or verbal

TABLE 7.2
Benefits, Barriers, and Possible Solutions of Digital Health in Medical Practice

Benefits	Barriers	Solutions
• Treatment effectiveness advance	• Lack of time	• Evidence-based solutions
	• More workload	• Practice guidelines
• Time saving	• Deficient resources and financial support	• Readiness of special training
• More patient satisfaction		
• Improve patient safety	• Poor reimbursements	• Sympathetic work environment
• Diagnostic ability upsurge	• Absence of technological knowledge	
		• Refining quality and safety of health technologies
• Improves productivity	• Lack of trained medical staff	
• Uplift physician-patient relationship	• Misinterpretation of technologies	• Simplifying regulations
		• Approvals from peers
• Improvements interpersonal communication	• Overdiagnosis	• Perceived practicality, and benefit
	• More health inequalities	
	• More administrative tasks	• User-friendly interfaces
• Reduce burden of routine check-ups	• Troubled patient data privacy	• Incentive structures
	• Resistance from physicians	• Positive attitudes
• Cost-savings	• Work culture declining innovation	• Innovation oriented work culture

mediums of several digital platforms. Globally, digital know-hows were expressively amplified efficiency and performance of any establishments. Dangers to confidentiality are countless, including mass surveillance a great apprehension for public and humanoid rights questions. Trustworthiness of facts is also a problem as data may simply be fake yet difficult to confirm, resultant torrent belongings through financial, communal and dogmatic inferences.

A countless research publication in AI, one of the goals of the digital revolution, is being driven by abundant additional existing computational power, upgraded techniques, huge capital funds in technology, and Big Data (cloud and open source) and is stirring rapidly in multiple of logarithmic trajectory.

Machine learning (ML) refers to supercomputer systems by means of algorithms and statistical models for everyday jobs without using obvious commands, depend on patterns and extrapolation as a substitute. This is the future of the digital revolution. Deep learning is one type of machine learning, founded on deep neural networks, deep belief networks, recurrent neural networks and convolutional neural networks etc. These were applied to arenas including computer vision, speech and audio recognition, natural language processing, social network filtering, machine translation, bioinformatics, drug design and medical image analysis where they are claimed progressively of outcomes similar to or higher to those grasped by human experts. Image omics (radio genomics or deep learning applied in radiology) is a very powerful tool to detect the molecular and phenotypic properties of the complete tumour, thereby improve the patient's treatment.

One pertinent topic in swift development regarding progress of 'digital scribe'. As per E. Coiera et al. [89], the electronic health record (HER) generates additional frustration for many doctors. Recent EHR suffer several hitches making them unproductive and poor clinical gratification. Digital scribes or intelligent documentation support systems with advanced technologies of speech recognition, language processing and AI, make the medical documentation task automatic. Though in its embryonic stage, digital scribes are expected to change a lot in clinical documentation. Amit Sokoo et al. [90] stated that the dashboard will play a major role in future monitoring the information captured for various systems that need to be monitored. Similarly, study of Chinmay et al. (2019) [91], Chinmay et al. (2015) [92] and Chakraborty et al. [93] mentioned a tele-wound monitoring (TWM) framework were used with smartphone for monitoring chronic wound status based on colour variation.

Precision Medicine or personalized medicine, a method in growth for illness treatment and anticipation considering individual unpredictability in genetic factor, atmosphere and lifestyle in each individual to forecast precisely which investigative, action and anticipation plans appropriate to a sickness. It is based on clinical medicine, as well as health psychology, bodily investigation and epidemiology. Bioinformatics and computational biology are important introductory gears of precision medicine and digital health.

Blockchain technology, a popular technology used to provide robust solution to healthcare sector issues like, to prevent data breaches and supply of medicine etc.

7.7 CONCLUSION

Digital health will support the future needs of medicine by analyzing the massive amounts of recorded patient's data that generate by high-tech devices from multiple sources. Digital care can transform disease-centred services towards patient-centred services. Many of the digital health solutions are still in their infancy and need to be improved. Furthermore, they need extensive and successful validation in human testing and improved clinical reliability. Medical professionals also need to be familiarized and adapt themselves with these advances for better healthcare delivery to the patients. Along with digital care growth, researchers, scientists, clinicians, payers, and regulators must accompany technology developers to reach the ultimate goal to support individuals living lengthier and sense well. Revolution in digital health appearances quite a lot of moral and strategy encounters.

First, information is the key and contains paramount reputation for digital health. Entry to appropriate and adequate quantities information is the prime ailment in progressing pioneering investigative, healing and regulating apparatuses.

Second, conformation with prevailing legal necessities concerning data safety, safekeeping and confidentiality are crucial for digital health revolution. Lawful contexts have most important influence in growth in this arena.

Third, strong and in addition translucent responsibility mechanisms should confirm the credentials, accountability regarding information usages and its significances on persons, relatives and societies.

Fourth, signal of security and usefulness is a substantial ailment in victory of digital health. To be a Registered digital health technologies or solutions, it has to be pass lots of valuation procedures to encounter cost-effectiveness prerequisite.

Satisfying the above necessities will substitute the *fifth* ailment of digital health revolution, which is trustworthiness equally for designers and controllers of digital health innovation.

Digital know-hows grasp abundant potential aimed at speaking injustices then barricades to healthcare excellence and admittance. Digital health likely diminishes medical treatment prices, renovate the systems for more precise and approachable care, and amalgamates with other segments. But then again uncertainties in digital skills consequential in human rights violations are factual of peoples previously question to judgement, communal downgrading and shadowing. In the coming days, more consideration should be given to the progress of community-based solutions, allied with moral values, with responsibility and impartiality. Moreover, administrations ought to yield benefit of the information providing by digital health for development of transparency and to authenticate the conclusions.

CONFLICT OF INTEREST

There is no conflict of interests.

FUNDING

There is no funding support.

DATA AVAILABILITY

Not applicable.

REFERENCES

1. Meskó B, Drobni Z, Bényei É, Gergely B, Győrffy Z. Digital health is a cultural transformation of traditional healthcare. *Mhealth*. 2017;3:38. doi: 10.21037/mhealth.2017.08.07
2. Miller EA, West DM. Where's the revolution? Digital technology and healthcare in the internet age? *J Health Polit Policy Law*. 2009;34:261–84.
3. World Health Organization. 2016. *Monitoring and Evaluating Digital Health Interventions: A Practical Guide to Conducting Research and Assessment*. Geneva: World Health Organization.
4. Fischell D, Fischell T, Harwood J, Johnson S, Turi G. Implantable device for vital signs monitoring. Google Patents. 2007

5. Serbanati LD, Ricci FL, Mercurio G, Vasilateanu A. Steps towards a digital health ecosystem. *J Biomed Inform*. 2011;44:621–36.
6. Swan M. Health: The realization of personalized medicine through crowdsourcing, the quantified self, and the participatory Biocitizen. *J Pers Med*. 2012;2:93–118.
7. Birnbaum F, Lewis D, Rosen RK, Ranney ML. Patient engagement and the design of digital health. *Acad Emerg Med*. 2015;22:754–56.
8. Greaves F, Joshi I, Campbell M, Roberts S, Patel N, Powell J. What is an appropriate level of evidence for a digital health intervention? *Lancet* 2019;392:2665–67.
9. WHO. *Report of the WHO Group Consultation on Health Telematics*. Geneva: World Health Organization; 1997. A Health Telematics Policy in Support of WHO's Health-For-All Strategy for GlobalHealth Development; pp. 11–6
10. Meister S, Deiters W, Becker S. Digital health and digital biomarkers–enabling value chains on health data. *Curr Dir Biomed Eng*. 2016;2:577–81.
11. Stanberry B Telemedicine: Barriers and opportunities in the 21st century. *J Intern Med*. 2000;247:615–28.
12. World Health Organization. *MHealth: New Horizons for Health Through Mobile Technologies*. Geneva: World Health Organization; 2011.
13. McAuley A Digital health interventions: Widening access or widening inequalities? *Public Health*. 2014;128:1118–20.
14. Bhavnani SP, Narula J, Sengupta PP. Mobile technology and the digitization of healthcare. *Eur Heart J*. 2016;37:1428–38.
15. Al-Durra M, Nolan RP, Seto E, et al. Nonpublication rates and characteristics of registered randomized clinical trials in digital health: Cross-sectional analysis. *J Med Internet Res*. 2018;20:e11924.
16. WHO. *WHO Guideline: Recommendations on Digital Interventions for Health System Strengthening*. Geneva: World Health Organization; 2019. Licence: CC BY-NC-SA 3.0 IGO.
17. Food and Drug Administration. Policy for device software functions and mobile medical applications, 2019. https://www.fda.gov/regulatory-information/search-fda-guidance-documents/policy-device-software-functionsand-mobile-medical-applications (accessed 26 October, 2019).
18. George PP, Zhabenko O, Kyaw BM, et al. Online digital education for post registration training of medical doctors: Systematic review by the Digital Health Education Collaboration. *J Med Internet Res*. 2019;21:e13269.
19. Kelsey, T, National director of patients and information, *NHS England, Digital health and Care Congress*, London, 2015 June.
20. Life Sciences Minister George Freeman MP, Keynote speech at the AXA PPP Health Tech & You Forum, 2014 October.
21. Lee RT, Seo B, Hladkyj S, Lovell BL, Schwartzmann L. Correlates of physician burnout across regions and specialties: A meta-analysis. *Hum Resour Health*. 2013 Sep 28;11:48. doi: 10.1186/1478-4491-11-48
22. Mulero A, Healthcare Dive. Bureaucracy tops causes of burnout among physicians, 2016 Jan 15. https://www.healthcaredive.com/news/bureaucracy-tops-causes-of-burnout-among-physicians/412227/ (accessed 2019-03-04)
23. Mesko B. Health IT and digital health: The future of health technology is diverse. *J Clin Transl Res*. 2017;3(S3):431–34. doi: 10.18053/jctres.03.2017S3.006
24. Goodridge D, Marciniuk D. Rural and remote care: Overcoming the challenges of distance. *Chron Respir Dis*. 2016 May;13(2):192–203. doi: 10.1177/1479972316633414

25. Balatsoukas P, Kennedy CM, Buchan I, Powell J, Ainsworth J. The role of social network technologies in online health promotion: A narrative review of theoretical and empirical factors influencing intervention effectiveness. *J Med Internet Res.* 2015 Jun 11;17(6):e141. doi: 10.2196/jmir.3662. Medline: 26068087.

26. Maher CA, Lewis LK, Ferrar K, Marshall S, De Bourdeaudhuij I, Vandelanotte C. Are health behavior change interventions that use online social networks effective? A systematic review. *J Med Internet Res.* 2014 Feb 14;16(2):e40. doi: 10.2196/jmir.2952

27. Laranjo L, Arguel A, Neves AL, Gallagher AM, Kaplan R, Mortimer N, et al. The influence of social networking sites on health behaviour change: A systematic review and meta-analysis. *J Am Med Inform Assoc.* 2015 Jan;22(1):243–56. doi: 10.1136/amiajnl-2014-002841

28. Ranney ML, Genes N. Social media and healthcare quality improvement: A nascent field. *BMJ Qual Saf.* 2016 Dec;25(6):389–91. doi: 10.1136/bmjqs-2015-004827

29. Rollin A, Ridout B, Campbell A. Digital health in melanoma posttreatment care in rural and remote Australia: Systematic review. *J Med Internet Res.* 2018 Sep 24;20(9):e11547. doi: 10.2196/11547. Medline: 30249578

30. deBronkart D. How the e-patient community helped save my life: An essay by Dave deBronkart. *BMJ.* 2013 Apr 2;346:f1990. doi: 10.1136/bmj.f1990

31. Gagnon MP, Ngangue P, Payne-Gagnon J, Desmartis M. m-health adoption by healthcare professionals: A systematic review. *J Am Med Inform Assoc.* 2016 Jan;23(1):212–20. doi: 10.1093/jamia/ocv052

32. Engel GL. The need for a new medical model: A challenge for biomedicine. *Science.* 1977 Apr 8;196(4286):129–36.

33. Mesko B. The role of artificial intelligence in precision medicine. *Expert Rev Precis Med Drug Dev.* 2017 Sep 20;2(5):239–41. doi: 10.1080/23808993.2017.1380516

34. Dassau E, Zisser H, Harvey RA, Percival MW, Grosman B, Bevier W, et al. Clinical evaluation of a personalized artificial pancreas. *Diabetes Care.* 2013 Apr;36(4):801–9. doi: 10.2337/dc12-0948

35. Ministry of Health, Denmark. *A Coherent and Trustworthy Health Network for All: Digital Health Strategy 2018–2022.* Copenhagen, Denmark: Ministry of Health, Denmark; 2018 Jan 21. https://www.sum.dkAktuelt/Publikationer/~/media/Filer%20-%20Publikationer_i_pdf/English/2018/A-coherent-and-trustworthy-health-network-for-all-jan-2108/A-coherent-and-trustworthy-health-network-jan-2018.pdf (accessed 2019-03-04)

36. Wallace EL, Rosner MH, Alscher MD, Schmitt CP, Jain A, Tentori F, et al. Remote patient management for home dialysis patients. *Kidney Int Rep.* 2017 Nov;2(6):1009–17. doi: 10.1016/j.ekir.2017.07.010

37. Digital Health, 2014. Available from: http://www.weforum.org/issues/digital-health

38. Lewis T, Synowiec C, Lagomarsino G, Schweitzer J. E-health in low- and middle-income countries: Findings from the center for health market innovations. *Bull World Health Organ.* (2012) 90(5):332–40. doi: 10.2471/BLT.11.099820.

39. Mcaskill R. State licensing a major hurdle for telehealth. Available online: http://mhealthintelligence.com/news/state-licensing-a-major-hurdle-for-telehealth (accessed April 21, 2017).

40. Hamel MB, Cortez NG, Cohen IG, et al. FDA regulation of mobile health technologies. *N Engl J Med.* 2014;371:372–9.

41. Rosenberg L. Are healthcare leaders ready for the real revolution? *J Behav Health Serv Res.* 2012;39:215–19.

42. Goodrich K. CMS Finalizes its Quality Measure Development Plan. US Centers for Medicare & Medicaid Services (CMS). Available online: https://blog.cms.gov/2016/05/02/cms-finalizes-its-quality-measure-development-plan/

43. WHO. *World Report on Ageing and Health*. Geneva, Switzerland: World Health Organization, 2015.

44. Pan X. Application of personal-oriented digital technology in preventing transmission of COVID-19, *China Ir J Med Sci*. 2020 Mar;27:1–2. doi: 10.1007/s11845-020-02215-5

45. Mackert M, Mabry-Flynn A, Champlin S, Donovan EE, Pounders K. Health literacy and health information technology adoption: The potential for a new digital divide. *J Med Internet Res*. 2016 Oct 4;18(10):e264. doi: 10.2196/jmir.6349. https://www.jmir.org/2016/10/e264/

46. Sim I. Mobile devices and health. *N Engl J Med*. 2019 Sep 5;381(10):956–68. doi:10.1056/NEJMra1806949

47. Gamble A, Pham Q, Goyal S, Cafazzo JA. The challenges of COVID-19 for people living with diabetes: Considerations for digital health. *JMIR Diabetes*. 2020 May 15;5(2):e19581. doi:10.2196/19581. https://diabetes.jmir.org/2020/2/e19581/

48. Nguyen A, Mosadeghi S, Almario CV. Persistent digital divide in access to and use of the Internet as a resource for health information: Results from a California population-based study. *Int J Med Inform*. 2017 Jul;103:49–54. doi: 10.1016/j.ijmedinf.2017.04.008.

49. Ferretti L, Wymant C, Kendall M, Zhao L, Nurtay A, Abeler-Dörner L, Parker M, Bonsall D, Fraser C. Quantifying SARS-CoV-2 transmission suggests epidemic control with digital contact tracing. *Science* 2020 May 8;368(6491):eabb6936. doi: 10.1126/science.abb6936. http://europepmc.org/abstract/MED/32234805.

50. Keesara S, Jonas A, Schulman K. Covid-19 and healthcare's digital revolution. *N Engl J Med*. 2020 Apr 2;382:e82. doi: 10.1056/nejmp2005835. https://www.nejm.org/doi/full/10.1056/NEJMp2005835

51. Muinga N, Magare S, Monda J, English M, Fraser H, Powell J, Paton C. Digital health systems in Kenyan Public Hospitals: A mixed-methods survey. *BMC Med Inform DecisMak*. 2020 Jan 06;20(1):2. doi: 10.1186/s12911-019-1005-7. https://bmcmedinformdecismak.biomedcentral.com/articles/10.1186/s12911-019-1005-7.

52. Kruse C, Betancourt J, Ortiz S, Valdes Luna SM, Bamrah IK, Segovia N. Barriers to the use of mobile health in improving health outcomes in developing countries: Systematic review. *J Med Internet Res*. 2019 Oct 09;21(10):e13263. doi: 10.2196/13263. https://www.jmir.org/2019/10/e13263/

53. Davis SLM, Esom, K, Gustav R, et al. A democracy deficit in digital health? *Health Hum Rights*. 2020 January 16. Available at https://www.hhrjournal.org/2020/01/a-democracy-deficit-in-digital-health/. See also S. L. M. Davis, "Contact tracing apps: Extra risks for women and marginalized groups," *Health and Human Rights Journal* (April 29, 2020). Available at https://www.hhrjournal.org/2020/04/contact-tracing-appsextra-risks-for-women-and-marginalized-groups/.

54. IEEE Global Initiative on Ethics of Autonomous and Intelligent Systems. *Ethically aligned design: A vision for prioritizing human wellbeing with autonomous and intelligent systems*, 1st edition. Piscataway: IEEE, 2019; T. Philbeck, N. Davis, and A. Engtoft Larsen, Values, ethics and innovation rethinking technological development in the big data, technology, fourth Industrial Revolution (World Economic

Forum, 2018). Available at http://www3.weforum.org/docs/WEF_WP_Values_
Ethics_Innovation_2018.pdf; European Commission, High Level Excerpt Group
on Artificial Intelligence, Ethics guidelines for trustworthy artificial intelligence
(Brussels: European Commission, 2019).

55. United Nations. Chief Executives Board for Coordination, First Version of a Draft
Text of a Recommendation on the Ethics of Artificial Intelligence, 2020 July.

56. National Commission for the Protection of Human Subjects of Biomedical and
Behavioral Research, US Department of Health, Education and Welfare, The
Belmont report: Ethical principles and guidelines for the protection of human
subjects of research (1979). PINION Open Access

57. Vayena E, Mastroianni A, Kahn J. Caught in the web: Informed consent for online health
research. *Sci Transl Med.* 2013;5(173):173fs6. doi: 10.1126/scitranslmed.3004798.

58. Gayle D, Topping A, Sample I, Marsh S, Dodd V. NHS seeks to recover from
global cyber-attack as security concerns resurface. *The Guardian*, 2017 May 13.
Available from https://www.theguardian.com/society/2017/may/12/hospitals-across-
england-hit-by-large-scale-cyber-attack

59. Information Commissioner's Office [Internet]. London: Information Commissioner's
Office; 2017 [cited 2017 Jul 20]; [about 3 screens].

60. Tasioulas J, Vayena E. The place of human rights and the common good in global health
policy. *Theor Med Bioeth.* 2016;37(4):365–82. doi: 10.1007/s11017-016-9372-x.

61. Kawamoto K, Houlihan CA, Balas EA, Lobach DF. Improving clinical practice using
clinical decision support systems: A systematic review of trials to identify features
critical to success. *BMJ.* 2005;330(7494):765. doi: 10.1136/bmj.38398.500764.8F.

62. Hsu W, Markey MK, Wang MD. Biomedical imaging informatics in the era of precision medicine: progress, challenges, and opportunities. *J Am Med Inform Assoc.*
2013 Nov–Dec;20(6):1010–13

63. Wen J, Kozak M, Yang S, Liu F. COVID.19: Potential effects on Chinese citizens'
lifestyle and travel. *Tour Rev.* 2021;76(1):74–87. doi:10.1108/TR-03-2020-0110.

64. Fagherazzi G, Goetzinger C, Rashid MA, Aguayo GA, Huiart L. Digital health strategies to fightCOVID-19 worldwide: Challenges, recommendations, and a call for
papers. *J Med Internet Res.* 2020;22:e19284.

65. World Health Organization (WHO). Coronavirus disease (COVID-2019) situation reports. https://www.who.int/emergencies/diseases/novel-coronavirus-2019/
situationreports/(2020).

66. Mahmood S, Hasan K, Colder Carras M, Labrique A. Global preparedness against
COVID-19: WeMust leverage the power of digital health. *JMIR Public Health
Surveill.* 2020 Apr 16;6(2):e18980. doi:10.2196/18980. https://publichealth.jmir.
org/2020/2/e18980/

67. Barasa E, Ouma PO, Okiro EA. Assessing the hospital surge capacity of the Kenyan
health system in the face of the COVID-19 pandemic. *PLoS One.* 2020;15:e0236308.

68. Rasmussen SA, Khoury MJ, Del Rio C. Precision public health as a key tool in the
COVID-19 response. *JAMA.* 2020;324:933–34.

69. Leung GM, Leung K. Crowdsourcing data to mitigate epidemics. *Lancet Digit
Health.* 2, e156–e57 (2020).

70. Murray CJL, Alamro NMS, Hwang H, Lee U. Digital public health and COVID-19.
Lancet Public Health. 2020;5:e469–e70.

71. Li LW, Chew AMK, Gunasekeran DV. Digital health for patients with chronic pain
during the COVID-19 pandemic. *Br. J. Anaesth.* 2020;125:657–60.

72. Wetsman N. The Verge. [2020-04-21]. Effective communication is critical during emergencies like the COVID-19 outbreak, 2020 Mar 04. https://www.theverge.com/2020/3/4/21164563/coronavirus-risk-communication-cdc-trump-trust.

73. World Health Organization. [2020-04-21]. WHO Health Alert brings COVID-19 facts to billions via WhatsApp. https://www.who.int/news-room/feature-stories/detail/who-health-alert-brings-covid-19-facts-to-billions-via-whatsapp.

74. Liu S, Yang L, Zhang C, Xiang Y, Liu Z, Hu S, Zhang B. Online mental health services in China during the COVID-19 outbreak. *Lancet Psychiat*. 2020 Apr;7(4):e17–e8. doi: 10.1016/S2215-0366(20)30077-8. http://europepmc.org/abstract/MED/32085841

75. Zhou X, Snoswell CL, Harding LE, Bambling M, Edirippulige S, Bai X, Smith AC. The role of telehealth in reducing the mental health burden from COVID-19. *Telemed J E Health*. 2020 Apr;26(4):377–9. doi: 10.1089/tmj.2020.0068.

76. Torous J, Jän Myrick K, Rauseo-Ricupero N, Firth J. Digital mental health and COVID-19: Using technology today to accelerate the curve on access and quality tomorrow. *JMIR Ment Health*. 2020 Mar 26;7(3):e18848. doi: 10.2196/18848. https://mental.jmir.org/2020/3/e18848/

77. Signorini A, Segre AM, Polgreen PM. The use of Twitter to track levels of disease activity and public concern in the U.S. during the influenza A H1N1 pandemic. *PLoS One*. 2011 May 04;6(5):e19467. doi: 10.1371/journal.pone.0019467.

78. Du J, Tang L, Xiang Y, Zhi D, Xu J, Song H, Tao C. Public perception analysis of tweets during the2015 measles outbreak: Comparative study using convolutional neural network models. *J Med Internet Res*. 2018 Jul 09;20(7):e236. doi: 10.2196/jmir.9413. https://www.jmir.org/2018/7/e236/

79. Stefanidis A, Vraga E, Lamprianidis G, Radzikowski J, Delamater PL, Jacobsen KH, Pfoser D, Croitoru A, Crooks A. Zika in Twitter: Temporal variations of locations, actors, and concepts. *JMIR Public Health Surveill*. 2017 Apr 20;3(2):e22. doi: 10.2196/publichealth.6925.

80. Liang H, Fung IC, Tse ZTH, Yin J, Chan C, Pechta LE, Smith BJ, Marquez-Lameda RD, Meltzer MI,Lubell KM, Fu K. How did Ebola information spread on twitter: broadcasting or viral spreading? *BMC Public Health*. 2019 Apr 25;19(1):438. doi: 10.1186/s12889-019-6747-8. https://bmcpublichealth.biomedcentral.com/articles/10.1186/s12889-019-6747-8.

81. Morin C, Bost I, Mercier A, Dozon J, Atlani-Duault L. Information circulation in times of Ebola: Twitter and the sexual transmission of Ebola by survivors. *PLoS Curr*. 2018 Aug 28;10:E1. doi:10.1371/currents.outbreaks.4e35a9446b89c1b46f8308099840d48f.

82. Tang L, Bie B, Park S, Zhi D. Social media and outbreaks of emerging infectious diseases: A systematic review of literature. *Am J Infect Control*. 2018 Sep;46(9):962–72. doi:10.1016/j.ajic.2018.02.010. http://europepmc.org/abstract/MED/29628293.

83. Ayyoubzadeh SM, Ayyoubzadeh SM, Zahedi H, Ahmadi M, Kalhori SRN. Predicting COVID-19 incidence through analysis of google trends data in Iran: Data mining and deep learning pilot study. *JMIR Public Health Surveill*. 2020 Apr 14;6(2):e18828. doi: 10.2196/18828. https://publichealth.jmir.org/2020/2/e18828/

84. Li C, Chen LJ, Chen X, Zhang M, Pang CP, Chen H. Retrospective analysis of the possibility of predicting the COVID-19 outbreak from Internet searches and social media data, China, 2020. Euro Surveill. 2020 Mar;25(10):pie=2000199. doi: 10.2807/1560-7917.ES.2020.25.10.2000199. http://www.eurosurveillance.org/content/10.2807/1560-7917.ES.2020.25.10.2000199.

85. Alessa A, Faezipour M. Flu outbreak prediction using twitter posts classification and linear regression with historical centers for disease control and prevention reports: Prediction framework study. *JMIR Public Health Surveill*. 2019 Jun 25;5(2):e12383. doi: 10.2196/12383.

86. Viboud C, Santillana M. Fitbit-informed influenza forecasts. *Lancet Digital Health*. 2020 Feb;2(2):e54–e5. doi: 10.1016/s2589-7500(19)30241-9. http://paperpile.com/b/Jwnkjq/b4gV.

87. Luo X, Zimet G, Shah S. A natural language processing framework to analyse the opinions on HPV vaccination reflected in twitter over 10 years (2008–2017). *Hum Vaccin Immunother*. 2019;15(7–8):1496–504. doi: 10.1080/21645515.2019.1627821.

88. Abd-Alrazaq A, Alhuwail D, Househ M, Hamdi M, Shah Z. Top concerns of tweeters during the COVID-19 pandemic: Infoveillance study. *J Med Internet Res*. 2020 Apr 21;22(4):e19016. doi:10.2196/19016. https://www.jmir.org/2020/4/e19016

89. Coiera E, Kocaballi B, Halamka J, Laranjo L. The digital scribe. *NPJ Digit Med*. 2018 Oct 16; 1:58. doi: 10.1038/s41746-018-0066-9. eCollection 2018. Review. Available from: https://ico.org.uk/action-weve-taken/data-security-incident-trends/e0236308.

90. Sookoo A, Garg L, Chakraborty C. Improvement of system performance in an IT production support environment. *Int J Syst Assur Eng Manag*. April 2021;12(5). DOI: 10.1007/s13198-021-01092-0.

91. Chinmay C. Mobile Health (m-Health) for Tele-wound Monitoring, IGI: Mobile Health Applications for Quality Healthcare Delivery, Ch. 5, 98–116, ISBN: 9781522580218. DOI: 10.4018/978-1-5225-8021-8.ch005, 2019.

92. Chakraborty C, Gupta B, Ghosh SK. Identification of chronic wound status under tele-wound network through smartphone. *Int J Rough Sets Data Anal*. 2015;2:58–77. doi:10.4018/IJRSDA.2015070104

93. Chakraborty C, Gupta B, Ghosh SK, et al. Telemedicine supported chronic wound tissue prediction using classification approaches. *J Med Syst*. 2016;40:68. doi:10.1007/s10916-015-0424-y

8 An Overview of Artificial Intelligence for Advanced Healthcare Systems

Akarsh K. Nair, EbinDeni Raj, and Jayakrushna Sahoo
Indian Institute of Information Technology, Kottayam, Kerala

CONTENTS

8.1   INTRODUCTION

Artificial Intelligence (AI) is a hotly discussed topic of the era due to its wide applicability and usefulness. AI does the process of prompting computer systems to do intelligent tasks, similar to humans. Previously, the major difference between humans and machines was related to cognition. With the introduction of AI, machines became capable of doing cognitive tasks which were previously limited to humans. AI makes use of datasets to make the system understand a particular pattern or make inferences that will help the system to achieve designated tasks. AI has a wide range of applications in all sorts of domains. An intelligent system has to go through certain steps to be able to achieve the aforementioned intelligent skills. They are acquisition, thinking and adaptive skills.

> **Acquisition process**: The basic step of AI aims at collecting data, generate a set of steps as to which will help in converting the data into valid information. Such generated steps are referred to as algorithms, which provide devices with formal directions as to how a task needs to be performed.
> **Thinking process**: They are also referred to as the reasoning process. The major task of AI is selecting the precise algorithm aiming for a peculiar outcome.
> **Adaptive process**: This stage of AI is the tuning stage where the algorithms undergo fine-tuning and make sure that the ideal result is provided as much as possible. Thus it is sometimes also referred to as self-correction process.

In the light of the current pandemic, healthcare workers and allied service sectors are facing unparalleled stress in all facets, including manpower shortage, organizational requirements, and so on. An effective solution for such issues, in the long run, is to incorporate efficient technology into the mix. Over the last few years, there has been considerable progress in the application of AI in the field of healthcare. It is predicted that the upcoming years will see a taking over of several tasks by AI applications that were previously performed by skilled medics and healthcare executives.

There is also an active debate on the applicability of AI on such highly sensitive tasks which require a high amount of cognitive and decision-making skills. With all this being said, along with the positive sides, AI does possess several ethical risks as well. The capability of AI applications to make changes to the inherent attributes that healthcare tasks possess is a thing of concern. Such modifications may give rise to ethical issues related to regularization, cognition, and so on giving rise to incomplete, enigmatic or misleading statements leading to prejudiced outcomes. To solve such issues, a clear and efficient methodology is required for the implementation of AI techniques in the healthcare domain that is capable of identifying the challenges and providing direct solutions. Mainly, such approaches should not be completely dependent on stringent administration measures, proving to be deficient to tackle the issue. Such regulation only provides an understanding of the processes and is not an easy way to surpass the allied issues.

The solution is to have a user-targeted focusing on their supposition, specific or basic requirements and privileges. The main hindrance is the lack of a sufficiently coherent method to perform such an analysis. However, the cognitive, regularized, and overarching issues related to the usage of AI in healthcare also happens on a much broader level with respect to the different levels of relationship among users. This may lead to several critical issues as the healthcare sector always needs to give prime consideration for accuracy in diagnostic problems. Therefore, whenever a virtuous analysis of an AI system for healthcare is performed, the authorities should always consider studying the origin of ethical issues at multiple levels and varying stages of the algorithmic lifecycle. For example, cognitive issues associated with erroneous corroboration and AI diagnosing systems could result in hazardous mishappenings for individuals whence the algorithm miscalculates the condition of a patient or visible symptoms.

Thus, such a step-by-step study is indispensable as it is possible to change the ethical influence of an algorithm in multiple ways at any given point of development. For example, a disease diagnosing algorithm developed in an ethical manner that has been tested individually may still vandalize a healthcare system when it is not able to manage the changing amount of data it has to accommodate during deployment. Such an ethical review of AI-based healthcare systems is a very relevant one and it cannot be taken lightly. Only whence such application satisfies these ethical reviews, society will be able to capitalize on the full potential of AI and its application in the healthcare industry. Else, it will remain a Pandora's box, never meeting desired functionalities.

These discussions are aiming for the future, and they lack to provide a detailed insight into the restriction AI faces in the healthcare sector in the current scenario. A detailed study will provide a clear idea of the application of AI in all aspects of the healthcare domain as well as their merits and demerits in real-life scenarios. This article will be providing an elite view of the above-mentioned topic. Figure 8.1 will give an abstract idea of the subdomain-based application of AI in healthcare which will be discussed in detail in the coming sections.

When the researchers are discussing AI in the healthcare context, another terminology should also be discussed briefly: Digital Health Transformation (DHT). It is because of the fact that such a proposal was the paving stone of all the technologies being discussed below. DHT is a gradual process where technology is positively revolutionizing the healthcare sector. When using the term 'technology', we are not employing AI alone but multiple technologies such as the Internet of Things, Big Data, Telemedicine, and so on. Amidst the technological advancements in every sector, the healthcare industry is still lagging behind when it comes to automation or adaptation of technologies. It may be due to several factors such as setup cost, rapidly changing requirements, or even ethical issues, but still, DHT can be said as the need of the hour when we consider the effects that the pandemic has done on the healthcare sector. DHT simply helps to bridge the gap between the patients and the service provided. Along with that, quality-of-service is ensured. It also ensures high delivery of services as well. DHT provides enhanced personal care for patients and allied treatments along with preparing the industry

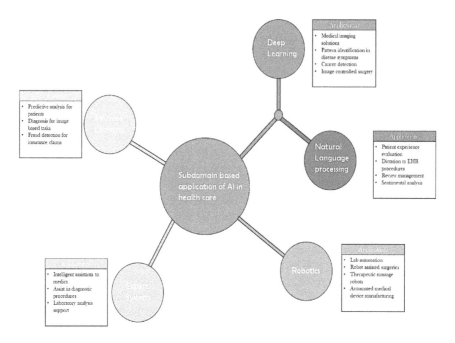

FIGURE 8.1   Subdomain-based AI application in healthcare.

for incorporating next-generation technologies into the scene. When talking about AI in DHT, some of the very common applications include tasks such as analysis of pathology images, image processing tasks as part of disease diagnostics, doctor–patient interactive system development, drug-related systems, and so on. These tasks will be separately discussed in the coming section at some stage. The context of our study is limited to AI in healthcare, thus the other domains which facilitate DHT are out of our scope.

AI is a very inclusive term that comprises of a group of technologies rather than a single one. The basic motto of all of them will be same but their area of application or methodology will vary. Some of the major subdomains of AI are Deep Learning (DL), Machine Learning (ML), Computer Vision, and Natural Language Processing (NLP). Most of these are directly relevant to the healthcare domain even though the technical support they offer may vary widely. In this study, we will be going through several subdomains of AI and their respective application in healthcare scenarios. Later on, we shift our study to various tasks related to healthcare that can benefit from AI-based applications. Some of the most recent advancements of AI combined with other technologies in health-related scenarios will also be discussed in the last sections. This chapter is further organized into a total of seven sections. Section 8.2 discusses the different subdomain-wise applications of AI in healthcare, including Machine Learning, Deep Learning, Natural Language Processing, Expert systems, and Robotics [1].

Then, we will be discussing AI in the context of healthcare with respect to its applicability in Section 8.3, followed by Section 8.4, presenting a study on combinational applications of AI with other technologies in the healthcare context. We present the outcomes and discussions made and discuss the future scope of the work in Sections 8.5 and 8.6 respectively. The paper is concluded with Section 8.7 discussing the conclusion arrived from our work.

The contributions we aim to provide through this study are the following:

- Perform a detailed study of application of AI-based technologies in advanced healthcare systems.
- Perform in-depth analysis of recent publications of AI in healthcare context from the last three years.
- Discuss various combinational applications of AI with upcoming technologies in healthcare scenario.
- Make necessary observations and scope for future improvements.

8.2   SUBDOMAIN-BASED AI APPLICATIONS IN HEALTHCARE SYSTEMS

In this section, we will be discussing the various subdomains of AI and their respective application in healthcare sector. We will be doing a detailed analysis going through some of the most recent works in each domain.

8.2.1   MACHINE LEARNING

Machine Learning is a subdomain of AI which helps us to build a model using statistical techniques with the aid of a dataset referred to as 'training data'. Such models in later stages are used for decision-making operations and to perform predictions without the need for explicit programming aiming for the particular task. ML is further divided into different types based upon the autonomy in their training process. these include Supervised ML, Unsupervised ML, Semi-supervised ML, Reinforced ML and Transfer Learning. ML is one of the most applied forms of AI due to its versatility and high applicability. Fast progression in ML has been enabled with the evolution of novel learning algorithms and methodologies as well as by the current development in the ease of availability of data and cheap computation. The espousal of data-demanding ML methodologies is now available at passim in all domains which has led to a decision-making process oriented on evidence. Such applications are widely used in different areas such as production, academics, finance, marketing, and healthcare [2]. In the healthcare domain, the most prevalent use of conventional ML is for precision medicine that is to predict the next step in treatment for patients from the previous history or condition of the diseased. Almost all instances of ML including precision medicinal applications require a dataset for training the system for which the output is known. Such a case comes under the category of supervised learning [3].

ML algorithms have widespread applications in the field of healthcare. There have been several works involving ML in direct healthcare tasks related to radiology, cardiology, ophthalmology, and so on. As with dermatology, ML has a huge role to play in tasks requiring oral vision. Diseases such as melanoma can be easily detected by ML algorithms when provided with a quality dataset [4]. On a broader scale, ML applications in dermatology can be used for multiple purposes like disease classification using clinical images as well as dermatopathology images, assessment of skin diseases, expediting extensive research on the epidemiology, and even for precision medicine [5]. As with cardiology, ML could be applied in several instances. For example, echocardiography can be combined with ML for the automated calculation of aortic valve areas in aortic stenosis. It can also be used for differentiating various prognostic phenotypes. ML has also been employed in automatic segmentation of different components of the heart for monitoring the cardiovascular system function. Cardiovascular disease detection is another application where ML has shown high potential [6]. ML-based algorithms have been applied for the detection of visual field progression as part of glaucoma and attained high performance compared to existing methodologies. Similarly, glaucomatous nerve fibre damage has also been detected using ML from optical coherence tomography images [7]. The above-mentioned are just a sample from a long list of ML applications in ophthalmology. ML also has the capacity to exponentially change the way data extraction from images is done in radiology as well. Not just images, it can also change the way several tasks such as clinical decision support systems, detection and interpretation of findings, post-processing and dosage estimation, examination quality control, and radiology reporting are performed [8–10]. ML techniques such as Naive Bayes, SVM, and CART have given highly accurate results for the diagnosis of heart disease, breast cancer and diabetic diseases respectively.

ML applications are not just limited to diagnosis and treatment-related tasks. They do play a vital role in allied tasks as well. Fraud detection is a major task performed by ML in all sorts of systems. In the context of healthcare, fraud detection helps to identify the real people in need and provide them with the necessary resources [11]. ML can also be used for improving the quality of life of patients and medical personnel by developing satisfaction determining models making use of regression or similar techniques. With the outbreak of DL, several deeper applications were devised which will be discussed in the coming section.

8.2.2 DEEP LEARNING

Deep learning is a subdomain of ML that facilitates high-level humanly functions in machines by processing data and inferencing patterns for decision-making. DL processes are unsupervised in nature and capable of making use of unlabelled as well as labelled data for processing. They are also referred to as Neural Networks

(NN). DL models usually consist of several layers whose purpose is to learn and draw inferences from data with several layers of contemplation. They have entirely changed the way applications such as speech recognition, object detection, medical image processing, and so on were perceived. DL models usually try to uncover deep-lying patterns in datasets by making use of backpropagation algorithms and denote the changes that need to be made at the parametric level in every single layer to attain an ideal output. Convolutional Neural Networks (CNN) are now being widely used in image, video, and speech processing applications as they are giving optimal output with minimal effort whereas recurrent NN are proving their applicability in tasks related to text and speech processing. Due to its applicability in the aforementioned tasks, DL is highly applicable for healthcare tasks as well. As of now, DL applications in healthcare are mostly related to image-intensive tasks related to radiology, pathology, ophthalmology, dermatology, cancer detection and image-controlled surgical procedures. It does such tasks with high precision, even better than human technicians.

Medical Imaging is a prominent domain where DL has a high potential of applicability. The estimation is that DL applications will eradicate the need for human intervention in image-related diagnostic tasks in near future. DL has been widely used on MRI scans and CT scan images to draw particular inferences. One such application is the usage of CNN and neural autoregressive distribution estimation (NADE) for brain tumour detection [12]. In the current pandemic situation, CT scan images are being used widely with DL techniques for COVID-19 detection as well [13]. Cancer detection is another major hurdle that has been cleared with the help of DL techniques. DL has been used in cardiology cases as well for the detection and characterization of myocardial delayed enhancement on MRI images which can be used for detection of myocardial disease and diagnosis of ischaemic and non-ischaemic cardiomyopathy [6]. With respect to radiology applications as well, CNNs have been employed to improve the performance of systems through protocol determination-making use of short-text classification [14].

When dealing with text-related tasks, DL also has its application. A recurrent neural network functions best for applications such as sequence modelling problems; for example, to predict the upcoming word from health record data. Such a model comprises of weighted connections which further facilitates such applications to combine findings over time and provide a consolidated output as well. Long Short-Term Memory (LSTM) is another DL model that can be used for text-related tasks. LSTM had been tested and proved for missing data prediction for ECG signals. It makes use of the capability to learn long-term dependencies for identifying the missing data and outperforms linear regression as well as Gaussian Process Regression. Even though the current application is limited to ECG, it has a high scope of applicability for other technologies like ECG, EEG, EMG, Phonocardiogram, and so on [15]. Another particular subdomain exists where the sole concentration will be given to text-based tasks only will be discussed in the coming section.

8.2.3 Natural Language Processing

NLP is a subdomain of AI which tries to make human language sensible for computers. Tasks mainly concerned with NLP are speech recognition, text data analysis, language translation and any other tasks which are directly related to languages. NLP tasks are performed based on two approaches, statistical methods and semantic methods.

Statistical NLP methodologies have their roots based on DL and have played a major role in the growth of recognitions tasks in terms of accuracy. A large dataset is needed for the learning process which is referred to as 'corpus'. NLP has a vast range of applications in the healthcare domain for text-related tasks. Some of the most prominent tasks include production, interpretation and categorization of clinical and allied data. They are also used for the analysis of unorganized clinical records of patients, preparing records from scientific data (scanning/test reports), decipher treatment-related conversations and even organize interactive AI applications.

Usage of Electronic health records (EHR) is getting wide acceptance today. With the outreach of NLP, knowledge mining from such unstructured EHR and other health-related data has become easier than ever. The development in noisy text processing techniques has opened up the wider area of utilizing unstructured data whereas previous applications were completely limited to ordered data [16]. When talking about knowledge mining from EHR, major applications of NLP related to oncology making use of such data should be discussed as well. One such application of NLP was to develop a quick learning healthcare system capable of reducing clinical inferences from EHRs for unstructured data usually related to cancer outcomes [17]. This was a very relevant endeavour as unstructured EHRs usage of cancer-related data is proving to be viable. Thus, DL-NLP methods were used to train models capable of predicting disease progression from the textual data available in radiology reports. It is just an example of a proven methodology for analysis of cancerous results from EHR records which can be applied to several other contexts as well.

Another prevalent application of NLP is for the detection of peripheral artery diseases from EHR. A particular case of Critical limb ischaemia (CLI) detection using symptoms with the aid of a dedicated CLI-NLP algorithm is such an example. The addition of NLP in such instances enables overcoming the limitation in detection procedures from EHRs due to the non-existence of a unified classification criterion for CLI cases [18]. NLP helps in achieving higher true positive results from descriptive clinical data available in EHRs helping to develop a higher accuracy model and automated diagnosis systems. Monitoring of healthcare-associated infections from EHRs and NLP for identification of neuropsychiatric symptoms authenticated by home healthcare clinicians are a few among many other direct applications. The former made use of semantic algorithms and expert rules whereas the latter used a set of terms included in the training vocabulary which directly pointed to Alzheimer's disease and related dementias or its allied symptoms for detection.

Even though NLP has multiple applications like the ones mentioned before, it has many issues for implementation as well. Clinical NLP is different from normal NLP, and it needs to be created from normal NLP systems as per the application requirements. Some of the various challenges faced during the same are related to corpus assembly, heterogeneity of report structures, variations in languages used, and so on [19]. Another set of observed challenges are related to data availability, evaluation workbenches and reporting standards. Even though their countermeasures are proposed, they need further studies and refinements to achieve an optimally stable system.

8.2.4   RULE-BASED EXPERT SYSTEMS

Rule-based expert systems are one of the most basic applications of AI and make use of ordained 'knowledge-based rules' for solving problems. Expert systems aim at devising a set of rules using knowledge obtained from human counterparts to be applied to input data. The role of such systems in healthcare is mainly limited to clinical decision support systems. Their applications are used in EHRs as well. They are limited to smaller systems as with the increase in rules, so does an increase occur in the difficulty to model outcomes. Rule-based expert systems (RBES) can be implemented as fuzzy or belief-based. It is generally stated that belief rule-based expert systems are to be considered as a generalized version of fuzzy RBES [20]. As a basic application of RBES, we can consider systems capable of managing tumorous growths. The system will be able to calculate the diameter of the growth with the aid of conditional arguments and the value will be used to determine whether the growth has reached an alarming stage requiring immediate attention or otherwise. Another simple application of RBES is for headache diagnosis along with a medication recommendation system. It is a backward rule-based system working as assistance for medical personnel using the information attained from them that is previously stored inside the system. Even though the applicability of the model is narrow, it can be extended to a vast range of other applications by bringing changes to the knowledge base of the system. Even though not directly related to healthcare tasks, the application of RBES is relevant in other allied sections as well. One such application is regarding medical billing for insurance claims. The task of going through and scrutinizing medical insurance claims is a tedious one and it can be efficiently done with the aid of RBES. The motto of RBES in such instances is to perform a task known as 'claim-scrubbing', that is, to identify applications with erroneous data and rejection of such applicants [21]. RBES does such tasks with utmost accuracy meaning that it is suited for similar other applications as well.

As mentioned earlier, the belief BRBES is one method of implementation of RBES which is used in all sorts of applications in the healthcare domain. BRBESs are extensively used in tasks requiring capture of unsure knowledge and to perform reasoning on unsure tasks by making use of belief rule base and proof-based reasoning. One such application of BRBES is for determining the predictableness of acute coronary syndrome. Such predictions are made with the system inference signs and symptoms related to the disease [22]. Tuberculosis disease diagnosis under uncertain conditions is another application where BRBES has proved its mettle. They use the previous history of TB patients to create the knowledge base and make use of symptoms to make the diagnosis. Being a potent disease, such systems are extremely relevant as it performs far better than the traditional methods and even fuzzy RBES in terms of efficiency. Another similar application of BRBES is for determining the severity of coronary artery disease using a combined belied-based approach. The results of BRBES are said to be as credible as their counterparts on the same mission that is Artificial NN and SVMs. If implemented properly, it has considerable accuracy and can be used for optimal decision-making procedures.

As with BRBESs, Fuzzy rule-based expert systems (FRBES) also have widespread application areas inside the healthcare domain. FRBES works well for the early diagnosis of orthopaedic disease affecting knee joints. One such application is used specifically for an inflammatory disease called Osgood Schlatter disease. Using symptoms, the system is capable of calculating the severity of the disease as well as prescribe medicines. Fuzzy logic works efficiently for such an application giving highly accurate results. A similar methodology is used for the identification of asthma severity in emergency care units. The FRBES makes use of the fuzzy logic principles for determining acute asthma and the system performs efficiently under all tasks. Extensive hybridization can enable the system to be extended to similar tasks without affecting the accuracy when correctly configured. Another application of FRBES can be for multiple allergy detection using fuzzy rules. The system enables patients to diagnose multiple allergic conditions with respect to their symptoms under the same umbrella with high accuracy [23]. Fuzzy logic-based systems are not limited to few applications. When they are configured properly and possess a strong knowledge base, their application scenarios can be drastically varied.

8.2.5 ROBOTICS

With the recent developments in technology, robots are becoming more common as supportive machineries aiding humans in different fields of work. Such devices are becoming more intelligent and being embedded with AI capabilities giving them different levels of autonomy in decision-making with respect to their applications. Their application in the healthcare domain is also rising to the occasion rapidly. 'Robotics' is a collective term, meaning that they refer to both physical robotics as well as robotic process automation applications. Physical robots have been used in the healthcare industry for several purposes. Surgical robots are one of the major applications. They aid medics in surgery-related tasks, providing them with needed help for tasks such as high precision invasive dissection, improving vision for remote locations inside the body, medication control, and so on. Some of the common departments making use of robotic surgical procedures are gynaecology, prostate-related surgeries, head and neck related surgeries and so on. Even therapeutic robots are nowadays being used for massaging applications. Motivated by the speedy advancements of medical imaging and mechatronics technologies, healthcare robots are being rapidly incorporated into every single medical procedure as possible by medics and therapists [24]. Robotic process automation (RPA) is another task coming under robotics that focuses on performing structured works on managerial grounds. Such applications are usually cost-effective allowing ease of programming and transparency in their processing. RPA doesn't make use of robots in the literal sense, but only computer programs. They are basically semi-intelligent in nature and uses an amalgamation of plans, business policies and the 'presentation layer' along with a computer system to perform specified tasks. Their area of application primarily concentrates on performing monotonous tasks such as advanced authorizations, amendment of patient details and so on. A combination of RPA with other technologies like image processing increases their strata of application as in the processing of receipts, billing, etc. Extensive studies state that the future of such technologies lies in their capability to be combined with other domains for getting more feasible applicability.

8.3   AREAS OF APPLICABILITY OF AI

The previous sections have already provided a clear explanation of subdomains of AI and their application for different purposes which suites them the best. In this section, we will be discussing in a broader perspective the domain-based applicability of AI in healthcare. The scope of applications of AI techniques in healthcare deliverance and allied tasks are clearly apparent. Figure 8.3 gives a basic overview of the different applications of AI in healthcare. Some of the major application areas that need AI the most, or are already using AI optimally, will be listed and discussed in the following sections.

8.3.1   ADMINISTRATIVE LEVEL APPLICATIONS

With the changing global business environments, the healthcare industry has also started shifting its concentration towards the way services are being offered. The current approach urges attaining quality-of-service as well as the quality of treatment for patients. The intensive shortage of human resources for such administrative tasks can be solved with the aid of AI applications [25]. Mundane tasks such as patient data entry or automated review of data from the laboratory can be easily handled with AI applications. AI techniques such as ML and NLP can be incorporated with EHRs for mining data and performing diagnostic operations extensively. This can in turn reduce the need for clinicians for such tasks. Also when it comes to data fetching from older health records as well, AI proves to be leagues ahead of its human counterparts. Similarly, NLP applications using voice capture and transcription services for reading and writing of health records have also proved efficient as it gives more time for clinicians for evaluation of the diseased [26]. Some of the other common tasks where AI can perform efficiently are patient scheduling for admission, insurance claim verification or devising interactive chat boxes making use of NLP, using predictive analysis for prediction medicine stock from previous data, and so on. There are several other applications as well which has surely revolutionized the administrative sector and the way healthcare administration is perceived.

8.3.2   DIAGNOSTIC SUPPORT

Another major application of AI in healthcare is to provide diagnostic support to healthcare professionals. AI is capable of doing diagnoses of multiple diseases or situations when trained with a proper dataset and performs efficiently and meticulously than humans. Even though they can't be treated as an alternative for human diagnostics, they surely do provide an additional support in most cases as false positives and false negatives can be minimized in AI applications with meticulous training whereas, with humans, there are always chances of erroneous decision-making.

Many research groups and labs are extensively working on such processes and every day, newer applications are being developed. This particular area is growing very rapidly and attaining high usability due to the caution with which research is being done [27]. ML has been widely used to provide personalized treatment for various sets of ailments such as coronary artery disease, liver diseases, and so on. An advanced version of ML, NN are now being used widely for diagnostic applications. When compared to traditional methods, NN provides superior performance in terms of accuracy and overall performance. For diagnosis of different types of cancerous growth, NNs have been employed making use of CT scan, MRI scan images, or some other methodologies [28]. Similarly, cardiac disease diagnostic attempts have also been made. Even though such applications do surpass human excellence, it is always best to consider them as support systems and a hybridized method making use of both human expertise and AI's discriminative power should be considered as we are still a long way from going for complete autonomy with such sensitive use cases.

8.3.3   OTHER APPLICATION AREAS

In the previous sections, a few major applications in the healthcare system which have the capability of extensive usage of AI were discussed. It cannot be concluded from any perspective that those are the only applications of AI in healthcare. Several other applications do exist which make use of combinations of AI with other technologies for working. Application of AI can be done in any tasks requiring automation and a state of improvement. AI is not limited to direct healthcare application; it can also be applied to allied services. ML has been used for assisting in the development and deployment of medicines at an industrial level [15]. Similarly, it has also been used for detecting the spreading of particular diseases based upon the symptoms and corresponding triggering situations leading to the spread. Such applications are even being used for tracking details of COVID-19 spreading [29]. Another prominent application of AI is robotics. As of

Administrative support
For maintaining data at administrative side, keep a track of the whole functioning of hospitals, medicine stock history updation and so on.

Diagnostic Support
Applications to take inferences from clinical data and perform diagnostic operation completely or as a supportive measure to medics.

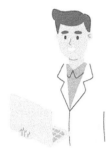

Patient welfare support
Chatbots to converse with patients, patient emotion tracking applications and so on.

Surgical support
Robot-aided surgery procedures or autonomous robotic surgeries.

Clinical Research
Accelerate research on drug discovery, disease symptom discovery, drug delivery and so on.

Electronic Health Record
Data extraction from unstructured text, running diagnostic algorithm from EHR.

Personalised medical care
Personal devices to keep track of bodily function and diagnosis of disease symptoms without the presence of a clinician.

FIGURE 8.2   Application of AI in healthcare tasks.

now, surgical robots are being used for sophisticated surgeries. Even though they are not autonomous, they still have a considerable degree of intelligence allowing them to be driven by surgeons according to the need of the situation [30]. Figure 8.2 provides an overview of different areas of application of AI in healthcare discussed above. The future of AI will be primarily based on robotics and the development of more efficient and user-friendly humanoid robots and virtual health assistants. The other half of the outreach of AI will be based upon its ability to incorporate other technologies into the mix for healthcare applications. We will be having a small discussion of such an application in the next section.

8.4   COMBINATIONAL APPLICATIONS OF AI

The current technological advances have seen an exponential growth of the IoT and blockchain technologies. A huge amount of data being generated by IoT devices has in turn increased the need for advances in the application of AI. Such data has various applications when combined with ML, DL or NLP techniques. To be precise, most of the current applications have centralized training procedures relying on a server for providing training and validating data. With the growth of IoT, many changes have been brought to this approach including Federated

Learning (a type of distributed ML). Similarly, security and authenticity issues of data are being cared for by incorporating various techniques including blockchain technology. Even though these technologies have various applications areas, in our particular discussion, we will be only dealing with such applications in the context of healthcare.

8.4.1 ARTIFICIAL INTELLIGENCE FOR IoT-BASED HEALTHCARE APPLICATION

With the fast growth of IoT technology, the healthcare industry has started widely implementing IoT-based technologies directly into different applications. Such IoT devices are combined with AI applications to develop a new generation of devices where the main motto is reduced cost along with performance efficiency. The era demands personalized healthcare applications, and the new technology just provides the same. Wearable smart senor devices that are capable of detecting body functions without expert care are becoming a trend. The technology has such a high applicability level that even a generalized diagnostic model can be constructed with such AI-enabled IoT networks [31]. Such devices are not just limited to diagnostic tasks but also perform other hospital-related tasks well. IoT-based AI applications are even used for human emotion and state of mind detection. Currently, both academia and industry are focusing on a developing terminology known as the Internet of Medical Things (IoMT) which is a term used to denote what we have discussed as a whole. IoMT on its own has the potential to emerge as a standalone domain needing extensive studies. Surely the future of healthcare is dependent on the optimal application of AI to such varying domains.

8.4.2 BLOCKCHAIN FOR AI IN HEALTHCARE APPLICATIONS

Blockchain has enabled a steady revolution for the creation of scalable and distributed systems incorporating several other popular technologies like AI, Cloud Computing, and so on. AI and blockchain are two hotly discussed topics, and the latter does help in enhancing and solving some of the major issues that the former faces. Even though AI is capable of efficiently working with huge datasets for classification and analysis in the healthcare sector, the presence of such huge volumes of raw medical data does raise questions of integrity due to its sensitive nature. The combination of AI and blockchain adds an additional layer of security to the data as well as brings considerable changes and aids for improvement as a whole [32]. Blockchain integrated AI technology for cardiovascular medicine, AI integrated with blockchain to devise measures for coronavirus spreading are some of the most recent applications among many others. Figure 8.3 shows the overview of AI combined with blockchain application in the healthcare sector at different stages.

As previously discussed, DHT is one of the prima facie of AI in healthcare. The combination of AI and blockchain has enabled an acceleration of DHT as a whole. The incorporation of blockchain into DHT has also enabled the transformation of

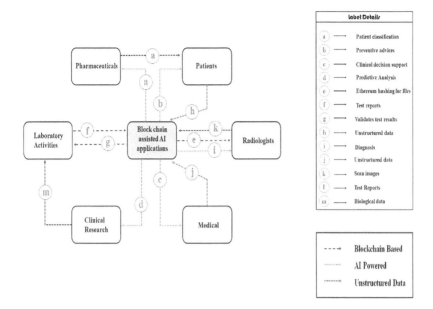

FIGURE 8.3   Overview of different stages involved in healthcare sector.

healthcare into more of a patient-centric system as well as mark an increase in the security, privacy and interoperability of the system. The system has also opened up new scopes for health information exchanges (HIE) via highly efficient, decentralized and secure medical record management procedures. The wide applicability of the technology has given rise to high demand for it in healthcare-based applications. The sensitive nature of data in healthcare application calls for a high degree of data confidentiality and such an approach guarantees it well. We will not be moving into a very detailed analysis of the technology as it is out of scope for our study.

8.4.3   OTHER MAJOR COMBINATION APPLICATIONS OF AI

Bioinformatics is another domain that makes use of AI extensively. Bioinformatics in healthcare mainly deals with the genetic level study of root causes of diseases and AI helps in performing it extensively. Various types of cancer diagnostics, COVID-19 management using bio-sensing applications, multi-disease diagnostics from DNA or RNA samples are some of the very common applications that use AI in bioinformatics [33]. Even cloud computing-based healthcare applications are making use of AI in the current day scenario. New models are being devised for chronic kidney disease diagnostics, electrocardiogram evaluation, and so on. The scope of AI in healthcare is unlimited on its own and when being applied with other technologies it increases manifold.

8.5 DISCUSSIONS

We have shown how healthcare applications are currently leveraging the AI techniques in multiple instances relating to diagnosis, treatment, support and so on, which are directly related to patients and organizational functionalities as well. By systematizing the related research, and likening with traditional techniques it can be inferred that there is a huge prospective for AIs in healthcare and becomes an integral part of it. Furthermore, this empirical study shows that the applicability decision support system can be extended to treatment and recovery stages of other critical diseases such as breast related diseases, Parkinson, diabetes and so on [6]. Moreover, it has been shown in dermatological applications ML models perform best for highly complex needing predictive application and are capable of anticipating future outcomes [4].

With the increasing amount of electronics data being generated, so does the possibility for applications of AI increases. There are many instances in which such applications provide better performance than their human counterparts, but the industry has not reached up to a level where it is technically and ethically feasible to move forward for a complete automation. It is best to implement an integrated system where constant interaction exists between AI applications and healthcare workers. The era of pure AI application is almost over, and we are getting fast forwarded to an era of individualized human health monitoring systems. Human health monitoring systems mainly make use of non-invasive sensors, wearable devices, implanted sensors and multiple combinations of all these. Such devices enable us for early detection as well as timely monitoring of body functions without the aid of a trained personnel. The wide usage of AI in the healthcare industry has revolutionized the way a large number of procedures have been perceived.

Not with just a couple of applications, but generally AI-based applications, have been subjected to extensive laboratory and real-life experimentations and only applications with high efficiency are made available for the general public.

8.6 CONCLUSION

Data is said to be the propellant of the future, and when it comes to healthcare data, it is a very costly and sensitive matter. Previously, healthcare data was dissevered and stored without considering the need for future use. Thus, these data were of least use for patients or organizations. The need for aggregation was always high as it was a convenient solution for optimal data usage. With widespread use of AI, as with all domains, the healthcare sector also started adopting AI techniques and this enabled the long-term need of data aggregation to be fulfilled and also increase accuracy for most of the healthcare tasks. This helps in developing powerful models capable of doing high-level tasks such as automated diagnostic of diseases and even enabled high precision methods for optimal usage of resources for designated tasks in a well-timed and dynamic manner.

Despite this, AI as of now is still not available at field for medical applications in reality. The main reasons contributing to this are: Firstly, the AI application are not designed to re-design the existing way of work. It is subject to a whole set of external factors and merely the addition of AI application into a meaningless distributed system will never bring relevant changes. Secondly, the lack of technological advancements for data collection, processing and training of AI applications or algorithms is a real issue in most healthcare institutes. Algorithms need constant updating with respect to the changing environments and constraints. For example, an algorithm devised for Asian ethnic people will never work with the same efficiency for another ethnic group. Thus to not lose their relevance, constant revaluation and adjustments need to be done throughout the lifetime of the system which requires dedicated settings. There are many other fundamental issues that need to be resolved prior to the above-mentioned ones. AI is all about the manipulation of data and in the healthcare industry, a major issue that arises is also related to the management of data. Basic questions such as possession of data, who is held responsible for the data, and even who is given the authority of its usage, and all are still unanswered. Multiple rules and regulation need to be devised to provide a solid answer for the same. Only when such issues are solved, can we move on to the real technical issues related to the domain [34].

The capabilities of AI are highly studied and discussed but in healthcare systems, it is faced with a dilemma like no other domain. With the devising of multiple combinational technologies such as Fog, Edge, IoT and Cloud, the ever-evident technological gap has been reducing gradually. It is hopeful that in near future, the complete potential of AI can be harnessed by the healthcare domain extensively. Even though it is still a several-mile-long journey, the industry is taking baby steps and being accelerated by extensive support from academia as well as research. Else it will always remain as it is: utilized opportunities.

8.7   FUTURE SCOPE

Currently, AI already is being applied in healthcare for multiple tasks. At the rate of current development, the future of AI and healthcare seems to be highly interlinked and closely related. The major issue that is still forbidding the rapid development of AI in healthcare is related to the ethical issues accompanied with it. Any technology applied to humans or living beings, in general, undergoes extensive trial runs and research prior to field implementation. This creates a considerably large amount of waiting time before the technology gets to the hands of the general public. Such issues are a major hurdle that the technology faces with respect to healthcare applications among other few already discussed. Future applications of AI in healthcare may undertake a wide variety of applications from simple tasks such as automated phone calls for treatment enquiries, population health-related tasks to high-end applications such as therapeutic applications, treatment schemes, and even systems to provide direct interaction with patients. Virtual assistants are one such technology that is expected to gain high popularity in the coming era. Even though already employed, they do lack a touch of human cognition as they are still being worked upon. The future developments are expected to be aiming at patients suffering from ailments such as Alzheimer's and so on who need a constant reminder system to lead a daily life. Robotics is another domain that is expected to show exponential growth in the healthcare sector. Already, they are employed as surgical assistants and even perform autonomous surgical procedures in some high-end applications. The industry is now expecting robotics to be applied to therapeutic applications as well in the near future. Similarly, technologies are being developed for better medical image processing and similar tasks which will directly affect the healthcare industry when it comes to scanning reports or such sorts of data analysis. Also, alternative methodologies in pharmaceutics as well are being developed. Technologies that are capable of understanding ailments from reports or clinical notes intelligently are being deployed in many cases. From the available status quo, it can be inferred that the future of AI in healthcare is bright if it is open to making adaptations and evolving with time.

REFERENCES

1. Diaz J.M., Shariq A.B., Edeh M.O., Chinmay C., Qaisar S., Emiro D.L.H.F., and Paola A.C., 2021. Artificial intelligence-based kubernetes container for scheduling nodes of energy composition, *International Journal of System Assurance Engineering and Management*, 1–14. 10.1007/s13198-021-01195-8.
2. Puaschunder, J.M., 2020. The potential for artificial intelligence in healthcare. *SSRN Electronic Journal*, Available at SSRN 3525037.
3. Paul, A.K., and Schaefer, M., 2020. Safeguards for the use of artificial intelligence and machine learning in global health. *Bulletin of the World Health Organization*, *98*(4), p. 282.
4. Du, A.X., Emam, S., and Gniadecki, R., 2020. Review of machine learning in predicting dermatological outcomes. *Frontiers in Medicine*, *7*, p. 266.
5. Al-Imam, A., and Al-Lami, F., 2020. Machine learning for potent dermatology research and practice. *Journal of Dermatology and Dermatologic Surgery*, *24*(1), p. 1.
6. Li, J.P., Haq, A.U., Din, S.U., Khan, J., Khan, A., and Saboor, A., 2020. Heart disease identification method using machine learning classification in e-healthcare. *IEEE Access*, *8*, pp. 107562–107582.
7. Sekimitsu, S., and Zebardast, N., 2021. Glaucoma and machine learning: A call for increased diversity in data. *Ophthalmology Glaucoma*, 8, pp. 339–342.
8. Mongan, J., Kalpathy-Cramer, J., Flanders, A., and Linguraru, M.G., 2021. RSNA-MICCAI panel discussion: Machine learning for radiology from challenges to clinical applications. *Radiology: Artificial Intelligence*, 3(5), e210118.
9. Abdul R.J., Chinmay C., and Celestine W., 2021. Exploratory data analysis, classification, comparative analysis, case severity detection, and internet of things in COVID-19 telemonitoring for smart hospitals, *Journal of Experimental & Theoretical Artificial Intelligence*, 1–24. doi:10.1080/0952813X.2021.1960634.
10. Amit K., and Chinmay C., 2021. Artificial intelligence and internet of things based healthcare 4.0 monitoring system, *Wireless Personal Communications*, 1–14. [SCI, IF-1.20., doi: 10.1007/s11277-021-08708-5.
11. Matloob, I., Khan, S.A., and Rahman, H.U., 2020. Sequence mining and prediction-based healthcare fraud detection methodology. *IEEE Access*, *8*, pp. 143256–143273.
12. Jia, Z., and Chen, D., 2020. Brain tumor identification and classification of MRI images using deep learning techniques. *IEEE Access*.

13. Chakraborty, C., and Abougreen, A.N., 2021. Intelligent internet of things and advanced machine learning techniques for COVID-19. *EAI Endorsed Transactions on Pervasive Health and Technology*, *7*(26), p. e1.

14. Chea, P., and Mandell, J.C., 2020. Current applications and future directions of deep learning in musculoskeletal radiology. *Skeletal Radiology*, *49*(2), pp. 183–197.

15. Rodrigues, T., and Bernardes, G.J., 2020. Machine learning for target discovery in drug development. *Current Opinion in Chemical Biology*, *56*, pp. 16–22.

16. Neumann, M., King, D., Beltagy, I., and Ammar, W., 2019. Scispacy: Fast and robust models for biomedical natural language processing. arXiv preprint arXiv:1902.07669.

17. Chen, P.H., Zafar, H., Galperin-Aizenberg, M., and Cook, T., 2018. Integrating natural language processing and machine learning algorithms to categorize oncologic response in radiology reports. *Journal of Digital Imaging*, *31*(2), pp. 178–184.

18. Lavingia, K.S., Tran, K., Dua, A., Itoga, N., Deslarzes-Dubuis, C., Mell, M., and Chandra, V., 2020. Multivesseltibial revascularization does not improve outcomes in patients with critical limb ischemia. *Journal of Vascular Surgery*, *71*(6), pp. 2083–2088.

19. Baclic, O., Tunis, M., Young, K., Doan, C., Swerdfeger, H., and Schonfeld, J., 2020. Artificial intelligence in public health: Challenges and opportunities for public health made possible by advances in natural language processing. *Canada Communicable Disease Report*, *46*(6), p. 161.

20. Cao, Y., Zhou, Z.J., Hu, C.H., He, W., and Tang, S., 2020. On the interpretability of belief rule based expert systems. *IEEE Transactions on Fuzzy Systems*.

21. Abdullah, U., Ligęza, A., and Zafar, K., 2017. Performance evaluation of rule-based expert systems: An example from medical billing domain. *Expert Systems*, *34*(6), p. e12218.

22. Ahmed, F., Chakma, R.J., Hossain, S., and Sarma, D., 2020, February. A combined belief rule based expert system to predict coronary artery disease. In *2020 International Conference on Inventive Computation Technologies (ICICT)* (pp. 252–257). IEEE.

23. Thukral, S., and Rana, V., 2019. Versatility of fuzzy logic in chronic diseases: A review. *Medical Hypotheses*, *122*, pp. 150–156.

24. Porkodi, S., and Kesavaraja, D., 2021. Healthcare robots enabled with IoT and artificial intelligence for elderly patients. *AI and IoT-Based Intelligent Automation in Robotics*, Wiley Online Library, pp. 87–108.

25. Meskó, B., Hetényi, G., and Győrffy, Z., 2018. Will artificial intelligence solve the human resource crisis in healthcare?. *BMC Health Services Research*, *18*(1), pp. 1–4.

26. Wang, W., Chen, L., Xiong, M., and Wang, Y., 2021. Accelerating AI adoption with responsible AI signals and employee engagement mechanisms in healthcare. *Information Systems Frontiers*, pp. 1–18.

27. Dias, R., and Torkamani, A., 2019. Artificial intelligence in clinical and genomic diagnostics. *Genome Medicine*, *11*(1), pp. 1–12.

28. Kleppe, A., Skrede, O.J., De Raedt, S., Liestøl, K., Kerr, D.J., and Danielsen, H.E., 2021. Designing deep learning studies in cancer diagnostics. *Nature Reviews Cancer*, *21*(3), pp. 199–211.

29. Garg, L., Chukwu, E., Nasser, N., Chakraborty, C., and Garg, G., 2020. Anonymity preserving IoT-based COVID-19 and other infectious disease contact tracing model. *Ieee Access*, *8*, pp. 159402–159414.

30. Haidegger, T., 2019. Autonomy for surgical robots: Concepts and paradigms. *IEEE Transactions on Medical Robotics and Bionics*, *1*(2), pp. 65–76.

31. Chakraborty, C., Roy, S., Sharma, S., Tran, T., Dwivedi, P., and Singha, M., 2021. IoT Based Wearable Healthcare System: Post COVID-19. In *The Impact of the COVID-19 Pandemic on Green Societies Environmental Sustainability* (pp. 305–321).
32. Salah, K., Rehman, M.H.U., Nizamuddin, N., and Al-Fuqaha, A., 2019. Blockchain for AI: Review and open research challenges. *IEEE Access, 7*, pp. 10127–10149.
33. Jindal, S., Marriwala, N., Sharma, A., and Bhatia, R., 2021. Methodological Analysis with Informative Science in Bioinformatics. In Marriwala N., Tripathi C.C., Jain S., Mathapathi S. (eds) *Soft Computing for Intelligent Systems* (pp. 49–57). Springer, Singapore.
34. Trishan, P., Mattie, H., and Celi, L.A., 2019. The "inconvenient truth" about AI in healthcare. *NPJ Digital Medicine, 2*(1), 77.

9 Future Trajectory of Healthcare with Artificial Intelligence

A. Siva Sakthi
Sri Ramakrishna Engineering College, Coimbatore, India

S. Niveda and S. Srinitha
Sri Ramakrishna Engineering College, Coimbatore, India

CONTENTS

DOI: 10.1201/9781003247128-9

9.1   INTRODUCTION

9.1.1   OVERVIEW OF AI IN HEALTHCARE

Artificial Intelligence (AI) is an intelligence demonstrated by machines, in which the machines learn from experience, adjust to the new inputs and perform tasks like humans. The term AI was coined by John McCarthy in 1956. Many expert systems have been developed due to the improvements in the field of AI over the last two decades. AI has enormous application in the field of healthcare, robotics, automation, manufacturing etc. AI systems constitute both hardware and software. Here, software represents the conceptual algorithms, and to execute these algorithms artificial neural networks (ANNs) are used. Neural networks are layered structures that generate output as responses to the external stimuli. AI responds to this stimulation and helps the system in making a decision, predicting the outcome, and resolving the issue.

Jiang et al. [1] proposed a transformational force in healthcare industry using AI. The American Medical Association defined the role of AI in healthcare as 'augmented intelligence', as AI is used to design and improves human intelligence, rather than replacing it. It has numerous applications in diagnosing and treating the disease effectively. AI provides endless opportunities to implement an efficient, precise and impactful intervention. It also brings a paradigm shift to the healthcare by digital automation and by compiling and analyzing the healthcare data effectively. Advancement in the field of healthcare helps to mitigate the mortality and morbidity. Chen et al. [2] proposed the consistency and the quality of data improve as most of the data is generated by the machine. AI integrated healthcare provides clinical effectiveness access and affordability of care. The primary aim of this chapter is to assimilate and explore various applications of AI in disease management.

This chapter is organized thus:

Section 9.1 gives an overview of AI, machine learning in the field of healthcare, robotics, automation etc.

Section 9.2 provides a development of Artificial Intelligence in medical field for surgeries using robots and cancer diagnosis with the help of machine learning and deep learning algorithms.

Section 9.3 gives an overview about Electronic Health Record (EHR) and various tools like Med2Vec, Deepr, mNotes, Data mining techniques.

Section 9.4 deals with the conclusion and discussion of integrating AI with other emerging technologies like Big Data which offers immense applications in healthcare field.

9.1.2   MACHINE LEARNING (ML) IN HEALTHCARE

Machine learning is a core subset of AI, which is used to determine the usage of data and algorithms and to imitate humans. It helps to improve accuracy by its self-learning capability. Shailaja et al. [3] suggested that ML brings more

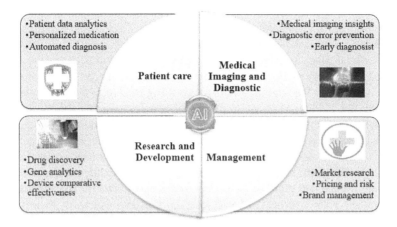

FIGURE 9.1   Applications of AI in healthcare.

powerful transformation in the field of healthcare as it is fuelled by efficacious machine learning techniques like deep reinforcement learning methodologies, Adversarial networks, Natural language processing, convolutional networks etc. There are four types of ML methodologies: Supervised Learning, Unsupervised learning, Semi-supervised learning and Enhanced learning. In supervised learning, the main task is to infer the function from the labelled training data that constitutes a set of training examples. But the models in the unsupervised learning are trained by unlabelled dataset and determine the correlation. And in reinforcement learning, the models are trained to make a sequence of decisions and it learns through interaction and feedback. ML brings more powerful transformation in the field of healthcare as it is fuelled by efficacious machine learning techniques like deep reinforcement learning methodologies, Adversarial networks, Natural language processing, convolutional networks etc., AI has numerous applications like early disease diagnosis, data analytics, medical imaging, automated diagnosis, personalized medication, gene analytics and drug discovery. Figure 9.1 demonstrates various applications of AI in the field of healthcare.

9.1.3   DEEP LEARNING (DL) IN HEALTHCARE

By having an immense capability, DL redefines the healthcare industry, in which it helps to assist the healthcare professionals in discovering the unique opportunities in data and provides path-breaking applications. By using annotated training data, DL helps to model an intelligent system. DL gathers data and applies its neural networks to increase the computational capability and to provide an accurate result. Robots assisted modern laparoscopic surgery integrated with the computer vision techniques helps in autonomous tele-operation which localize the position of the instrument and its orientation in its vicinity. DL techniques enhance the adaptability and robustness of robotic-assisted surgeries, and by using reinforcement algorithms, it learns from a surgeon's physical motion. By employing CNN, image level diagnostics of diseases becomes easier, and the disease can be detected at the early stage. Recurrent neural networks are used in processing the speech, language and time series data which is helpful in healthcare domain.

Reddy et al. [4] proposed EHRs are considered as the backbone of digital healthcare system. Maintaining EHRs requires Big Data tools for next generation data analytics. Adding AI or ML tools, with this, helps to improve the automation and intelligent decision-making capability. By using these tools, the data can be gathered, processed and a well-defined output is produced that leads to intelligent data analysis. ML algorithms are used to recognize the pattern and create the logic on its own. These ML models will be trained by employing huge amounts of data. These algorithms will evaluate the patient record and predict the risk for a disease based on the collective data. AI will leverage this data and assist them for the effective treatment. Strachna et al. [5] proposed decision-making in diagnosing and confirming the disease is the critical process in healthcare, which involves careful decision and subsequent treatment recommendation. AI and IoT integrated healthcare systems help to diagnose the disease in real time, and provide support to patients without healthcare workers. In order to augment these processes, AI and ML tools can be implemented.

Using AI in the healthcare field decreases the cost of disease diagnosis and provides better prediction for treatment. The objective of AI in healthcare is not to replace clinicians, but to provide assistance in performing their jobs effectively and with high accuracy. As clinical data keeps on increasing in healthcare, it provides new pathways for computerized clinical decision support systems (CDSSs). AI-based CDSS helps to generate a case specific decision or advice based on the patient data present in the active knowledge system. These system models learn from the statistics and ML from the data. These learning processes involve two phases: to estimate the unknown dependencies from the given input of a system and the output prediction based on the estimated dependencies. The huge amount of data will be processed, and a feasible recommendation will be given to the patient. Maadevaiah et al. [6] proposed AI-based CDSS mitigates unwanted cost, resource use and unwarranted variations.

9.1.4 REAL-TIME HEALTH MONITORING

Hameed et al. [7] suggested that AI assisted medical robots are used in rehabilitation, surgical operations and assisted living. These robots analyse the health records of the patient and assist the surgeon in real time. By using suitable wearable devices and IoT sensors integrated with AI technology helps to monitor the patients continuously in real time. With the help of a wearable device, the data will be collected and transmitted to the cloud by using AI tools for analysis. Real-time healthcare analytics enhance the quality of care by automatically collecting and processing the patient data. Data mining and knowledge discovery plays the major role in real-time monitoring system. The data from EHRs and the real-time data will be processed and analyzed using AI predictive analysis technique. Kaur et al. [8] proposed that the AI-powered health monitoring systems monitor the patient activities continuously and send the collected data to clinicians in real time. From the collected data, if something unusual is sensed, an immediate alert is sent to clinicians for treatment.

Disease prognosis plays the major role in prediction of likelihood of future occurrences of disease which is essential for the doctors to provide better treatment for the patients. By analyzing various data retrieved from the samples, features and structured images of the patient, AI helps in early prognosis and treatment procedures. A device with the help of AI algorithms, the disease like stroke can be predicted early. Disease prognosis also helpful in oncology, by screening the budding cancer, before the development of visible symptoms at an early stage. By using various classifiers and algorithms, AI offers prognosis to cancer patients. For better precision and high accuracy in the detection of cancer cells, the algorithms like support vector machine, naive bayes are used. AI also has the potential to diagnose the cardiovascular diseases earlier by using the cardiac image data such as ECG, CT scan etc., AI is also helpful in examining all the cataract diseases by using ocular image data [9–12].

Automated disease diagnosis is a pivotal phenomenon and a challenging process. AI helps clinicians for studying various complex diseases by parallel comparing the various stages of a disease by using the huge data. Diabetes mellitus affects our human body adversely that causes long term damage which leads to chronic disorders, cardiovascular diseases, nephropathies, dysfunction and failure of multiple organs. With the help of AI tools and various classification and regression algorithms, diabetes can be automatically diagnosed by using an automated artificial pancreatic system that enhances the accuracy of both glucose monitoring and insulin controlling. In this system, AI application helps in diagnosing hyper-and hypo-glycaemia, plasma glucose levels, glycaemic variability detection and provides lifecycle support by estimating the amount of carbohydrate in the unpackaged foods. The clinical diagnosis not only involves clinical data, but it also collects the patient's current situation, lifestyle, biometric and genetics related data [13–15]. For diagnosing the disease using ML algorithms, a systematic review is done based on which an effective methodology and the algorithm can be taken for analysis [16–20]. AI provides support, feedback, guidance for the patients and healthcare professionals for better understanding of the disease and its implications. AI won't replace healthcare professionals; rather, it just enhances the role and effectiveness of clinicians for providing better treatment with the help of AI-powered healthcare system. The complete literature survey is shown in Table 9.1

9.2 ROLE OF AI IN ROBOTIC SURGERY, CANCER DIAGNOSIS AND BCI

9.2.1 ROLE OF AI IN ROBOTIC SURGERY

Daniel et al. [30] proposed that the concept robotic surgery starts with the invention of laparoscopic surgery in the late 1990s. It has an advantage of minimal hospital stays, less pain, and cosmetically appeal, when compared to traditional

TABLE 9.1
Literature Survey

S. No.	Reference Paper	Inferences
1.	[1–3]	Describes the overall improvements in healthcare using AI
2.	[4, 7]	An AI-IoT integrated prognosis system using neural networks
3.	[5, 6]	Clinical decision support systems
4.	[8]	AI-based predictive and prescriptive analytics techniques
5.	[9–12]	Cancer diagnosis using imaging and stroke diagnosis using cardiac imaging with AI
6.	[13, 14]	Methodologies used in diagnosing diabetes
7.	[15, 17–20]	AI algorithms and methodologies used in healthcare
8.	[21]	Gastrointestinal bleeding of patients is recorded using deep neural network
9.	[22]	The patient's visit is recorded with the Med2Vec
10.	[23]	The occurrence of stroke using data mining technique is recorded
11.	[24]	To monitor patients in remote areas mNotes are used
12.	[25]	To secure the patient's data k-nearest Neighbour classification algorithm is used
13.	[26]	Voice services and commands for saving patient's health
14.	[27]	m-Health technique helps in sharing patient's health record
15.	[28]	Data is secured with the help of STRIDE modelling tool
16.	[29]	eKartonisweb application improves efficiency for quality healthcare

operations. With advancements in technology, the surgeries were assisted using the partially computer-controlled device called robots. In robot-assisted surgery, the robots act as a remote extension where it has all the surgical instruments connected to its arms and the master surgeon who controls it through the console. The robots will provide a HD image of the inner body and the surgeon who sits at a computer console will remotely operate the robots to perform surgeries. With robots, one can make minimally invasive surgery possible for almost all situations. With the advent of AI in the medical field, it also finds its application in surgeries. Xiao-Yun et al. [31] proposed that the AI enabled robots can solve problems and make decisions during the surgery. AI in robotic surgery is used in three main decision-making steps: 1. Pre-operative planning; 2. Intra-operative guidance; and 3. Surgical Robots. The overview of AI in surgery is shown in Figure 9.2

9.2.2 PRE-OPERATIVE PLANNING

Pre-operative planning is a foremost step in any kind of surgery, especially in knee replacement. Jiabang Huo et al. [32] suggested that pre-operative planning should include anatomical classification, detection, segmentation and registration.

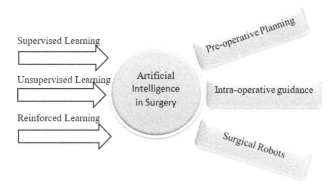

FIGURE 9.2   Overview of AI in surgery.

It is previously done using the images of the knee obtained by various imaging modalities and developed with Mimics software. Nowadays, AI enabled software are used for locating the anatomical structures of the surgical site. This reduces the time and increases the precision. Various neural networks are trained for performing such tasks efficiently. The steps involved in pre-operative planning is shown in Figure 9.3.

Anatomical classification is the main step in pre-operative guidance in which the robots are trained to identify the anatomical structure of each and every part of the body to perform the surgery accurately along with the guidance of the surgeon. Once the robots classified the anatomical structures, the next task is to detect the abnormalities in the surgical site. ML based algorithms are used for this to train the robot based on the images acquired from the various imaging modalities. Then the robots have to use appropriate surgical tool to dissect the organ or remove any abnormal findings in the surgical site. Convolutional Neural Network (CNN) is commonly used to segment the abnormal lesions. Registration is an important step in both pre-operative planning and intra-operative guidance, it acts

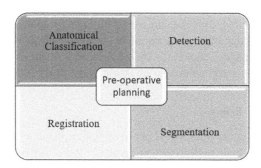

FIGURE 9.3   Steps involved in pre-operative planning.

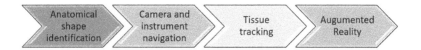

FIGURE 9.4   Process involved in intra-operative guidance.

as the alignment between two medical images or modalities. Deep regression models are used for registration of images from various modalities, which is less time consuming when compared to other traditional methods.

9.2.3   INTRA-OPERATIVE GUIDANCE

Lack of visual perception and misjudgement of anatomical dissection leads to various serious threats. This can be overcome by implementing DL during the surgery to provide intra-operative guidance. This substantially reduces the adverse effects during the operating procedure. The intra-operative guidance is based on four main categories: anatomical shape identification, camera and instrument navigation, tissue tracking and Augmented Reality (AR). In traditional methods 3D reconstruction of organs is done using various imaging modalities. With AI, 3D shapes of an organ are acquired real-time during the phase of surgery. Bishoy Morris [33] proposed Convolutional Neural Network (CNN) based approaches are used for navigation of camera and surgical instruments and it also helps in dept estimation and visual odometry during the surgical procedure. The role of AI in intra-operative guidance during surgery is clearly stated in Figure 9.4

During intra-operative guidance, the robots have to identify the shape of each organ to dissect it and to perform surgery. The robot assisted surgical equipment has many arms embedded in it based on the design. Each arm holds a surgical instrument to perform the operation. An important instrument in this computer assisted surgery is camera, the robotic arm which has camera has to advance the surgical site at first to have a clear vision of the surgical site to the surgeon. The navigation of camera and instrument during the surgery may get blocked due to any liquid interaction. The navigation of camera should be done with utmost care. For this the robots are trained using various ML algorithms. Once the instruments and the camera are inserted, then the surgeon at the console operate the robot to perform surgery by initially removing the outer membrane of the organ. The surgical site is being continuously monitored by the surgeon through the images provided by the robots. AR is used to enhance the vision of surgical site for better results.

9.2.4   SURGICAL ROBOTS

With the increased success rate of AI in pre-operative planning and intra-operative guidance, AI now finds application in surgical robots. It plays a major role in four main categories during surgery: 1. Perception; 2. Localization and Mapping; 3. System Modelling and control; and 4. Human–robot interaction. Xiao-Yun

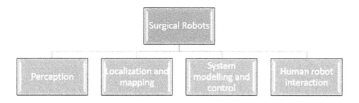

FIGURE 9.5   Major functions of surgical robots.

et al. [31] proposed surgical robots are mainly used for minimally invasive surgery, where the robot gives a high-definition images of the surgical site and the surgeon sitting at the console will operate the robot. The functions of AI in surgical robots are shown in Figure 9.5.

9.2.5   ROLE OF AI IN CANCER DIAGNOSIS

Cancer is one of the deadliest diseases in the world. The mortality rate of lung cancer is more predominant as it cannot be diagnosed in its early stages. Early diagnosis of cancer will increase the life expectancy of victims in many ways. AI plays a major role in predicting cancer at its earlier stage. Integration of AI in cancer research will lead to better health outcomes by precisely detecting the cancer site. It also helps in speedy disease diagnosis and aids in decision-making [34–36]. DL, a part of AI is used for cancer diagnosis. The radiological images of normal and cancer cells are feed to the DL model, and it is trained to identify the cancer cells at its earliest stage. It spots the tumour site more precisely and accurately. Luis et al. [37] concluded that AI has gained a 65% more accuracy in detecting lung cancer, which is the highest accuracy rate that radiologist would achieve. Slowly AI will find way in predicting other cancers also. The role of AI in diagnosing lung cancer is depicted in Figure 9.6.

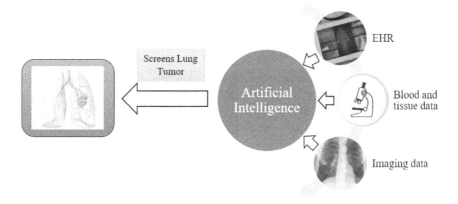

FIGURE 9.6   AI in diagnosing lung cancer.

AI is feed with EHR, Blood and tissue samples report, risk factors and imaging data to detect lung cancer. EHRs includes the vital signs like blood pressure, temperature, ECG, heartrate etc. of the patient, previous history of disease and treatment, patient general information etc. The blood and tissue samples reports consist of lung function test report and the biopsy reports of the cancer. The imaging data includes CT, MRI of the lungs for the identification of the tumour site. It also looks for risk of getting the lung cancer such as age, gender and their smoking habits are also assessed for decision-making. These data are fed to the ML algorithm to train the model for predicting the lung cancer. The AI model will correlate all the data given to it and conclude whether the identified lesion is tumorous or non-tumorous. It uses CNN and regression models to predict the lung cancer efficiently and it also achieved a reasonable success rate.

9.2.6 ROLE OF AI IN BRAIN COMPUTER INTERFACE

BCI is an emerging field in science and technology, where it decodes the neural activity of the brain. Rafeed et al. [38] suggested the main aim of BCI is to restore the neuromuscular activity of the disabled people by analyzing neuro potentials. It can be used to treat cerebral palsy, neuro degenerative disorder, Amyotrophic Lateral sclerosis and so on. By introducing AI in BCI, early diagnosis of neurological disease is possible. The combination of AI and ML in Brain computer interface has more advantage in data collection and training to predict the disease diagnosis and treatment at the earliest. With AI and brain computer interface, EEG enabled prosthetic limbs are possible. Jerry et al. [39] proposed AI and ML in BCI is meant for neuroimaging in neurofeedback and neuromodulation. In prosthetic limb, the EEG signals are used to activate the fatigue muscles of the amputation site to restore the limb functions. AI helps in collecting the strong EEG signals and train them to control the prosthetic limb for its degree of freedom. It also finds applications many other domains like neurorehabilitation, disease diagnosis and prognosis, gaming etc.

9.3 ROLE OF AI IN MAINTAINING THE PATIENT DATABASE

9.3.1 OVERVIEW OF ELECTRONIC HEALTH RECORD

Electronic Medical Record contains the physician fitness details, surgery notes, progress notes, nursing notes, drug formulation notes, allergy details related to their medication. The electronic Health note using AI consists of details about doctor, patient, labs, pharmacy which leads to quality treatment, better decision-making, improved doctor efficiency, precise medicine and significant cost reduction. AI is the key indicator which learns from data stored on health record system and analyses them. The electronic prescription helps the doctor to pick the medicine and it alerts the patient to take medicine on time. It also intimates the patient whether the prescribed drug is safe or not to the patient. The components of EHR are depicted in Figure 9.7.

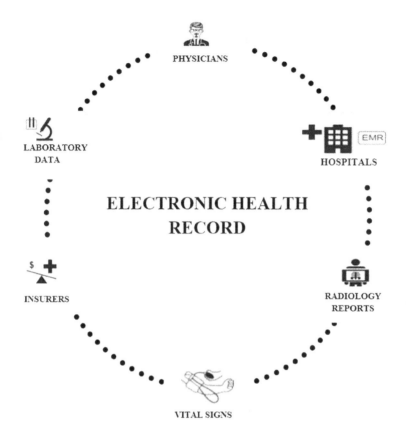

FIGURE 9.7　Components of electronic health record.

Electronic Health Record (EHR) provides the health information about individual patients and their feedback in real time. It provides medical history of the patient and alert the doctor about health needs of the patient which helps to track the decisions on future treatment. It helps to build collaboration between patient and doctor. Some of the tools in EHR are Personal Health record, Clinical Decision support, computerized physician order entry and info-buttons. The computerized order entry allows to enter the data electronically in the hospital or in patient settings. This helps to avoid handwritten records. The Clinical Decision support provides patient information about diseases or allergies, illness, immunization, medicine taken and records of appointment. The computerized physician order entry helps to enter orders about the drugs, laboratory tests, therapy to monitor the patient's health. The Health Information Exchange (HIE) is the method of sharing information about the patient between diverse organizations which helps to provides improvement in their health. This helps to reduce the cost and develops in quality care.

9.3.2 TECHNOLOGIES INVOLVED IN EHR

The technologies involved in EHR are picture archiving and communication system, barcoding, Automated dispensing medicines, Radio frequency identification and electronic medication administration records. The picture archiving and communication system is an integration of input devices from x-ray, CT, MRI or ultrasound and stores the data and disseminates the information in the medical record. The barcoding technology electronically captures information encoded on the product (medicines) with the help of optical scanner. With this barcoding, the nurse can verify the patient's record and their drug intake. Radio frequency identification technology track the patient details, their medication, hospital appointments through wireless communication module. Automated dispensing medicine is a drug storage device which is used to store and dispense the medicines.

Electronic Medication Administration Record alerts the nurse about the next medication for the patient. The main use of Electronic Health Record is that the documentation time spent on the medical record is reduced, quality time spent for the patients, communication between physician and patient is increased, reduced error. Natural Language processing and ML helps to organize the patient's medical experience, medical records regarding the diseases or allergies, patient feedback which will be useful for large database. Some of the Artificial Intelligence (AI) applications in EHR systems are data extraction (patient data from different source like fax, medical record), Predictive analysis using image algorithms, clinical documentation based on the patient's treatment and medications, fetching data from wearables.

To forecast the occurrence of diseases or problem related to medication, EHRs applied using ML method contribute to a greater healthcare quality. With the help of deep neural network (classification and feature extraction), gastrointestinal bleeding for patients hospitalized in taking anticoagulants or antiplatelet drugs is recorded. The record contains the details of individual patient at the time of enrolment like demographic measurements (gender, age), medication measurement (steroids, painkillers), laboratory measurements (haemoglobin levels in the past records). Hung et al. [21] proposed that by implementing early fusion algorithms, the accuracy of predicting the gastrointestinal bleeding achieved greater success.

9.3.3 TOOLS USED IN EHR

The Electronic Health Record (EHR) tools available in market are deep patient, Med2Vec, Deepr, Doctor AI. To predict the risk of the patient, Deepr tool is used to identify regular clinical motifs of irregular data. Stacked Denoising Auto encoders (SDA) is used to learn data from multi-domain clinical data and deep patient frame. The disease diagnosing is done in two ways, classification of disease and tagging of the patient disease which collects the inpatient and outpatient visits. Med2Vec is a simple algorithm to learn real world Electronic Health Record. Caroprese et al. [22] proposed, AI is an application of Recurrent Neural Network which helps in diagnosing the disease with medical prescription. This helps to predict the patients next visit to the hospital.

Data mining is used to predict the occurrence of stroke based on a patient's record. The inputs are gender, patient identification, age, whether the patient is suffering from hypertension and/or heart disease or not, occupation type, residence (rural/urban), marital status, glucose levels, smoker status, and if a stroke has been suffered in the past or not. Nwosu et al. [23] proposed the classification algorithms used for predicting stroke are decision trees, random forest and neural network. The multi-layer perceptron model (Neural network approach) provides good accuracy of 75.02%. Here the binary response variable 1/0 is used for predicting the stroke condition. For a stroke condition, 1 is indicated, and for not, 0. The patient record is indicated by a point in sub-space. These sub-spaces are done by the Principal Component Analysis (PCA).

For metabolic disorder and lifestyle diseases which is treated by nutrient supplementation m-notes are created for Remote Patient Management system. The mNotes consists of appointment scheduling, demographics, SOAP notes, Billing, Follow-up reminders and pharma interaction. The appointment scheduling is implemented with the help of embedded calendar, demographics (name of the patient, date of birth, contact address, contact number, mail-ID and patient's photograph). The patient information which is automatically imported into lab orders is the main feature of using demographic data. Kadambi et al. [24] proposed SOAP (Subjective Objective Physical examination) notes, containing various fields such as history, allergies, family history, treatment and medications/prescriptions. The prescriptions are created with name of the medicine, dose, timing with their doctor treated. Pharma tracker is used to track the dosage of medicines is completed or not and reminds the patient to order the medicine. The model is built for chronic health and wellness problems related to patients for future treatment.

9.3.4 Security in EHR

Data security plays a vital role in Electronic Health Record (EHR) system. Due to data storage issue, the patient's data and their medical history are stored in two different cloud servers. To secure the personal data of the patient, k-Nearest Neighbour classification algorithm is used. The main advantage of HER is that the data of the patient can be accessed and updated from any place. The data is analyzed by the physician or clinician and knows about the health condition of the patient. For securing the data in EHR, data security and encryption algorithms are used. Dalal et al. [25] suggested that EHR architecture is a centre point in which different healthcare centres are engrossed. These are connected through a central server and communicated the data to the hospital. The data of the patient is generated after every visit. The data is then transmitted through secret sharing method. For each patient detail uploaded in EHR, an identification number will be generated.

Vuppalapati et al. [26] suggested a voice generation outpatient data driven EHR consists of Voice Service API, Alexa Voice Service APIs, Alexa Skill Kit, Apple SiriKit, International Classification of Diseases (ICD), Sanjeevani

Electronic Health Records, Edge Processing, ML. The voice service API's enable voice connected products via speaker and microphone. Alexa Voice Service APIs contains mobile, web like volume control, voice recognition, audio. Application Programming Interface contains grouped messages called events (Sent from EHR client to cloud) and directives (messages from EHR client to cloud). Alexa Skills Kit (Sets alarm, play music, medicine notification) helps to interact with voice service apps and customer device through voice commands. Apple SiriKit inter-acts with the mobile app and iOS to control the behaviour of app using voice command. Sanjeevani Electronic Health stores the patient details, treatment and medications. Edge Processing voice services converts the patient voice into text. Thus, the EHR is integrated with voice services which helps in saving the life of the patient.

Mandel et al. [40] proposed that the healthcare system consists of a legislative base, staff groups of different medical institutions, and a group to carry out the actions of medical care. There are three types of medical care: primary, emer-gency and specialized, which comes under treatment and prophylactic care. Treatment and prophylactic care are divided into inpatient, outpatient, emergency, sanatorium resort and rehabilitation medical care. Depending on the requirement, they classify into first aid, medical and specialized care. These are stored and managed in large hospitals.

9.3.5 M-Health in EHR

Maganti et al. [27] suggested to avoid the outflow of patient's health records stored in the cloud, a mobile healthcare application is implemented known as m-health. This provides security in sharing their health record to the service pro-viders of healthcare. It generates a secret key for users of the system, in which the patient has to register first and then enter their details. The patient can share their health record details to the doctors securely. Then the doctors decrypt the data with the secret key and provide medications based on Identity-Based Broadcast Encryption (IBBE), with constant size cipher texts and private keys algorithm to provide security. Hence this application securely handles the health record of patients.

Huang et al. [28] suggested to provide integrity, availability, confidentiality of health records a security framework is modelled using STRIDE modelling tool. To protect the data from unauthorized users, sensitive data is stored on the cloud. To encrypt patient's health record, attribute-based encryption (ABE) is used. The attributes are name of the healthcare institute, designation of the doctor, health Department and experience of the doctor. To access the patient data from a particu-lar hospital, user has to grant access to that person. Here, salting methods are used to improve the security and makes it difficult for the attacker to access the data.

The major challenge is to compile different sets of data into a single group. The data is collected from different domains and aggregated into the same standard. This is done by significant schemas. For each type of data, data schemas enumer-ate the format and content. Some of the examples are heart rate readings, blood pressure values, EHRs of diagnose of disease, medications, lab results, treatment. Koren et al. [29] suggested to utilize the data properly, schemas need to be defined distinctively for each clinical measure. Privacy and security play a major role in e-health solutions. An EHR named eKartonis a web application used to view the medical data of a patient. To access the patient's data, clinicians use their smart-card and pin number. The model aims to merge healthcare data collected from wearable and non-wearables into a standard format within the central health information system. Many hybrid optimization and ML algorithms are proposed in healthcare to improve the efficacy and quality of the healthcare system [41–46].

9.4   CONCLUSION

AI continues to enhance the healthcare expertise and patient experience; various ML algorithms are used in the field of healthcare to diagnose human diseases and for indispensable intelligent data analysis. It is also essential in understanding the potential risks associated with the usage of the technologies like ML, NLP etc. To provide the patient privacy and to increase the security against hackers is important to improve the trust among the patient. This chapter mainly focuses on understanding the applications of AI in healthcare, to diagnose the disease at an early stage, to prevent and to treat them accordingly. It also explains about the major role of AI algorithms in diagnosing the cancer and effectiveness of robotic surgeries and about EHR in detail. It identifies the patterns and detects any deviation in the patient's behaviour and feasible treatment will be suggested. AI shows promising results in care delivery by providing better productivity and efficiency in taking care of patients and it also improves accessibility and helps in early diagnosis.

By integrating AI with other emerging technologies like Big Data, it offers immense applications in healthcare field. With this integrated methodology, it offers more targeted healthcare with useful insights. Due to the larger availability of complex data in the healthcare field, AI plays the major role in evaluating and storing the information. But the major challenge in implementing AI in healthcare is its adoption in daily clinical practice and the extra care that is needed to safeguard the exponential growth of healthcare data. For adopting AI in clinical practice, AI systems will be integrated with EHR systems and approved by regulated committees and it should be standardized.

AI systems cannot replace the clinicians at a larger scale, but have the capability to augment their efforts in taking care of the patient. With better predictions, AI could help to combat serious illnesses. Recent advancements and breakthroughs in AI will push the frontier continuously and widen the scope of AI application and fast developments are envisioned in the near future.

Various applications of AI in disease management are addressed with different technologies. ML and DL algorithms play a vital role in improving the accuracy of the result with the help of surgical robots for providing the treatment. EHR provides the Doctor with the patients database to monitor the patient's health data regularly using different tools like SOAP (Subjective Objective Physical examination) notes, Pharma tracker, Alexa Skill Kit, Apple SiriKit, voice recognition etc. This improves the data security. AI systems cannot replace the clinicians at larger scale, but it has the capability in augmenting their efforts for taking care of the patient.

CONFLICT OF INTEREST

There is no conflict of interests.

FUNDING

There is no funding support.

DATA AVAILABILITY

Not applicable.

REFERENCES

1. Jiang F, Jiang Y, Zhi H, Dong Y, Li H, Ma S & Wang Y (2017) Artificial intelligence in healthcare: past, present and future. *Stroke and Vascular Neurology* 2(4), 230–243.
2. Chen, M & Decary M (2020) Artificial intelligence in healthcare: An essential guide for health leaders. *Healthcare Management Forum* 33(1), 10–18.
3. Shailaja K, Seetharamulu B & Jabbar MA (2018) Machine learning in healthcare: A review. In *2nd International Conference on Electronics, Communication and Aerospace Technology (ICECA)*, 910–914, IEEE.
4. Reddy JEP, Bhuwaneshwar CN, Palakurthi S & Chavan A (2020) AI-IoT based healthcare prognosis interactive system. In *IEEE International Conference for Innovation in Technology (INOCON)*, 1–5, IEEE.
5. Strachna O & Asan O (2020) Reengineering clinical decision support systems for artificial intelligence. In *IEEE International Conference on Healthcare Informatics (ICHI)*, 1–3, IEEE.
6. Mahadevaiah G, Rv P, Bermejo I, Jaffray D, Dekker A & Wee L (2020) Artificial intelligence-based clinical decision support in modern medical physics: Selection, acceptance, commissioning, and quality assurance. *Medical Physics* 47(5), e228–e235.
7. Hameed K, Bajwa IS, Ramzan S, Anwar W & Khan A (2020) An intelligent IoT based healthcare system using fuzzy neural networks. *Scientific Programming*, 2020, 1–15.
8. Kaur J & Mann KS (2017) AI-based healthcare platform for real time, predictive and prescriptive analytics using reactive programming. *Journal of Physics: Conference Series* 933, 012010.
9. Dilsizian SE & Siegel EL (2014) Artificial intelligence in medicine and cardiac imaging: harnessing big data and advanced computing to provide personalized medical diagnosis and treatment. *Curr Cardiol Rep* 16:441.
10. George L (2020) AI & medicine releases biomarker discovery and targeted proteomics services for researchers, www.clinicalresearchnewsonline.com.

11. Huang S, Yang J & Fong S et al. (2020) Artificial intelligence in cancer diagnosis and prognosis: opportunities and challenges. *Cancer Letters* 471, 61–71.
12. Villar JR, Gonzalez S & Sedano J et al (2015) Improving human activity recognition and its application in early stroke diagnosis. *International Journal of Neural Systems* 25(4), 1450036.
13. Alfian G, Syafrudin M, Ijaz MF, Syaekhoni MA, Fitriyani NL & Rhee J (2018) A personalized healthcare monitoring system for diabetic patients by utilizing BLE-based sensors and real-time data processing. *Sensors* 18(7), 2183–3208
14. American Diabetes Association (2020) Classification and diagnosis of diabetes: standards of medical Care in Diabetes-2020. *Diabetes Care* 43 (Suppl 1), S14
15. Bothe MK, Dickens L, Reichel K, Tellmann A, Ellger B, Westphal M & Faisal AA (2013) The use of reinforcement learning algorithms to meet the challenges of an artificial pancreas. *Expert Review of Medical Devices* 10(5), 661–673.
16. Caballé-Cervigón N, Castillo-Sequera JL, Gómez-Pulido JA, Gómez-Pulido JM & Polo-Luque ML (2020) Machine learning applied to diagnosis of human diseases: A systematic review. *Applied Sciences* 10(15), 5135.
17. Dhomse Kanchan B & Mahale Kishor M (2016) Study of machine learning algorithms for special disease prediction using principal of component analysis. In *International Conference on Global Trends in Signal Processing Information Computing and Communication (ICGTSPICC)*, 5–10, IEEE.
18. Ferdous M, Debnath J & Chakraborty NR (2020) Machine learning algorithms in healthcare: A literature survey. In *11th IEEE International Conference on Computing, Communication and Networking Technologies (ICCCNT)*, 1–6, IEEE.
19. Qayyum A, Qadir J, Bilal M & Al-Fuqaha A (2020) Secure and robust machine learning for healthcare: A survey. *IEEE Reviews in Biomedical Engineering* 14, 156–180.
20. Siddique S & Chow JC (2021) Machine learning in healthcare communication. *Encyclopedia* 1(1), 220–239.
21. Hung C-Y et al. (2019) Predicting gastrointestinal bleeding events from multimodal in-hospital electronic health records using deep fusion networks. In *41st Annual International Conference of the IEEE Engineering in Medicine and Biology Society (EMBC)*, IEEE.
22. Caroprese L et al. (2018) Deep learning techniques for electronic health record analysis. In *9th International Conference on Information, Intelligence, Systems and Applications (IISA)*, IEEE.
23. Nwosu CS et al (2019) Predicting stroke from electronic health records. In *41st Annual International Conference of the IEEE Engineering in Medicine and Biology Society (EMBC)*, IEEE.
24. Kadambi V et al. (2018) Review of an electronic health record model to facilitate remote patient management in metabolic and lifestyle diseases. In *10th International Conference on Communication Systems & Networks (COMSNETS)*, IEEE.
25. Dalal, KR (2019) A novel hybrid data security algorithm for electronic health records security. In *2019 4th International Conference on Computational Systems and Information Technology for Sustainable Solution (CSITSS)*, vol. 4, IEEE.
26. Vuppalapati JS et al. (2017) The role of voice service technologies in creating the next generation outpatient data driven Electronic Health Record (EHR). In *Intelligent Systems Conference (Intelli Sys)*, IEEE.

27. Maganti PK & Chouragade PM (2019) Secure application for sharing health records using identity and attribute-based cryptosystems in cloud environment. In *3rd International Conference on Trends in Electronics and Informatics (ICOEI)*, IEEE.

28. Huang Q, Yeu W, He Y & Yang Y (2018) Secure identity-based data sharing and profile matching for mobile healthcare social networks in cloud computing. *IEEE Access Special Section on Cyber-Threats and Countermeasures in the Healthcare Sector* 6, 36584–36594.

29. Koren A, Jurčević M & Huljenić D (2019) Requirements and challenges in integration of aggregated personal health data for inclusion into formal electronic health records (EHR). In *2nd International Colloquium on Smart Grid Metrology (SMAGRIMET)*, IEEE.

30. Hasimoto DA, Rosman G & Meireles OR (2018) Artificial intelligence in surgery: Promises and perils. *Annals of Surgery* 268, 70.

31. Zhou X-Y, Guo Y, Shen M & Yang G-Z (2020) Artificial Intelligence in surgery. *Frontiers of Medicine*, 1–50.

32. Huo J, Huang G, Dong H, Wang X, Yufan B, Chen Y, Cai D & Zhao C (2021) Value of 3D pre-operative planning for primary total hip arthroplasty based on artificial intelligence technology. *Journal of Orthopaedic Surgery and Research* 16(1), 1–13.

33. Morris B (2005). Robotic surgery: Applications, limitations and impact on surgical education. *Medscape General Medicine* 7(3), 72.

34. Svoboda E (2020) Artificial – intelligence systems look set to make early detection of Lung cancer more accurate and widely available. *Nature* 587(7834).

35. Liang G, Fan W, Luo H & Zhu X (2020) The emerging roles of Artificial Intelligence in cancer Drug development and precision therapy. *Biomedicine and Pharmacotherapy* 128, 110255.

36. Savage N (2020) Artificial intelligence's ability to detect subtle patterns could help physicians to identify cancer types and refine risk prediction. *Nature*, 579, S14–S16.

37. Espinoza JL & Dong LT (2020) Artificial intelligence tools for refining lung cancer screening. *Journal of Clinical Medicine* 9(12), 3860.

38. Alkawadri R (2019) Brain computer interface applications in mapping of epileptic brain networks based on intracranial EEG: An update. *Frontiers in Neuroscience* 13, 191.

39. Shih JJ, Krusienski DJ & Wolpaw JR (2012) Brain computer interfaces in medicine. In *Mayo Clinic Proceedings*, Elsevier.

40. Mandel A et al. (2019) Electronic medical records as a tool of a large hospital management. In *25th International Conference Management of Large-Scale System Development (MLSD)*, IEEE.

41. Amit K, Chinmay C, Wilson J, Kishor A, Chakraborty C & Jeberson W (2020) A novel fog computing approach for minimization of latency in healthcare using machine learning. *International Journal of Interactive Multimedia and Artificial Intelligence* 1, 1–11. Available from: 10.9781/ijimai.2020.12.004

42. Sarkar A, Khan MZ, Singh MM, Noorwali A, Chakraborty C, Pani SK (2021) Artificial neural synchronization using nature inspired whale optimization, *IEEE Access* 9, 1–14. Available from: 10.1109/ACCESS.2021.305288

43. Chinmay C (2019) Computational approach for chronic wound tissue characterization. *Elsevier: Informatics in Medicine Unlocked* 17, 1–10. Available from: 10.1016/j.imu.2019.100162

44. Gupta A, Chinmay C & Gupta B (2021) Secure transmission of EEG data using watermarking algorithm for the detection of epileptic seizures. *Traitement du Signal* 38(2), 473–479. Available from: 10.18280/ts.380227

45. Manpreet K, Mohammad ZK, Shikha G, Abdulfattah N, Chinmay C & Subhendu KP (2021) MBCP: Performance analysis of large-scale mainstream blockchain consensus protocols, *IEEE Access* 9, 1–14. Available from: 10.1109/ACCESS.2021.3085187

46. Sachin D, Chinmay C, Jaroslav F, Rashmi G, Arun KR & Subhendu KP (2021) SSII: Secured and high-quality Steganography using Intelligent hybrid optimization algorithms for IoT, *IEEE Access* 9, 1–16. Available from: 10.1109/ACCESS.2021.3089357

10 Artificial Intelligence and Public Trust on Smart Healthcare Systems

Ajitabh Dash
Jaipuria Institute of Management Indore, MP, India

CONTENTS

DOI: 10.1201/9781003247128-10

10.1   INTRODUCTION

The emergence of artificial intelligence (AI) has the ability to transform and improve the efficiency of any system which is surrounded with complexities and uncertainties [1]. The introduction of AI in healthcare industry is rapidly evolving because of its capability to translate a complex and uncertain data into a robust clinical decision [2, 3]. Unceasing innovations in the domain of AI and their productive implementation in healthcare sector is not only transforming the present clinical decision-making system but also paving the path for early disease detection before their manifestation [4]. The advantages of AI in healthcare are not limited to the clinical diagnosis, but facilitate better experience to the public at diminished healthcare cost [5]. Traditionally, all sorts of clinical diagnoses were done manually by human beings, but the outbreak of the coronavirus pandemic (COVID-19) changed the mindset of healthcare service providers, and has brought prominence of AI for the review of medical histories, surgical procedures and diagnosis for all sort of clinical decisions [6, 7]. Efficacious application of computer vision and deep learning in oncology, machine learning in radiology, NLP (natural language processing) in psychiatry and chat-bots for telemedicine are a few of the prominent examples of AI implementation in Indian healthcare industry [8, 9].

The healthcare sector of India has embraced the power of AI to improve its efficiency and quality much before the pandemic situation. The healthcare industry powered by AI was projected to register an impressive growth rate of 40% in 2021, and to cross $6.6 billion US [10]. As per the report of NITI Aayog [11], there are 3,225 start-ups in the healthcare sector who have embraced AI, and it is also projected that its market size will touch $170 billion US by 2025. This indicates the acceptance of AI-empowered smart healthcare system across the country. The judicious distribution of healthcare services is acknowledged as a key challenge for the government of India where the doctor–population ratio is 0.62:1,000, which is less than the standard of 1:1,000 suggested by the World Health Organization [12]. Hence, the promotion of AI-based smart healthcare system turns out to be unavoidable in India.

But unfortunately, people are reluctant to rely on its accuracy as it is an automated system and lacks human integration. Many recent studies have reported that trust plays a significant role in influencing the human–computer interaction, including AI [13, 14]. Although there is a diverse range of users of AI in AI based healthcare sector, ranging from the public, to doctors, to insurance companies, this study is limited to the beneficiaries of healthcare: the public. A limited number of studies were conducted in Indian contexts to explore the dynamics between human trust and AI integration in the healthcare industry. Outcomes of this empirical research will reinforce the existing literature on human–computer interaction and will also help policymakers and service providers in crafting their strategy for promoting AI-powered smart healthcare sector in India.

Subsequent to the introduction section, this study emphasizes framing a set of hypotheses grounded on the in-depth literature review in the next section. The third section of the paper stresses the method of research, and is followed by the results of this study in the fourth section. Subsequently the fifth section of the paper highlights the findings of the study, and the last section concludes with the implications, limitations and scope for further study.

10.2 LITERATURE REVIEW

10.2.1 Artificial Intelligence

AI is an expansive field incorporating information and communication technology to accomplish certain activities which normally requires human intelligence in terms of visual inspection, language recognition and processing, and voice recognition [1, 15]. The concept AI is defined as 'the recreation of humanoid intelligence by a device, specifically computers with the help of a machine learning algorithm. These procedures comprise learning, thinking, and self-correction'[1]. AI has a universal applicability today, ranging from recommending what an individual should add next to his or her electronic shopping cart to drive a driver less vehicle on the road. It relies on certain computer programs like deep learning, machine learning, natural language processing and artificial neural networking to process both structured and unstructured data for making a robust decision [2, 16]. Modern literature accepts AI as a group of algorithms ready to play out all assignments similarly as well as, or perhaps stunningly better than the normal human being [3].

10.2.2 AI in Healthcare

The healthcare sector has for some time been full of significant expenses, symptomatic blunders, work process failures, expanding managerial intricacies, and lessening time among publics and their doctors [3]. These expanding costs are convoluted by the way that in any event 1 of every 20 public across the globe experiences a diagnostic error which can possibly prompt genuine harm [2]. These inadequacies have roused healthcare services pioneers and the AI people group to cooperate to investigate the job that AI may play in improving consideration conveyance and diminishing expenses [17]. Computer based AI has shown critical potential for mining clinical records, devising treatment plans, advanced robotics intervened medical procedures, clinical administration and supporting emergency clinic activities, clinical information understanding, visual diagnostics along with virtual nursing [3]. AI in medical care has two likely focal points. In the first place, AI can gain from huge information more effectively than clinicians. A fruitful AI framework can productively separate pertinent data to help with improving execution of healthcare activities and help clinicians in settling on educated choices continuously. Second, AI frameworks can perform predefined undertakings with higher accuracy. This component of AI can possibly reform confounded medical procedures [3].

10.2.3 ANTECEDENTS OF TRUST

The most referred definition for 'trust' was suggested by Mayer et al. [18], who contended that trust is

> a party's readiness to be vulnerable to the acts of another party in the anticipation that the other will do a certain activity that is vital to the trustor, regardless of the ability to monitor or control that other party.
>
> [18]

Attention on issues of trust permits us to address not just the use of any innovation, yet in addition its dismissal, or its abuse [19]. Trust can anticipate the degree of dependence on innovation, while the degree of correspondence between client's trust and the innovation's abilities, known as adjustment, can impact the real results of innovation use. Low trust in profoundly competent innovation would prompt neglect and significant expenses as far as lost time and work proficiency, as well as could be expected maltreatment, though high trust in unfit innovation would prompt over-trust and abuse, which thus may cause a break of wellbeing and other unwanted results [20].

Although AI is rapidly altering the healthcare sector [3], numerous individuals actually find it difficult to trust in AI. Different studies uncover that the dread is broader, for instance, 42% of individuals need general trust in AI, and 49% of individuals couldn't name a solitary AI item they trusted [3]. Trust is considered as the foundation for developing an affirmative relationship between human and any computer mediated technology including AI [8]. In the context of healthcare trust is considered as a vital influencer of public–physician–facilities relationship [2]. Previous studies on human–computer interaction have described trust as a blanket term and can be segregated into cognitive and affective trust [21]. It signifies that trust not only includes one's knowledge, but also his/her emotions. If knowledge forms the basis of cognitive trust, affective trust is grounded on mutual care. Furthermore, in few of the recent studies, affective trust is deliberated as sincere, welfare and caring behaviour towards others in the community.

In the context of AI, all kind of communication and interaction between the physician-public and facility is performed through technology which may develop a sense of ambiguity regarding healthcare; for which, the, AI-empowered healthcare settings necessitate the public to form a sensible opinion about the same (cognitive trust). In the meantime, the public–doctor connection is an inimitable relationship necessitating regular interactions where both may develop an emotional association. Accordingly, it becomes imperative to split trust into affective and cognitive in the context of integration of AI in healthcare and analyse them as two distinct variables. Past studies done in the context of trust described expertise, product performance and firm reputation as the integral element of cognitive trust [22]. Similarly, integrity and benevolence were described as the two vital elements of affective trust [21].

Using the results of past studies as a basis, we proposed few hypotheses in support of the relationship highlighted in the model.

10.2.4   AI-Empowered Healthcare's Expertise and Public Trust

Public perception of AI-empowered healthcare's expertise reveals the pertinent abilities allied with it. Expertise is commonly evaluated as far as a specialist co-op's degree of knowledge and experience concerning the central act [3]. Studies in the past has exhibited that a person's apparent degree of expertise upgrades his/her source believability and accordingly their cognitive trust [20]. Therefore, in our study we expect that public's perception of AI-empowered healthcare's expertise can have an affirmative effect on cognitive trust. Hence it is hypothesized that:

> H_1: Public's perception of AI-empowered healthcare's expertise has a positive effect on his/her cognitive trust.

10.2.5   AI-Empowered Healthcare's Performance and Public Trust

Performance of a product or service is described as a person's valuation of its performance with respect to its core benefits [23]. Since the AI-empowered healthcare service is extended to the publics through the integration of technology, it is possible that its performance with respect to core attributes can be ascribed to the service provider, and can affect the public's trust [17]. As the evaluation of product or service performance follows the conventional cognitive dimension of attitudes, no connection can be expected between affective trust and performance of AI-empowered healthcare service. But it can be hypothesized that:

> H_2: Public's perception of AI-empowered healthcare's performance has a positive effect on his/her cognitive trust.

10.2.6   AI-Empowered Healthcare's Reputation and Public Trust

Reputation has been described as an individual's confidence that a system or process is transparent and honest [23]. Reputation is both an image of significant response and an outflow of sympathy for the client [20]. An individual's evaluation of the reputation of a process or system will positively affect his/her evaluation of the trustworthiness of the same [22]. An individual who is not yet acquainted with the system may develop his/her perception from its reputation. Thus in the context of AI-empowered healthcare system it can be assumed that the reputation of the healthcare service provider can affect his/her cognitive as well as affective trust.

> H_3: Public's perception of AI-empowered healthcare's reputation has a positive effect on his/her cognitive trust.
> H_4: Public's perception of AI-empowered healthcare's reputation has a positive effect on his/her affective trust.

10.2.7   AI-Empowered Healthcare's Integrity and Public Trust

Integrity alludes to acknowledgement and adherence to predefined set of rules and principles followed to accomplish certain activity [24]. In the context of

AI-empowered healthcare system integrity refers to the perception of a public the AI-powered healthcare system can sincerely perform its promised activity. In the AI-powered healthcare setting, service providers ought to do what they guarantee when a public buys their offering, that is, they ought to give publics an ideal wellbeing experience [25]. At the point when a service provider's reactions are not ideal, it will impact the public's view of their integrity. Since research shows that for an individual, affective trust of an individual is firmly identified with their integrity [22], in the context of AI-empowered healthcare system it can be hypothesized that:

H₅: Public's perception of AI-empowered healthcare's integrity has a positive effect on his/her affective trust.

10.2.8 AI-EMPOWERED HEALTHCARE'S BENEVOLENCE AND PUBLIC TRUST

Benevolence is defined as 'the degree to which a person feels that he or she will not only look out for his or her own interests, but will also help others' [21]. In the context of AI-powered healthcare systems, benevolence can be described as the inclination of the healthcare service providers' earnest efforts to take care of publics welfare, while solving the problem faced by them [24, 26]. Findings of the past research revealed that, though benevolence denotes the degree to which a public assumes the AI-empowered healthcare service to do well, this anticipation is not grounded on cautious or cognitive evaluation of the AI-powered healthcare service [27]. Thus it can be hypothesized that:

H₆: Public's perception of AI-empowered healthcare's benevolence has an affirmative effect on his/her affective trust.

Outcomes of the past studies advocate that both affective and cognitive trust plays a vital role to determine the behavioural intention of individuals in terms of their willingness to adopt, especially technologically sophisticated products and services [19, 21]. Trust is also described as an indispensable mechanism for diminishing uncertainty associated with adoption decision especially in the technological environment [20, 21]. As AI-empowered healthcare service is a technological product, we assume that both cognitive and affective trust will affect the public's willingness to adopt the same. Therefore, we propose:

H₇: Cognitive trust of the public has an an affirmative effect on their willingness to adopt AI-powered healthcare system.

H₈: Affective trust of the public has an affirmative effect on their willingness to adopt AI-powered healthcare system.

10.3 RESEARCH METHOD

The methodology encompassed for this research is analytical in nature and executed in two levels. In the initial level, an extensive review of literature was done to develop knowledge about the varied facets of human trust towards AI-empowered healthcare system, and its effect on their willingness to adopt the same. In the subsequent level, primary data were collected with the help of a predesigned electronic questionnaire from 462 sample respondents who had experienced the AI-powered healthcare system in India using judgemental sampling method. The objective of using judgemental sampling method was to make sure that respondents with self-motivation and eagerness were involved in this study [28]. Data for this study was gathered over the months of August–December 2020. For data analysis, the Statistical Package for Social Sciences (SPSS) version 20 and Analysis of Moment Structure (AMOS) were used. Statistical tools like exploratory factor analysis, confirmatory factor analysis and structural equation modelling were used to derive an insightful conclusion.

10.3.1 SAMPLING TECHNIQUE

Former studies steered in the perspective of technology in healthcare industry have used the view of active beneficiaries (mostly the public) as their sample respondent. Therefore, sample for the purpose of this research had been carefully chosen from the publics with prior experience of AI in health care via a judgemental sampling system [28]. To diminish the inaccuracy of judgemental sampling, data collection was done as per the guidelines of Judd et al. [29]. The questionnaire consisted of a filtering question towards enquiring whether the public has exposed to AI-empowered healthcare system in the recent past or not. Those who responded adversely to this question were dropped from the study.

10.3.2 DATA COLLECTION

The current study is essentially grounded on primary data and to collect the data from the selected respondents an electronic questionnaire was circulated through Google form. The questionnaire developed for this study was consisting of 45 statements and respondents were asked to rate their level of agreement on a five-point Likert scale, with 1 representing 'Strongly Disagree' and 5 representing 'Strongly Agree'. The items in the questionnaire were adapted from existing literature. Three items measuring public's willingness to adopt AI-empowered healthcare system were modified from [17], items measuring cognitive and affective trust were modified from McAllister [30]. A short explanation of the reason for the investigation was additionally given to each respondent, and the respondent has right not to take part in the study as it is done on a wilful premise. At last, information acquired from 462 sample respondents were appeared to be adequate for the further analysis [31].

10.3.3 DATA ANALYSIS

EFA as well as CFA were done in this study to evaluate the validity of the survey instrument employed in this study. Empirical analysis of the collected data was executed in three steps in three steps. Initially EFA was executed to examine the validity of the latent constructs. In the consequent step, CFA was performed to authorize the measurement model and substantiate the outcome of EFA. As a final point, structural equation modelling was incorporated to perform the path analysis. The prominent benefit of structural equation modelling over the conventional regression analyses is the greater statistical power with higher probability of rejecting a false null hypothesis [32].

10.4 RESULTS

Demographic characteristics of the sample respondents considered for this study are presented in the Table 10.1 as below.

Descriptive statistical analysis of the data collected from the respondents regarding their gender uncovered that dominant part of them i.e., 55.84% were male and the rest 44.16% were females. Correspondingly, in terms of their age it was uncovered that significant segment of the sample respondents i.e., 26.27% were underneath the age of 25 years followed by 26.41% were in the age section of 35–44, 25.76% were in the age section of 26–35 and just 20.56% were beyond 45 years old. Similarly, in terms of educational qualification, it was uncovered that 39% of the respondents were graduates, 31% were postgraduates, 16% were intermediate and just 15% were having certain other degree/diploma with them.

TABLE 10.1
The Sample Respondents' Demographic Profile

Demographic Attributes	Frequency	Percentage
Gender		
Male	258	55.84%
Female	204	44.16%
Age		
Less than 25	126	27.27%
26–35	119	25.76%
36–45	122	26.41%
Above 45	95	20.56%
Qualification		
Undergraduates	74	16%
Graduates	178	39%
Postgraduates	142	31%
Others	68	15%

Source: Field Data.

10.4.1 EXPLORATORY FACTOR ANALYSIS

EFA was executed to check whether things fitted suitably to the resultant develop as foreseen or not. Because of the EFA, variables with meagre psychometric property were put beside additional investigation. The value of Kaiser-Meyer-Olkin (KMO) was figured to be 0.814 showing the wellness of the example for executing EFA [33]. Besides, all the builds accomplished a total difference of 71% which is a lot over the recommended base estimation of 0.60 [34]. As the value of Cronbach's alpha for all the constructs were more than 0.70, all constructs were recognized as being dependable for the examination [35].

10.4.2 INDICATORS OF MODEL FIT FOR MEASUREMENT MODEL

The data presented in Table 10.2 revealed that the CFI (comparative fit index), GFI (goodness fit index), NFI (normal fit index), AGFI (Adjusted Goodness of Fit Index), and IFI (Incremental Fit Index) were computed above 0.9. Similarly, the calculated value of RMSEA (root mean square of error approximation) was also less than 0.1, which specifies that the measurement model is robust [36]. Therefore, it is suitable to assess the discriminant validity and convergent validity of the model and appraise the assumed associations through path analysis (Table 10.3).

10.4.3 CONSTRUCT VALIDITY

To set up legitimacy of the construct, CFA has been executed. Convergent validity was affirmed for the proposed model as 'CR (Composite reliability) > 0.7, CR > AVE (Average variance explained) and AVE > 0.5' [37]. Moreover, discriminant validity of the model was additionally affirmed as the MSV (Maximum Shared Variance) < AVE and ASV (Average shared Variance) < AVE [38].

TABLE 10.2
Indicators of Model Fit for Measurement Model

Indices	Suggested Value	Calculated Value
χ^2/df	<5	3.258
GFI	>0.9	0.901
RMSEA	<0.1	0.054
IFI		
AGFI	>0.90	0.923
NFI	>0.90	0.914
CFI	>0.90	0.903

Source: Compiled up from the AMOS output

TABLE 10.3

The Constructs' Convergent and Discriminant Validity

	CR	AVE	MSV	ASV	Convergent Validity	Discriminant Validity
Expertise	0.745	0.625	0.278	0.211	Yes	Yes
Product performance	0.802	0.587	0.323	0.258	Yes	Yes
Reputation	0.785	0.658	0.347	0.187	Yes	Yes
Integrity	0.778	0.559	0.356	0.119	Yes	Yes
Benevolence	0.845	0.517	0.331	0.145	Yes	Yes
Cognitive trust	0.712	0.568	0.236	0.202	Yes	Yes
Affective trust	0.798	0.591	0.272	0.177	Yes	Yes
Willingness to adopt	0.879	0.523	0.344	0.179	Yes	Yes

Source: Output of Gakingston toolbox.

10.4.4 Results of Path Analysis

The path analysis results presented in the Table 10.4 uncovers the hypotheses testing results and gauges the relationship strength among constructs.

The value of R^2 (squared correlation) computed with respect to willingness to adopt AI-powered healthcare system is 0.587 which uncovers that both affective and cognitive trust of a public are responsible for 58.7% variation in a public's willingness to adopt AI-powered healthcare system. In addition to this, it was also uncovered that both cognitive ($p = 0.001$, $\beta = 0.425$) and affective trust ($p = 0.001$, $\beta = 0.326$) had a positive and significant effect on public's willingness to adopt AI-powered healthcare system. These outcomes of path analysis brought support for Hypothesis 7 and Hypothesis 8. Furthermore, the value of R^2 computed with respect to cognitive trust was 0.569, which uncovers that 56.9% variation in cognitive trust of a public with respect to AI-powered healthcare system is explained by expertise, performance and reputation. Additionally, it was also uncovered that these factors – expertise ($p = 0.001$, $\beta = 0.312$), product performance ($p = 0.001$, $\beta = 0.122$), and reputation ($p = 0.001$, $\beta = 0.268$) – had a positive and statistically significant relationship with the affective trust of a public with respect to AI-powered healthcare system. These outcomes of path analysis brought support for Hypotheses 1, 2 and 3. Lastly, the R^2 value of 0.541 relating to affective trust of public regarding AI-powered healthcare system uncovered that 54.1% variation in affective trust of public regarding AI-powered healthcare system is caused due to reputation, benevolence and integrity dimensions. Since the p-value with respect to reputation and integrity were less than 0.05, a statistically significant relationship between reputation, integrity and affective trust was concluded. These outcomes of path analysis brought support for Hypotheses 4 and 5. Finally it was also observed that benevolence is not significantly associated with the affective trust of a public with respect to AI-powered healthcare system. Thus Hypothesis 6 was not supported in this study.

TABLE 10.4
Results of Path Analysis

Hypothesis	Path	Estimate	t-Statistics	P-Value	Remark
H1	Expertise → Cognitive trust	0.312	3.217	0.001	Supported
H2	Performance → Cognitive trust	0.122	2.365	0.001	Supported
H3	Reputation → Cognitive trust	0.268	3.116	0.001	Supported
H4	Reputation → Affective trust	0.125	2.204	0.001	Supported
H5	Integrity → Affective trust	0.032	3.098	0.006	Supported
H6	Benevolence → Affective trust	−0.199	1.987	0.181	Not Supported
H7	Cognitive trust → Willingness	0.425	6.589	0.001	Supported
H8	Affective trust → Willingness	0.326	4.254	0.001	Supported

Source: Compiled from AMOS output.

10.5 CONCLUSION

Results of our study brought certain affirmative evidence supporting the hypothesized relationship between components of trust and public's willingness to use AI-powered healthcare system. These findings of our study are also in line with the findings of previous studies done in the context of human-technology relationship. This paper concluded that both cognitive and affective trust have an affirmative effect on the public's willingness to adopt AI-powered healthcare services which substantiates the findings of past studies done in this context. As per the finding of this study, it was also uncovered that cognitive trust results are the better predictor of a public's decision to adopt an AI-powered healthcare system in comparison to the affective trust. In light of the cognitive judgement the public may perceive services to be reliable. Thus, we can arrive at a conclusion that the higher the publics' cognitive trust in the AI-powered healthcare system, the more likely eagerness to pick this service will rise. Furthermore, results of our study also revealed that expertise of the healthcare service provider over AI, product performance and reputation of the AI-powered healthcare service provider has an encouraging effect on the cognitive trust of the beneficiaries of AI-powered healthcare services. This result substantiates the findings of previous studies done in the context of online health consultation adoption. The results of the study also uncovered that expertise and reputation are the stoutest predictor of cognitive trust. Affective trust of a public has emerged as the second important predictor of public's decision to adopt AI-powered healthcare services. Two major determinants of affective trust, namely reputation and integrity, have a positive and significant relationship with it, but the third element, benevolence, has no effect on affective trust. Thus it can be inferred that in order to boost the public's willingness to AI-powered healthcare services, the service providers should emphasize developing a good reputation and integrity.

The significant limitation of this investigation is that it is restricted to the opinion of 462 respondents of India, making it hard to generalize its outcomes. Also, this study has utilized a judgemental sampling technique. This investigation is a cross-sectional examination for which essential information was gathered distinctly during the period August–December 2020. Another significant limitation of this study is that it does exclude those respondents who have not experienced the AI-powered healthcare system. This study has just underscored on investigating the directing impact of 'trust' on the willingness of publics to use AI-powered healthcare system. Finally, opinion relating to a particular AI-powered healthcare service provider isn't collected, so in future, a particular healthcare service provider might be considered for the comparable sort of study.

Thus, future investigation may go through a longitudinal strategy to accompany a robust finding. In future comparative sort of studies can be directed utilizing moderately larger sample size chosen utilizing random sampling technique. Comparative studies can be done between the opinion of user's and non-user of AI-powered healthcare system incorporating few other factors into the model as moderator or mediator of the relationship between trust and willingness to use AI-powered healthcare system. Consideration of these factors may bring new dimensions into the study.

CONFLICT OF INTEREST

There is no conflict of interests.

FUNDING

There is no funding support.

DATA AVAILABILITY

Not applicable.

REFERENCES

1. R. Mitchell, J. Michalski and T. Carbonell, *An artificial intelligence approach*, Berlin: Springer, 2013.
2. T. Davenport and R. Kalakota, "The potential for artificial intelligence in healthcare," *Future Healthcare Journal*, vol. 6, no. 2, p. 94, 2019.
3. O. Asan, A. Bayrak and A. Choudhury, "Artificial intelligence and human trust in healthcare: focus on clinicians," *Journal of Medical Internet Research*, vol. 22, no. 6, p. 15154, 2020.
4. C. Chinmay, "Computational approach for chronic wound tissue characterization," *Informatics in Medicine Unlocked*, vol. 17, no. 1, pp. 1–10, 2019.
5. A. Kishor, C. Chakraborty and W. Jeberson, "A novel fog computing approach for minimization of latency in healthcare using machine learning," *International Journal of Interactive Multimedia and Artificial Intelligence*, vol. 1, pp. 1–11, 2020.

6. K. Gurumurthy and A. Mukherjee, "The bass model: A parsimonious and accurate approach to forecasting mortality caused by COVID-19," *International Journal of Pharmaceutical and Healthcare Marketing*, vol. 14, no. 3, pp. 349–360, 2020.

7. S. Dhawan, C. Chakraborty, J. Frnda, R. Gupta, A. Rana and S. Pani, "SSII: Secured and high-quality steganography using Intelligent hybrid optimization algorithms for IoT," *IEEE Access*, vol. 9, pp. 16–21, 2021.

8. Y. Agarwal, M. Jain, S. Sinha and S. Dhir, "Delivering high-tech, AI-based healthcare at Apollo Hospitals," *Global Business and Organizational Excellence*, vol. 39, no. 2, pp. 20–30, 2020.

9. A. Gupta, C. Chakraborty and B. Gupta, "Secure transmission of EEG data using watermarking algorithm for the detection of epileptic seizures," *Traitement du Signal, IIETA*, vol. 38, no. 2, pp. 473–479, 2021.

10. K. Belcher, "From $600 M to $6 billion. Artificial intelligence systems poised for dramatic market expansion in healthcare," 5 January 2016. Available: https://ww2.frost.com/news/press-releases/600-m-6-billion-artificial-intelligence-systems-poised-dramatic-market-expansion-healthcare/. [Accessed 25 December 2020].

11. NITI Aayog, "National strategy for artificial intelligence," NITI Aayog Government of India New Delhi 2018.

12. V. Chellaiyan, A. Nirupama and N. Taneja, "Telemedicine in India: Where do we stand?," *Journal of Family Medicine and Primary Care*, vol. 8, no. 6, p. 1872–1876, 2019.

13. C. Meske and E. Bunde, "Transparency and trust in human-AI-interaction: The role of model-agnostic explanations in computer vision-based decision support," in *Artificial Intelligence in HCI*, Copenhagen, Denmark, 2020.

14. E. Glikson and A. Woolley, "Human trust in artificial intelligence: Review of empirical research," *Academy of Management Annals*, vol. 14, no. 2, pp. 627–660, 2020.

15. K. Manpreet, Z. Mohammad, G. Shikha, N. Abdulfattah, C. Chinmay and K. Subhendu, "MBCP: Performance analysis of large-scale mainstream blockchain consensus protocols," *IEEE Access*, vol. 9, pp. 1–14, 2021.

16. S. Arindam, Z. Mohammad, M. Moirangthem, N. Abdulfatta, C. Chinmay and K. Subhendu, "Artificial neural synchronization using nature inspired whale optimization," *IEEE Access*, vol. 9, pp. 1–14, 2021.

17. W. Fan, J. Liu, S. Zhu and P. Pardalos, "Investigating the impacting factors for the healthcare professionals to adopt artificial intelligence-based medical diagnosis support system (AIMDSS)," *Annals of Operations Research*, vol. 294, no. 1, p. 567–592, 2018.

18. R. Mayer, J. Davis and F. Schoorman, "An integrative model of organizational trust," *Academy of Management Review*, vol. 20, no. 3, pp. 709–734, 1995.

19. A. Bauman and R. Bachmann, "Online consumer trust: Trends in research," *Journal of Technology Management & Innovation*, vol. 12, no. 2, pp. 68–79, 2017.

20. O. Gillath, T. Ai, M. Branicky, S. Keshmiri, R. Davison and R. Spaulding, "Attachment and trust in artificial intelligence," *Computers in Human Behavior*, vol. 115, no. 1, p. 106607, 2021.

21. Y. Wan, Y. Zhang and M. Yan, "What influences patients' willingness to choose in online health consultation? An empirical study with PLS–SEM," *Industrial Management & Data Systems*, vol. 120, no. 12, pp. 2423–2446, 2020.

22. B. Božič, S. Siebert and G. Martin, "A grounded theory study of factors and conditions associated with customer trust recovery in a retailer," *Journal of Business Research*, vol. 109, no. 1, pp. 440–448, 2020.

23. D. Johnson and K. Grayson, "Cognitive and affective trust in service relationships," *Journal of Business Research*, vol. 58, no. 4, pp. 500–507, 2005.

24. Y. Xie and S. Peng, "How to repair customer trust after negative publicity: The roles of competence, integrity, benevolence, and forgiveness," *Psychology & Marketing*, vol. 26, no. 7, pp. 572–589, 2009.

25. F. Gille, A. Jobin and M. Ienca, "What we talk about when we talk about trust: Theory of trust for AI in healthcare," *Intelligence-Based Medicine*, vol. 1–2, no. 1, p. 100001, 2020.

26. X. Zhang, M. Malik, Y. Cui and X. Peng, "How to use apology and compensation to repair competence-versus integrity-based trust violations in e-commerce," *Electronic Commerce Research and Applications*, vol. 40, no. 1, p. 100945, 2020.

27. J. Zhao, S. Ha and R. Widdows, "Building trusting relationships in online health communities," *Cyberpsychology, Behavior, and Social Networking*, vol. 16, no. 9, pp. 650–657, 2013.

28. J. Grossnickle, *The handbook of online marketing research: knowing your customer using the Net*, New York: McGraw-Hill, 2001.

29. C. Judd, E. Smith and L. Kiddler, *Research methods in social relations*, Bloomington: Holt, Rinehart, and Winston, 1991.

30. D. McAllister, "Affect-and cognition-based trust as foundations for interpersonal cooperation in organizations," *Academy of Management Journal*, vol. 38, no. 1, pp. 24–59, 1995.

31. J. Hair, W. Black, B. Babin, R. Anderson and R. Tatham, *Multivariate data analysis*, 7th ed., New Jersey: Prentice Hall, 2010.

32. S. Sharma, R. Durand and O. Gur-Arie, "Identification and analysis of moderator variables," *Journal of Marketing Research*, vol. 18, no. 3, pp. 291–300, 1981.

33. H. Kaiser, "An index of factorial simplicity," *Psychometrika*, vol. 39, no. 1, pp. 31–36, 1974.

34. A.B. Costello and J.W. Osborne "Practical assessment, research & evaluation," *The Journal of Consumer Marketing*, vol. 10, no. 7, pp. 1–9, 2005.

35. J. Nunnaly, *Psychometric theory*, New York: McGraw-Hill, 1978.

36. R.P. Bagozzi and Y. Yi, "Specification, evaluation, and interpretation of structural equation models," *Journal of the Academy of Marketing Science*, vol. 40, pp. 8–34, 2012.

37. J.F. Hair, W.C. Black, B.J. Babin, R.E. Anderson and R.L. Tatham, *Multivariate data analysis*, Upper Saddle River, NJ: Pearson Prentice Hall, 2010.

38. J.F. Hair, W.C. Black, B.J. Babin, R.E. Anderson and R.L. Tatham *Multivariate data analysis*, Upper Saddle River, NJ: Pearson Prentice Hall, 2006.

11 Role of Artificial Intelligence-Based Technologies in Healthcare to Combat Critical Diseases

Abhinay Thakur and Ashish Kumar
Lovely Professional University, Phagwara, India

CONTENTS

11.1 INTRODUCTION

Artificial intelligence (AI) is more than just a technology; it is a set of capabilities. AI is steadily assuming control of the healthcare infrastructure. It automates the mechanized health system, wherein humans execute regular work tasks in clinical

DOI: 10.1201/9781003247128-11

practice to maintain physicians and health resources (Bohr and Memarzadeh, 2020; Chandrasekaran and Fernandes, 2020). There are an estimated 6,000–8,000 recognized infrequent diseases, including an estimated 400 million human beings worldwide suffering from all of these diseases. This is estimated that it will take 5–10 years to cure an infrequent disease. As a consequence, patients suffering from infrequent diseases must expend a significant period of time, commitment and economic assets in order to obtain a precise treatment. 3Billion, a biotech company that provides DNA diagnosis facilities for infrequent diseases confirmed that AI was used to diagnose approximately 1,200 patients with rare diseases. Moreover using AI for health remediation, 7,000 rare diseases could be tested that impact over 300 million people globally. A recently medicated physician was given a distinct diagnosis by a doctor than the AI-based technique recommended. "Since the healthcare staffs are not having expertise in all ailments, they should concentrate solely only on minor diseases being familiar with," says the CEO of 3Billion. Throughout this time, the patient may lose time transiting from hospital to hospital for 'diagnosis explorations' (Omoruan et al., 2009). It's a challenge faced by people with rare infections all across the world. The ability of a doctor to care for a significant number of people is constrained. AI can safeguard thousands of thousands of lives globally if it is used in healthcare.

Rapid technological developments, particularly in the fields of AI and robotics, can help supplement the healthcare industry (Gerke et al., 2020). AI and robotics in healthcare are rapidly evolving, particularly for early diagnosis and medical applications, as shown in Figure 11.1. At the same time, AI has become more potent. It

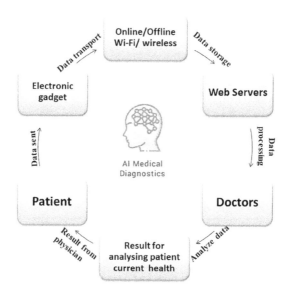

FIGURE 11.1 Schematic representation of the m-health scenario based on AI functionality.

empowers them to perform tasks that humans do often more effectively, effortlessly and at a lower cost. Nowadays, numerous entrepreneurs (for example, Freenome, a San Francisco-based AI genomics biotech firm; Recursion Therapeutics in Lake City or Cam at Israel and Benevolent AI in the United Kingdom) should use AI-based technologies to provide healthcare solutions and services. The most widely used AI application in the healthcare sector is IBM's 'Watson for Oncology', which assists doctors by proposing therapeutic targets. The foremost goal of AI-based health-related applications is to investigate the co-relations among treatment and diagnosis methods, plus clinical care. Prognosis, therapeutic protocol advancement, drug advancement, precision treatment, and hospital care and management are all examples of how AI programs are being used (Omoruan et al., 2009). For disease identification and cure, AI algorithms could be utilized in evaluating the huge quantity of data from electronic medical data. AI algorithms for medical care have been created by large technology corporations such as Google and Microsoft. AI has the potential to significantly enhance patient care while also lowering healthcare costs. Some of these technologies, such as machine learning are commonly utilized in healthcare. Machine learning is a subset in which you train models utilizing pre-existing data so when someone feeds the data that you are using for testing, it could recognize the test input based on prior learning. Machine learning is a type of AI Technology often being utilized widely. Furthermore, healthcare institutions are turning to AI technologies to help with administrative interventions which decrease costs, improve patient satisfaction and meet staff and workplace standards. The US government has committed to investing billions in AI in medical care (Mahomed 2020). Businesses are developing solutions to aid healthcare executives in raising utilization, decreasing patient admission, reducing service time and optimizing personnel levels in order to improve corporate operations.

This chapter aims to provide a critical overview on the efficacious role of artificial intelligence-based technologies being used in the healthcare industry against severe diseases such as cancer detection, monitoring, diagnosis and prevention. The role of medical imaging, deep learning following ANN, machine learning in the effective detection of heart failure and related issues have been discussed. The major influence of digital health transformation using AI and blockchain has been discussed with a view on recent literature. The applications of AI in the current pandemic COVID-19 have been deeply enlightened with an exploration of industrial innovations in the field of AI and several challenges and future perspective related to it.

11.2 WHAT AI CAN DO FOR HEALTH

Artificial intelligence in medical and healthcare infrastructure is now a possibility. Image analysis is becoming more sophisticated owing to AI-based devices. Deep learning algorithms are presently utilized in radiography to detect breast cancer, computed tomography (CT) to diagnose colon cancer, chest radiographs to recognize pulmonary nodules, and MRI to segment brain tumours and diagnose neurologic illnesses like Alzheimer's disease. Dermatologists can use algorithms to help them make more accurate diagnoses, such as detecting 95% of melanoma cancers using large datasets of medical pictures (Deepa et al., 2021; Laï et al., 2020). In radiology, AI provides an instantaneous privilege by smoothing and expediting processes that allow for traditional imaging interpretation, although it is on track to do even more, resulting in more specific and reliable illness understanding. In the coming years, anticipating the prognosis of cancer from imaging data might become standard practice. It might contribute to a more precise understanding of illness status, such as prediction of progression of the disease relying on previously underutilized imaging data. AI vastly simplifies image reconstruction using imaging data and radiological monitoring. Apart from that, critical quantities and characteristics could be determined with greater precision and speed. Lung nodules and tumour foci could be properly evaluated, lung capacities can be computed instantly, and calcium scoring can be expedited. Unwanted hospital visits are reduced as AI systems remotely monitor a patient's ailments as well as send information to physicians mostly when patient care is required. It can also relieve medical practitioners of some of their responsibilities. By minimizing visits, AI can save nurses up to 20% of their time (Kasperbauer, 2021). Individual patients will benefit from the advances as well as healthcare systems as a whole. Innovative digital-technology-based solutions can help facilitate changes in the organization of healthcare and long-term healthcare services. AI and supercomputing, according to the European Commission, "provide new prospects to change healthcare systems." Nina Schwalbe and Brian Wahl (2020) in their article, discussed the potential of AI for future global health by stating some known facts. They asserted that the global health society, along with several significant donor organizations, has become progressively aware of the importance of tackling these concerns in order to ensure that populations in middle and lower-income countries benefited from advances in digital health and AI. Since 2015, several global meetings have occurred. The World Health Assembly passed a resolution on digital technology for universal healthcare in May 2018. The UN Secretary-High-Level General's Committee on Digital Cooperation suggested in 2019 that 'by 2030, each individual must have accessible direct exposure to digital networks, and also digitally facilitated the health and financial assistance, as methods of making a significant participation to the achievement of the SDGs'.

11.2.1 PREVENTION AND DIAGNOSIS USING AI

In the healthcare industry, AI is progressively being used to create treatment regimens for patients. AI can develop greater techniques for the treatment of patients and assessing treatment programmes by studying data from prior patients. AI can spot indicators of disease more precisely and quickly with the usage of medical imagery like CT, MRI, X-rays, ultrasonography, etc. It benefits patients by allowing for a more precise diagnosis of disease and more specific therapy options. Watson, IBM's AI system, has recently gotten a lot of press for its capacity to specialize in precision medicine, particularly early cancer detection (Vatandsoost and Litkouhi, 2019; Kassam and Kassam, 2020; Lee and Yoon, 2021). Various types of AI approaches, such as neural network models, supporting vector machines and decisions planes are being utilized to diagnose various diseases. ANN (Artificial neural network) exhibited greater accuracy in identifying diabetes and CVD. Cancer, encephalitis, cardiac failures, brain tumours, lung diseases or seizures, renal failure, liver fibrosis, and a variety of other infectious disorders are all successfully diagnosed as a result of this well-known factor. People can quickly find information about their symptoms on the Internet due to the advancement of diagnostic procedures and systems; assuming that one does not become deceived by ordinary symptoms and concludes that it might be so-and-so sickness, but rather sees a doctor as soon as the symptoms become severe. Practitioners now often prescribe either an antibiotic or a tranquilizer depending on the patient's scenario in order to stabilize their health for a set amount of time. Some infections, such as meningitis, must be treated right away rather than waiting for serious symptoms to appear because it should be diagnosed promptly and accurately using a CT scan and lumbar biopsy to determine if it is induced by virus or bacteria. Machine learning is being used in diagnoses with automated systems using many data sources like CT, MRI, genomes and proteome, patient information, or even written medical document records to identify a disease or its progression. AI systems will be critical in distinguishing between healthy, malignant, and cancerous lesions/patterns, allowing doctors to make inferences based on the prognosis. Ahn et al. (2021) remarked how AI may be used to diagnose and cure liver disorders. Machine learning algorithms (MLA) featuring superior diagnostic ability and the capability to find novel biomarkers could be developed using advanced molecular analysis from multi-omics investigations. The Cirrhosis Risk Score, constituting seven single nucleotide polymorphisms was found to be better for clinical criteria in forecasting cirrhosis progression when applied to genome-wide sequencing of 420 HCV individuals. Reduced Error Pruning Tree study of HCV patients' genome sequencing found the IL28B SNP as a stronger marker of advanced fibrosis than FIB-4 or APRI. An SVM study of the spectrum variations among regular and HBV serum revealed 100% sensibility, 98% diagnostic efficiency and 95% selectivity for HBV diagnosis by Raman spectroscopy.

Patel et al. (2021) presented their findings in order to educate medical professionals on the essential features of artificial intelligence in order to minimize the emergence of AI-enabled technological advancements while demonstrating how machine learning might improve the treatment of neurological illnesses. They discovered that neurology is currently confronted with several obstacles in terms of diagnostic and treatment options. This includes everything from basic issues like identifying healthy sleep cycles to more sophisticated concerns including early detection and shortening the time it takes to recover from an acute ischaemic stroke. Integrating numerous epileptic features and inter-observer variability in interpreting EEG, or diagnosing unusual types of epilepsy, also preventing sudden unexpected death in epilepsy. Urvish et al. focused on machine learning terms to be an important part of AI (MI). In patients suffering from unidentified TSS (wake-up strokes), Machine learning (ML) has demonstrated that it predicts stroke risk one year after a mild stroke and is a better substitute for the existing DWI–FLAIR mismatch, assisting physicians in developing better treatment options. Smart devices including apps, as well as more accurate handheld electrocardiograph recorders, have been used to evaluate heart rate variability, as well as screening for asymptomatic atrial fibrillation, that effectively prevents embolic stroke.

Similarly, Zhang et al. (2021) demonstrated the value of AI by presenting an article on the use of chest radiography to diagnose coronavirus illness 2019 pneumonia. CV19-Net, a deep neural network, was investigated on chest radio imaging in persons with and without symptoms of COVID-19 pneumonia in this observational investigation. Between February 1, 2020, and May 30, 2020, patients having positive RTC-PR findings for SARS-2 and observations positive for pneumonia were enrolled in chest radiographs positive for COVID-19. The CV19-Net and three different thoracic radiologists evaluated CV19-Net's performance using a spontaneously selected test sample set of 500 chest radio imaging in 500 patients. This complied with a sensitivity of 88% (95% CI: 87, 89) and a high accuracy of 79% (95% CI: 77, 80) when using a high-sensitivity operating threshold, or sensitivity of 78% (95% CI: 77, 79) and a specificity of 89% when using a low-sensitivity operating threshold (95% CI: 88, 90). CV19-Net surpassed competent thoracic radiology in distinguishing coronavirus infection 2019-related pneumonia from various forms of pneumonia.

11.2.2 Monitoring and Detection of Diseases

Patient monitoring is essential in hospitalized patients, operating rooms, nursing homes, and cardiac wards, wherein clinical verdict is determined in seconds. Routine monitoring equipment creates a tremendous amount of data in such high-acuity scenarios, which presents an excellent potential for AI-assisted alarm systems. A cardiac arrest model was formulated utilizing vital signs and the Revised Early Warning Score. Cardiac arrest, transfers to the critical care unit, and death can all be predicted using demographics, test results, and vital signs. Furthermore, a comprehensible machine-learning framework can help anaesthesiologists anticipate hypoxia all through surgery. This shows that raw patient-monitoring data might be effectively utilized with deep learning algorithms to minimize information overloading and alert overloading while allowing more efficient diagnostic prediction and timely decision-making (Ullah et al., 2020). Nowadays, several researchers such as Chakraborty (2019) present an automated diagnostic method for continual chronic wound status assessment, that is critical for effective wound care and especially advantageous for the elderly, in order for physicians to make medication decisions. In his article, he proposed fuzzy c-means clustering enabling wound image segmentation, where he combined standard computational learning algorithms like Nave Bayesian (NB), Decision Tree (DT), Random Forest (RF) and Linear Discriminant Analysis (LDA). These methods are helpful in determining the percentage of injured tissue in a segmented zone. The suggested methodology yielded a 93.75% total efficiency, while he achieved 84.29%, 85.67%, and 78.66% efficiency and accuracy respectively by employing the Random Forest scheme with LDA, Decision Tree and Nave Bayesian, respectively, using manual segmentation as ground truth. Kwon et al. (2020) used electrocardiography (ECG) to build and verify an AI system for forecasting pulmonary hypertension (PH). An ensemble neural network was utilized to create and test an AI technique based on a 12-lead ECG output and biographical data using a derivation database in this study. During internal and external validation, the AI system's region of the transmitter operational characteristics graph for recognizing PH was 0.859 and 0.902, respectively. During the follow-up phase, those patients who were classified as having a greater risk by the AI (31.5% vs 5.9%, p 0.001) had a considerably greater risk of getting PH than that of in low-risk group (31.5% vs 5.9%, p 0.001). Using 12-lead and single-lead ECGs, the AI engine demonstrated promising PH detection efficiency. Gupta et al. (2021) created an AI-based method to predict epileptic seizures. They employed IoT in this scenario. The combination of IoT and healthcare systems allows for the resolution of challenges such as security, seizure recognition, and real-time tracking. This study investigates the efficacy of a Bacterial Foraging Optimization (BFO) oriented discrete wavelet transforms – discrete cosine transforms (DWT-DCT) strategy for watermarking two-dimensional EEG data. Peak Signal to Noise Ratio (PSNR) of 49.50 for class Z and 49.61 for class S EEG data, as well as Normalized Cross-Correlation (NCC) of 0.0039 for both classes of EEG data, indicated that watermarking efficiency was satisfactory.

Mansour et al. (2021) presented a disease diagnostic concept for smart healthcare platforms that combines the Internet of things and AI. The key objective of this article is based on the usage of AI and IoT fusion approaches to create a disease detection framework for heart disease and diabetes. Data collecting, preprocessing, categorization, and variable adjustment are all stages of the described model. For disease detection, the suggested method employs a Crow Search Optimization algorithm-based Cascaded Long Short-Term Memory (CSO-CLSTM) model. CSO is used to fine-tune the CLSTM platform's 'weights' and 'bias' factors in order to improve medical data classification. This study also uses the isolation Forest (iForest) technique to reduce outliers. The investigation outcome reported that the CSO-LSTM model had a peak overall accuracy of 96.16% in detecting heart disease and 97.26% in diagnosing diabetes, respectively. As a result, the presented CSO-LSTM model is being employed in smart healthcare services as a disease diagnosis device.

Deepa et al. (2021) suggested a Ridge-Adaline Stochastic Gradient Descent (RASGD) Classifier-based artificial intelligence-based optimization method for early disease prediction. The proposed strategy to improve the regularization of the classification process, RASGD employs weight decay techniques such as minimum absolute shrinkage and assortment operators, as well as regression-based procedures. The RASGD uses an unbounded optimization framework to reduce the classifier's cost value. The original data is pre-processed for generalization using the RASGD, which involved two stages: The min-max method is used for data normalization, while weight decay approaches like the ridges regression algorithms and LASSO are used for feature extraction. The data was then divided into two groups: a test set and a training set, which are each used to create the system and assess the outcomes. The Adaline Stochastic Gradient Descent classifier was used to create an AI-based intelligent platform. With a 92% recognition rate, the Ridge-Adaline Stochastic Gradient Descent classifier outperforms previous approaches. In any healthcare dataset, the proposed model could be utilized to predict disease.

11.2.2.1 Detection of Cancer

Cancer is a serious health issue worldwide, and it is still the second biggest cause of human death. Early identification of cancer may improve the odds of effective therapy and a positive patient fate. Predicting initial cancer and treatment approaches is an important aspect of cancer patients' personalized treatment (Abhinav and Naga Subrahmanyam, 2019; Randhawa and Jackson, 2020). AI is a domain of computer engineering which intends to design algorithms or computer systems that can perform complicated analytical or predictive tasks. Incorporation of AI technology into cancer early screening might increase precision diagnosis, enhance clinical decision-making, and change diagnostics and therapy in the long term. AI technology offers the potential to change a number of aspects of cancer treatment. Forecasting, scanning, assessment, analysis of large data sets, medication discovery and verification in a clinical domain are just a few examples. The ability to diagnose cancer early and with a better likelihood of therapy and cure is made possible by screening tumour targets in both healthy and large populations. Moreover, skin cancer is a severe diagnostic challenge since the deadliest variety, melanoma, is responsible for 75% of skin cancer mortality. Melanoma represents just 3–5% of the 1.5 million per annum skin cancer diagnoses in the United States. Early detection of melanomas is crucial, and since detection can be done on photographic images, there are currently programmes that allow people to submit their phone photographs for dermatological study. Furthermore, the identification of melanomas in screening exams is restricted – primary care physicians have a sensitivity of 40.2% and a specificity of 86.1% (Horgan et al., 2020).

The findings of a previous presentation of automated skin cancer detection that utilized a convolutional neural network algorithm were remarkable. The researchers used photos annotated by over 125,000 dermatologists from 18 distinct Internet resources as a training set. Biopsies were used to label two thousand of the photos. All of the dermatologist-labelled photos were used to run the experiment, which included 757 disease classes and nearly 2000 disorders. The taxonomy's highest tiers. The method has 72.1% accuracy in identifying at the first-level I (3 subgroups: benign, malignant and non-neoplastic) when compared to 66.0 and 65.56% for two dermatologists. The algorithm's accuracy in categorizing for the 2nd level (nine illness classes) was 55.4%, compared to 53.3% and 55.0% for the two dermatologists. The algorithm's functionality is very probably restricted by the sensitivity and precision with which images in the training sets are labelled.

Ullah et al. (2020) used AI to investigate the early identification and treatment of cancer. They showed how AI precision algorithms may aid precision medicine by selecting the right patient for the optimal treatment at the correct moment. Ki-67, a proliferation marker, is critical for early-stage breast cancer diagnosis, categorization, treatment and prognosis. Automated brain tumour segmentation techniques involve computer algorithms that produce tumour segmentation and are currently a useful diagnostic tool in precision medicine. For six different genetic mutations in lung cancer (EGFR, STK11, FAT1, KRAS, TP53 and SETBP1), gene mutation predictions and confirmation utilizing raw input digitized histopathology yield encouraging results. Tumour protein P53, KRAS mutations and the detection rate of these markers could be utilized to diagnose cancer at an earlier stage. Using AI, clinicians have established an early signature that can forecast the efficiency of cancer treatment.

Dlamini et al. (2020) highlighted next-generation sequencing (NGS) platforms that have transformed precision oncology's prospects. They discovered that NGS has various clinical uses, including risk prediction, early disease monitoring, genomic and medical imaging diagnosis, precise prediction, biomarker discovery, and therapeutic target acquisition for innovative drug discovery. NGS generates huge datasets that necessitate the use of sophisticated bioinformatics tools to examine the therapeutically useful data. Cancer diagnosis and prognosis prediction are improved using NGS and high-resolution medical imaging due to these AI applications. With recent technological advancements, it is projected that NGS systems would have lower costs, better sensitivity, and faster high throughput data available for diagnostic and therapeutic applications. AI has had a substantial influence on healthcare and precise chemotherapy, and it will continue to do so.

11.3 ROLE OF MEDICAL IMAGING AND DEEP LEARNING

Medical imaging is a set of procedures for creating visual depictions of the interiors of the human body for clinical examination and surgical treatment. Medical imaging, which aims to expose underlying structures concealed by the muscles and bones for evaluating and treating diseases, serves an essential role in clinical diagnosis, therapy, and therapeutic applications. AI is utilized in medicine to identify diagnoses and make treatment suggestions. Artificial neural networks (ANNs) are utilized in medical diagnosis to obtain the diagnosis outcome. In the healthcare profession, ANN gives an exceptional level of performance. For instance, work done by Sarkar et al. (2021) wherein for the production of the key exchange protocol, a whale optimization-based neural synchronization has been presented. A unique neural network design termed the Double Layer Tree Parity Machine (DLTPM) is proposed for brain synchronization. Dual DLTPMs use the same input but have dissimilar weight vectors, which they upgrade by trading output using neural learning methods. It achieves absolute synchronization in a few stages, and the masses of the two DLTMs are equal. The unique data is generated using these identical weights. Furthermore, there has been relatively little research on using a nature-inspired technique to optimize neural weight vectors for faster neural synchronization. ANN is being used in a variety of medical fields, including disease detection, biochemical tests, imaging analysis, and so forth. In recent years, ANNs have been used in medical image processing to analyze medical images. Medical picture object identification and classification, healthcare segmentation techniques and medical data processing are the major elements of medical image processing that rely heavily on ANNs (Gille et al., 2020; Macrae, 2019). Ultrasonography, MRI, interventional radiology, CT, spectroscopy, cardiograph, and other AI imaging technologies are used to investigate various aspects of the human body. Due to its high superior efficiency in categorization and pattern classification, NN algorithms and approaches have been applied in medical image processing in recent decades. Image preparation (creation and preservation), segment, recognition, and identification are all applications of NN approaches. Throughout the clinical analysis, image segmentation is critical for defining the boundaries of organs and tumours, as well as for visualizing human tissues. Medical image segmentation is critical for clinical data processing, diagnosis, and implementations, necessitating the use of strong, dependable, and adaptive segmentation approaches. Edge detection and image segmentation are widely employed following image processing in multi-step medical image analysis and could be used as an alternative preprocessing phase.

Subiksha and Ramakrishnan (2021) presented a deep learning AI-based platform of smart healthcare data analytics. They discovered the optimal features and classification architecture for a Deep Learning Healthcare Diagnosis System to detect endothelial dysfunction. The deep learning platform shares prototype architecture for data analysis generalizations that is available on the Internet and maybe improved by changing parameters. Employing semi-supervised machine learning approaches, variables in EHR are minimized depending on their type of association and assessed by ML techniques classifier, which achieves 97% accuracy and surpasses other current prediction models, improving illness prediction efficiency. Briganti and Le Moine (2020) discussed a long-awaited meta-analysis that contrasted the effectiveness of the deep learning model in respect to radiologists in the research area of imaging-based diagnosis: While deep learning appears to be quite as effective as a radiologist in diagnosis, the authors point out that 99% of studies have been found to be erroneous; moreover, just one-thousandth of the publications evaluated and verified their findings. Such findings highlight the importance of conducting broad clinical trials to validate AI-based technology.

11.4 ROLE OF MACHINE LEARNING (ML)

ML is a quantitative method of adapting a model to inputs in order to derive insights from the data using training models. According to a Deloitte survey of 1,100 US managers whose organizations already were working with AI in 2018, 63% of those polled used ML in their company operations. It's a broad technique that is at the root of a lot of AI approaches, and it comes in a variety of forms. The foremost common use of classical ML in medicine is precision medicine, which involves estimation of the treatments that are prone to have an effective impact on a patient based on certain patient attributes and the therapy situation. A substantial number of ML and precision medicine applications require a trained database in which the end parameter (for example, sickness onset) is defined; this is known as supervised learning (Alloghani et al., 2020). Kishor et al. (2020) presented an innovative fog computing methodology for minimizing latency in medical care utilizing ML, wherein they portray an innovative Intelligent Multimedia Data Segregation (IMDS) strategy implemented in the fog computing setting which separates multimedia data as well as the prototype that employed to determine the overall latency. They obtained a 92% model classification precision, a 95% decrease in latency when comparing to the previous model, and increased the reliability of e-healthcare services using the simulated results.

Guo et al. (2020) discussed heart failure readmission, diagnosis and mortality forecasting by employing ML systems. In their work, they used varied factors collected through EHR data, such as demographics, clinical notes, labs, and imaging data, to generate a series of MLA for HF diagnosis and treatment planning, and they reached expert-comparable prediction outcomes. From January 2015 to August 2020, they did a comprehensive evaluation of the published studies by searching the PubMed online databases for pertinent papers. After filtering matches from the previous two screenings, 374 unique articles were found. There were 335 publications published after 2015 that were relevant. Clinical EHR data has a variety of characteristics, such as a changeable data interface, data noise, the evaluation of several components of illnesses, and the prevalence of unstable HF compared to control study group samples. Model prediction dependability could be revolutionized by new machine learning algorithms for systematic data collection, integration, and predictions.

Using AI for the COVID-19 chest x-ray treatment, Borkowski (2020) proved the utility of AI and ML methods in evaluating COVID-19 CXRs. They used the Custom Vision automatic image segmentation and object recognition system to initially train it to distinguish instances of COVID-19 from pneumonia caused by other pathogenesis and also usual lung CXRs. Then researchers put the model to the experiment on patients from Tampa's James A. Haley Veterans Hospital. In distinguishing the three cases, the programme attained 100% sensitivity (recall), 95% specificity, 97% accuracy, 91% positive predictive value (precision), and 100% negative predictive value. They then proceeded to construct a website that might help with COVID-19 CXR diagnosis using a trained ML model. Both desktop and mobile gadgets can access the website. A healthcare practitioner can take a CXR snapshot or send the picture file using a mobile phone. The machine learning system could evaluate if the patient had non-COVID-19, COVID-19, or a healthy lung condition.

11.5 DIGITAL HEALTH TRANSFORMATION USING AI

Medical care and inpatient hospital care have deeply maintained the potential of being mostly administered digitally, but the digital transformation has indeed been moderate gradually. The truth of system inertia and delayed widespread adoption based on a variety of hurdles relating to reimbursements, licensing, and human factors have to temper expectations regarding digital transformation. Digital health encompasses a wide range of topics, including AI, the Internet of things, eHealth, and telemedicine, as well as the investigation and application of Big Data. It also opens up new opportunities for providing care to a bigger population.

Digital health (e-health), according to the WHO, could play a 'distinctive and crucial role in attaining global healthcare cover' in many countries as it 'expands the possibilities, accountability, and ease of access of healthcare and medical data, extending the massive community deserving of primary healthcare assistance and providing advancement and improvements.' Jones et al. (2020) provides an overview of their research into the influence of digital health technology in addressing issues of healthcare accessibility and affordability. The US National Institutes of Health (NIH) Research Plan on Rehabilitation, launched in 2017, recognizes the importance of information and communications technology (ICT) to revitalize healthcare remediation with cell phone apps, which include: 'illness tracking, real-time availability to data about patients, traversing the society', according to their paper. The emergence of digital health applications will greatly extend rehabilitation opportunities for persons with impairments as the ICT industry continues to progress. Mobile health solutions have been released by major ICT firms and a slew of health-focused start-ups to enable the recording, preservation, and analysis of user health, activity, and metadata as well as management platforms to promote community and self-based activities other rehabilitation practices (e.g., Datu).

Palanica et al. (2020) described a quite precious feature of digital therapeutics that distinguishes it from conventional medications or therapeutic: the use of AI to observe and anticipate specific health symptoms and data in a responsive diagnostic feedback mechanism via digital biological markers, resulting in a highly precise medicine strategy to healthcare. Digital therapeutics, in combination with AI enable more efficient clinical monitoring and treatment at the societal scale for a range of health diseases and groups. This important distinction between digital medicines and other types of therapeutics allows for a more personalized kind of healthcare which proactively responds to patients' unique clinical requirements, objectives, and behaviours. AI technologies allow for better effective and convenient patient symptom diagnosis and monitoring, as well as more time for clinicians to interact with their patient on sensitive, sympathetic, and personal topics. In a way that no conventional medicines, digitized or not, can attain, digital therapeutics combined with AI may adjust in real-time to the patient's current and expected health status. Similarly, Khemasuwan et al. (2020) presented a review to assist pulmonary experts as well as other individuals with knowledge on the application of AI in lung treatment. They began by explaining AI and some of the prerequisites for ML and artificial intelligence. They subsequently reviewed some of the publications on computer vision in medical imaging, predicting model with ML, and using AI to combat the new severe acute respiratory syndrome-coronavirus-2 pandemic. Furthermore, AI-based statistics enable extremely precise predictive analysis and create the groundwork for true data-driven precision medicine, reducing our need on human resources. As computing power improves, algorithms would be able to absorb and usefully analyse large amounts of data even faster, more precisely, and with less effort than human brains.

In a couple of weeks, the COVID-19 epidemic dramatically altered all of this technology. The potential of digital health technologies to shield patients, clinicians, and the wider community from infection has been widely recognized, resulting in unprecedented adoption of these tools. To facilitate healthcare delivery with minimal physical encounters, several countries have embraced digital-first initiatives, remote monitoring, and telehealth systems. The United Kingdom's primary care has embraced telehealth to a wide extent, implementing a new digital-first method to handle the deliverance of healthcare to the right location. In COVID-19, Peek et al. (2020) addressed their research on digital health and care, emphasizing that data sharing is critical for the digital health system to thrive in this pandemic era. To recreate and afterward potentially anticipate the growth and behaviours of the COVID-19 outbreak, large volumes of data were immediately acquired and collated from a variety of sources, including Facebook, Twitter, local media outlets, and global health data. Apple and Google teamed up to create an app to help people track down others they've met online. This app uses a decentralized strategy, storing data securely on each user's phone.

Additionally, The Internet of things (IoT) is a new digital technology that could be employed in ophthalmology to devise AI. IoT is a region where enormous data is transferred every second (Dhawan et al. 2021). The IoT allows any gadget linked to the Internet to exchange data in a completely automated manner, eliminating the requirement for human-human or human-computer interactions. By integrating imaging data with patient data not only within clinics, but also between health centres in a province or clusters, or even anywhere around the world, the internet of things has the potential to change eye care. AI algorithms or next-generation data analytics could evaluate images and clinical data. One key example is the work of Mansour et al. (2021), where his team proposed an intelligent healthcare system with a revolutionary AI and IoT convergence-based illness diagnosis approach. The main purpose of this paper was to use AI and IoT convergence approaches to create disease prediction models for diabetes and heart disease. Data collecting, processing, categorization, and parameter optimization are all stages of the described model. For disease diagnosis, the suggested method employs a Crow Search Optimization algorithm-based Cascaded Long Short-Term Memory (CSO-CLSTM) paradigm. CSO is used for improving the segmentation of medical information by fine-tuning the 'weights' and 'bias' variables in the CLSTM model. In addition, to minimize outliers, this study used the isolation Forest (iForest) methodology. The CLSTM model's diagnostic findings are greatly improved when CSO is used. The CSO-LSTM model's effectiveness was verified with healthcare data. The reported CSO-LSTM model achieved maximal accuracies of 97.26% and 96.16% in diagnosing diabetes and heart disease, respectively, as during experiments. As a result, the suggested CSO-LSTM model could be used in smart healthcare as a disease diagnostic tool.

11.6   DIGITAL HEALTH TRANSFORMATION USING BLOCKCHAIN

Blockchain is basically an accessible and decentralized database with key features like decentralization, tamper resistance, and transparency. As a result, it has the potential to be utilized as a database to help commodity proprietors recognize and charge resource consumers. A blockchain is a distributed database that stores transactions in a peer-to-peer network safely. Furthermore, it ensures that transactions are both secure and verified. The basic goal of blockchain technology is to enable two individuals to perform safe transactions eliminating the need for a middleman. However apart from blockchain, smart technologies like ML, Internet of Things (IoT), VR technology, and AI have redefined a variety of industries and sectors, including construction, automobiles, computer technology and electronics, aerospace, corporate and financial reporting, finance, defence, and healthcare (AI). The following are some of the advantages of blockchain technology in healthcare data management:

- Health data accuracy
  Medical information about a patient is frequently dispersed among many organizations, medical care facilities, and health insurance companies. To accurately acquire a patient's entire healthcare record, all of a patient's information should be merged in an autonomous approach. It could be achieved by storing all of a patient's health information on blockchain, which ensures that records are always up-to-date, verifiable, and tamper-proof. This enables healthcare providers to provide patients with effective, timely, and appropriate treatment. Healthcare professionals can get a detailed picture of a patient's medical record utilizing blockchain technology. On blockchain, all data is eternal, accessible, verifiable, and safe.
- Health data interoperability
  The capacity to communicate data across systems from various manufacturers is referred to as interoperable. The major portion of EHR/EMR systems have been built on a combination of clinical technology, technological standards, and functionality. Because of these disparities, compiling and transmitting data in a single format is difficult. In some circumstances, EHR systems developed on same platform are not really compatible since they are tailored to a health institution's individual requirements and interests. Transmission messages must be founded on standardized coded info to generate two EHR systems interoperable. However, a critical barrier that restricts the capability to communicate data electronically for patient care is the lack of standardized data. This obstacle can be removed by using a blockchain-based healthcare information administration infrastructure. All EHR/EMRs saved in the blockchain network have the same data coding, making them easily accessible and used by any healthcare professional.
- Health data security
  Many healthcare organizations have been victims of avoidable cyberattacks in the last decade. The large proportion of healthcare organizations depend on hand-operated systems that rely on centralized facilities to transfer digital health records. Because such processes are no longer in use, they can be easily fiddled for malicious purposes. Furthermore, medical records may be destroyed in the case of a catastrophic since standardization is

subject to a single point of failure. Blockchain's security model, which is based on cryptographic principles, could assist to eliminate the danger of data theft or mistreatment. Health data stored on blockchain is also safe from harm caused by disasters or medical facility collapse because the same data is saved in several locations so there is no solitary spot of failure. As previously mentioned, blockchain technology has improved accessibility and interaction among patients and healthcare professionals in the healthcare industry. The influence of blockchain technology on the healthcare industry has been studied by a number of researchers. Veeramakali et al. (2021) presented his insights on a safe healthcare system built on the intelligent Internet of things that uses blockchain technology and an optimal deep learning model. Three important processes are included in the developed framework: secure transactions, hash code encryption, and clinical analysis. For the secure communication of medical data, the ODLSB technique uses the orthogonal particle swarm optimization (OPSO) algorithm. In particular, the neighbourhood indexing sequence (NIS) technique is used to encrypt the hash value. Finally, to identify the ailment, the optimum deep neural network (ODNN) is used as a classification model. The OPSO-DNN model produced superior results during the diagnosis process, with maximum sensitivity (92.75 %), selectivity (91.42 %), and precision (93.68 %).

Similarly, Hasselgren et al. (2021) demonstrated the significance of block chain in enhancing faith in virtual healthcare activities. This research aims to lay a conceptual justification for a sophisticated healthcare system interference which intends to utilize a cryptographically secure facilities for forming and sustaining trust in virtualized care contexts, and to show a proof of concept that meets the necessary requirements based on that theoretical foundation. For the design and assessment of complex intervention research in healthcare, the following framework is used: For technological forecasting, a survey of the literature and expert consultation are required. In a virtualized healthcare environment, this study determined and outlined the critical functional and non-functional needs and standards for improving trust between providers and patients. The use of blockchain technology is the cornerstone of this architecture. The proposed decentralized system provides a novel trust model with an innovative governance structure. A concrete implementation of an Ethereum-based platform called VerifyMed backs up the presented theoretical design principles.

Tanwar et al. (2020) proposed a system design and algorithm for users to use in order to accomplish patient data security and privacy in the EHR system. The development of a blockchain-based EHR sharing system is also outlined. The proposed attempt minimizes the central control of the network as well as a single point of failure. Because no one can change the blockchain, irreversible ledger architecture assures data security. The calliper has been used to analyse the proposed system's efficiency by defining block, block creation duration, endorsement policy, and suggested improvement for evaluation measures such as traffic, bandwidth, and network monitoring. By improving its efficiency, the suggested system's effectiveness was enhanced ×1.75 and its congestion was lowered ×1.5. This highlights the blockchain's utility and importance in a multitude of sectors, indicating that it has the capacity to become the next technological breakthrough to replace present healthcare systems.

Yaqoob et al. (2021) discussed how utilizing blockchain for healthcare data management systems may promote innovations and result in significant benefits. They discussed the major advantages of blockchain technology as well as the potential for the health sector. They noted that while blockchain and AI are two growing concepts on their own, integrating the two can result in increased fuel economy in healthcare data analytics. Blockchain technology may be able to assist in overcoming some of the core difficulties that the healthcare industry faces, such as data quality, transparency, and privacy. Healthcare businesses can use blockchain to record variations in their data in real time, allowing them to make rapid choices without the need for human intervention, owing to AI's ability to enable new analytics. Two major factors that may influence the efficacy of analytics are data quality and interoperability. Blockchain-based healthcare data management helps to address both quality and integration issues, allowing AI solutions to enhance the precision of analytics outputs even further. The healthcare business could be transformed if blockchain and AI are combined. Furthermore, strict laws must be established in order for blockchain technology to be widely adopted in the healthcare industry. Regulations are divided into two categories: restrictive and permissive. An effective policy must establish a balance between these two extremities. The strategy must be written in such a manner that it can meet all of the authorities' goals. It must not be in conflict with government programmes or national legislation. In addition, the strategy should be adaptive enough to reflect both lessons learned and a quickly evolving technical and worldwide landscape. The immense promise of blockchain technology will never be realized unless national regulations that are consistent are enacted.

11.7 AI APPLICATIONS FOR COVID-19

The medical sector is seeking innovative tools to identify and mitigate the transmission of the COVID-19 (Coronavirus) pandemic in such global health disasters. AI becomes a tool for tracking the virus's transmission, identifying high-risk individuals, and assisting in real-time infection management. It may also be able to anticipate death rates by thoroughly analyzing the patients' historical data. Such a technique offers great ability to improve COVID-19 patients' prognosis, therapy, and appropriate decisions as an evidence-based medical aid. Medical imaging methods such as magnetic resonance imaging (MRI) and computed tomography (CT) images of human body components could help AI identify infected individuals.

Mendels et al. (2021) designed and tested smartphone software (xRCovid) that utilizes ML to categorize SARS-CoV-2 serological RDT findings and eliminate reading ambiguity. When contrasted to reading by sight, the app provided 99.3% accuracy across 11 COVID-19 RDT models. The application replaces the ambiguity of optical RDT interpretations with a lower image classification error, giving physicians and laboratory personnel more confidence when utilizing RDTs and allowing patients to self-test. Also, Chandrasekaran and Fernandes (2020) presented a presentation at COVID-19 about the impact of AI on management and prevention. AI is a viable and useful tool for recognizing early coronavirus infections and tracking the status of those who have been infected. It could improve treatment consistency and verdict by developing useful algorithms. AI is useful not only in the treatment of COVID-19 patients, but also in the close monitoring of their health. It might keep track of the COVID-19 outbreak on a variety of levels, notably medical, genomic, and epidemiologic ones. It is beneficial to assist viral research by analyzing the existing data. AI could assist in the creation of effective treatment regimens, preventative initiatives, as well as drug and vaccine formulation. From this analysis we can justify the impact of AI and its components on this epidemic management and also for other previously discussed diseases.

11.8   INDUSTRIAL INNOVATION IN THE FIELD OF AI

Clinical decision support technologies account for a significant proportion of the healthcare industry's AI adoption strategy. ML algorithms improve as additional data is collected, allowing for more reliable responses and suggestions. Many organizations are investigating the possibility of incorporating Big Data into the medical and healthcare sector. Several companies are looking at the business opportunity for data assessment, collecting, maintenance, and analytics technologies, which are major elements of the healthcare industry.

Instances of significant organizations which has made a significant contribution to AI for healthcare applications include:

- IBM's Watson Oncology has been developed with Memorial Sloan Kettering Cancer Center and Cleveland Clinic. To discover potential drug development pathways, IBM is collaborating with CVS Health and Johnson & Johnson on scientific document analytics on AI in chronic illness care. IBM and Rensselaer Polytechnic Institute cooperated on a project called Health Empowerment by Learning, Analytics, and Semantics in May 2017 to examine how AI can help with healthcare.
- Microsoft's Hanover initiative, in collaboration with the Knight Cancer Institute at Oregon Health & Science University, analyses patient records to forecast the safest and potentially successful cancer medication therapy therapeutic possibilities. Two other approaches are medical image processing of cancer and the development of programmable cells.
- Deep learning software was developed by Kheiron Medical to identify breast cancer in mammography.

11.8.1 Types of Commercial-based AI technologies

- Path AI
  PathAI is working on ML systems to help pathologists make better diagnoses. Two of the company's primary considerations include reducing cancer detection errors and developing solutions for customized medical treatment. PathAI has collaborated with pharmaceutical companies like Bristol-Myers Squibb and non-profits like the Bill and Melinda Gates Foundation to broaden their AI technology into other healthcare fields.
- Buoy health
  Buoy health offers an artificial intelligence-powered symptom and therapy analyzer which uses algorithms to detect and cure diseases. A chatbot answers to the patient's ailments, then arise medical feedback before sending all data to the right care depending on the chatbot's assessment. Buoy's AI is used by a number of medicine and healthcare institutes, notably Harvard Medical School, to help prevent and diagnose patients promptly.
- Berg health
  Berg is a diagnostic AI-based biotech technology that tracks diseases to speed up the identification and establishment of innovative treatments. By combining its 'Interrogative Biology' method with traditional R&D, BERG could develop highly efficient treatment possibilities for rare diseases. At the Neuroscience 2018 event, BERG presented their findings on Parkinson's Disease treatment, in which they used AI to establish formerly undiscovered correlations between compounds in the human body.

11.9 CHALLENGES AND FUTURE OUTLOOKS

Although there has been significant development in healthcare, there are numerous problems and drawbacks related to deep learning. The volume of data is one of the most critical aspects in making deep learning work. A neural network requires a large number of network configurations as well as a large amount of data to do this. Typically, the number of parameters required for every neural network must be ten times the average of samples. Relating to safety issues, companies rarely obtain many patients willing to work in providing data in the healthcare profession. Furthermore, comprehending the diversity of diseases in each individual is far more difficult than in other AI disciplines. Other AI domains, such as vision, voice, and languages, will also have pristine, structured data, while healthcare data is imprecise, unpredictable, and inadequate. As AI-based technologies and systems rely on large datasets, ethical issues about data collecting and distribution arise. Since patient records include personal information, it is extremely difficult to communicate and control disease-related data across several systems. This implies that software developers must follow strict secrecy guidelines, which might inhibit AI progress. According to Mohammad Reza Davahli et al. (2021) the biggest challenge is security which is tied to AI systems' harmful and wrong behaviours and suggestions. In response to the requirement to tackle safety

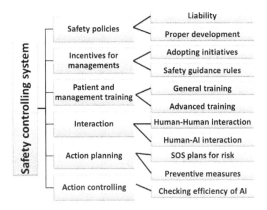

FIGURE 11.2 The first and second level attributes of the SCS.

issues, this study intends to create a safety controlling system (SCS) paradigm to minimize the threat of possible healthcare-related incidents. The framework was built using a multi-attribute value technique (MAVT), which has four symmetrical parts: extracting attributes, producing attribute weights, constructing a rating scale, and summarizing the approach. The framework comprises a number of qualities organized into many layers and could be utilized to validate AI models in hospitals. The SCS's primary first-level aspects are (1) Safety policies; (2) Incentives for clinicians; (3) Clinician and patient training; (4) Communication and interaction; (5) Planning of actions, and (6) Control of actions (Figure 11.2).

As AI is growing rapidly in a variety of industries such as in healthcare, it has the potential to have a significantly positive influence on clinicians and patients as some of its positive aspects have been shown in Figure 11.3. AI could provide far faster and more efficient diagnoses for a larger portion of society due to its potential to collect and evaluate a massive amount of data.

11.10 CONCLUSION

AI, DL and ML may aid us in providing optimal treatment, such as facilitating surgeries and early detection of diseases such as cancer. AI will serve as an enormous component in future health technology. Precision medicine, which is unanimously recognized as a much-required innovation in healthcare, is based on this skill. Researchers estimate that AI would ultimately master diagnosis and therapeutic prescriptions, despite early attempts being tough. As AI advances, it will revolutionize how doctors perceive their patients, expand the possibility for diagnosing and curing diseases, lessen healthcare costs, and improve medical treatment in locations where it is limited. It is one of the fastest-growing technologies, and it has grown in prominence as a result of its distinctive features, as per Manpreet Kaur's article (Kaur et al. 2021). Blockchain is a publicly open database that is distributed across multiple nodes that don't automatically trust one

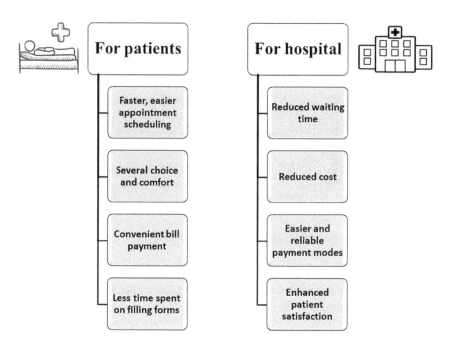

FIGURE 11.3   AI service benefits in accordance to the patients and hospital.

another with reliably based on AI. As these nodes use an append-only database structure, updated information and transactions could only be added to the block-chain. This type of framework needs enhancing for the credibility of AI and it is broadening its usage among individuals at the global level. Without significant organizational investment, growth potential outcomes may be difficult to come by in the future, but there is a great possibility for progressive development in the AI area of healthcare. As per a recent Accenture analysis, AI applications in the healthcare sector do have the capability to save the United States $150 billion per year by 2026. In the coming years, significant equity financing and equity partnerships are expected, with AI in healthcare investment at record levels of $600 million (Q2′18). Particularly in healthcare, machine learning (ML) would become extremely relevant due to its potency to enhance practitioner and clinician efficiency and standard of healthcare, strengthen patient engagement in their very own care and simplify patient access to medical care, expedite the speed and lower the cost of developing new pharmaceutical therapies, and personalize medical treatments by utilizing a data set.

Despite significant advances in AI for image interpretation, the bulk of radiological and pathology imaging will be examined by a machine at some point. Patient communication and medical record collecting are already using voice and language processing, and this evolution is expected to expand. First and foremost, a legislative framework for information dissemination and exchange for AI applications must be established. To improve AI effectiveness in healthcare, real-time data collecting and sharing is essential. Considering 'the higher the information/data reliability, the more trust users would have in the outcomes being generated, minimizing risk in results and boosting potency', data quality is critical. To promote AI innovation, a common infrastructure for exchanging standardized cancer datasets is required. In many healthcare sectors, the most difficult challenge for AI is ensuring its adoption in regular medical practice not if the technology will be sufficiently competent to be useful at all. AI systems should be authorized by authorities, incorporated with EHR systems, regulated to the point that similar items work in a similar way, explained to physicians, funded by publicly or privately insured institutions, and upgraded throughout time in the area in order for successful implementation to occur. These challenges need to be conquered as soon as possible, although it will take much longer than the technological advancement itself. While each AI tool has tremendous value on its own, the greater promise resides in the synergies that can be achieved by combining them across the full patient journey, from diagnosis to treatment to follow-up.

> We always overestimate the change that will occur in the next two years and underestimate the change that will occur in the next ten.
>
> (Bill Gates, 1996)

CONFLICT OF INTEREST

There is no conflict of interest.

FUNDING

There is no funding support.

DATA AVAILABILITY

Not applicable.

REFERENCES

Abhinav, G.V.K.S., and S. Naga Subrahmanyam. 2019. "Artificial Intelligence in Healthcare." *Journal of Drug Delivery and Therapeutics* 9 (5-S): 164–66. doi:10.22270/jddt.v9i5-s.3634.

Ahn, Joseph C., Alistair Connell, Douglas A. Simonetto, Cian Hughes, and Vijay H. Shah. 2021. "Application of Artificial Intelligence for the Diagnosis and Treatment of Liver Diseases." *Hepatology* 73 (6): 2546–63. doi:10.1002/hep.31603.

Alloghani, Mohamed, Dhiya Al-Jumeily, Ahmed J. Aljaaf, Mohammed Khalaf, Jamila Mustafina, and Sin Y. Tan. 2020. "The Application of Artificial Intelligence Technology in Healthcare: A Systematic Review." *International Conference on Applied Computing to Support Industry: Innovation and Technology*: 248–61. doi:10.1007/978-3-030-38752-5_20.

Bohr, Adam, and Kaveh Memarzadeh. 2020. The Rise of Artificial Intelligence in Healthcare Applications. *Artificial Intelligence in Healthcare*. doi:10.1016/b978-0-12-818438-7.00002-2.

Borkowski, Andrew. 2020. "Using Artificial Intelligence for COVID-19 Chest X-Ray Diagnosis." *Federal Practitioner* 37 (9): 398–404. doi:10.12788/fp.0045.

Briganti, Giovanni, and Olivier Le Moine. 2020. "Artificial Intelligence in Medicine: Today and Tomorrow." *Frontiers in Medicine* 7: 1–6. doi:10.3389/fmed.2020.00027.

Chakraborty, Chinmay. 2019. "Computational Approach for Chronic Wound Tissue Characterization." *Informatics in Medicine Unlocked* 17: 100162. doi:10.1016/j.imu.2019.100162.

Chandrasekaran, Baskaran, and Shifra Fernandes. 2020. "Artificial Intelligence (AI) Applications for COVID-19 Pandemic." *Diabetes Metab Syndr.* 14(4): 337–39.

Davahli, Mohammad Reza, Waldemar Karwowski, Krzysztof Fiok, Thomas Wan, and Hamid R. Parsaei. 2021. "Controlling Safety of Artificial Intelligence-Based Systems in Healthcare." *Symmetry* 13 (1): 1–25. doi:10.3390/sym13010102.

Deepa, N., B. Prabadevi, Praveen Kumar Maddikunta, Thippa Reddy Gadekallu, M. Thar Baker Ajmal Khan, and Usman Tariq. 2021. "An AI-Based Intelligent System for Healthcare Analysis Using Ridge-Adaline Stochastic Gradient Descent Classifier." *Journal of Supercomputing* 77 (2): 1998–2017. doi:10.1007/s11227-020-03347-2.

Dhawan, Sachin, Chinmay Chakraborty, Jaroslav Frnda, Rashmi Gupta, Arun Kumar Rana, and Subhendu Kumar Pani. 2021. "SSII: Secured and High-Quality Steganography Using Intelligent Hybrid Optimization Algorithms for IoT." *IEEE Access* 9: 87563–78. doi:10.1109/access.2021.3089357.

Dlamini, Zodwa, Flavia Zita Francies, Rodney Hull, and Rahaba Marima. 2020. "Artificial Intelligence (AI) and Big Data in Cancer and Precision Oncology." *Computational and Structural Biotechnology Journal* 18 (1): 2300–11. doi:10.1016/j.csbj.2020.08.019.

Gerke, Sara, Timo Minssen, and Glenn Cohen. 2020. Ethical and Legal Challenges of Artificial Intelligence-Driven Healthcare. *Artificial Intelligence in Healthcare*. doi:10.1016/b978-0-12-818438-7.00012-5.

Gille, Felix, Anna Jobin, and Marcello Ienca. 2020. "What We Talk about When We Talk about Trust: Theory of Trust for AI in Healthcare." *Intelligence-Based Medicine* 1–2: 100001. doi:10.1016/j.ibmed.2020.100001.

Guo, Aixia, Michael Pasque, Francis Loh, Douglas L. Mann, and Philip R. O. Payne. 2020. "Heart Failure Diagnosis, Readmission, and Mortality Prediction Using Machine Learning and Artificial Intelligence Models." *Current Epidemiology Reports* 7 (4): 212–19. doi:10.1007/s40471-020-00259-w.

Gupta, Akash Kumar, Chinmay Chakraborty, and Bharat Gupta. 2021. "Secure Transmission of EEG Data Using Watermarking Algorithm for the Detection of Epileptical Seizures." *Traitement Du Signal* 38 (2): 473–79. doi:10.18280/ts.380227.

Hasselgren, Anton, Jens Andreas Hanssen Rensaa, Katina Kralevska, Danilo Gligoroski, and Arild Faxvaag. 2021. "Blockchain for Increased Trust in Virtual Healthcare: Proof-of-Concept Study." *Journal of Medical Internet Research* 23 (7): 1–15. doi:10.2196/28496.

Horgan, Denis, Mario Romao, Servaas A. Morré, and Dipak Kalra. 2020. "Artificial Intelligence: Power for Civilisation – And for Better Healthcare." *Public Health Genomics* 22 (5–6): 145–61. doi:10.1159/000504785.

Jones, Mike, Frank Deruyter, and John Morris. 2020. "The Digital Health Revolution and People with Disabilities: Perspective from the United States." *International Journal of Environmental Research and Public Health* 17 (2). doi:10.3390/ijerph17020381.

Kasperbauer, T. J. 2021. "Conflicting Roles for Humans in Learning Health Systems and AI-Enabled Healthcare." *Journal of Evaluation in Clinical Practice* 27 (3): 537–42. doi:10.1111/jep.13510.

Kassam, Adam, and Naila Kassam. 2020. "Artificial Intelligence in Healthcare: A Canadian Context." *Healthcare Management Forum* 33 (1): 5–9. doi:10.1177/084047041987 4356.

Kaur, Manpreet, Mohammad Zubair Khan, Shikha Gupta, Abdulfattah Noorwali, Chinmay Chakraborty, and Subhendu Kumar Pani. 2021. "MBCP: Performance Analysis of Large Scale Mainstream Blockchain Consensus Protocols." *IEEE Access* 9: 80931–44. doi:10.1109/ACCESS.2021.3085187.

Khemasuwan, Danai, Jeffrey S. Sorensen, and Henri G. Colt. 2020. "Artificial Intelligence in Pulmonary Medicine: Computer Vision, Predictive Model and Covid-19." *European Respiratory Review* 29 (157): 1–16. doi:10.1183/16000617.0181-2020.

Kishor, Amit, Chinmay Chakraborty, and Wilson Jeberson. 2020. "A Novel Fog Computing Approach for Minimization of Latency in Healthcare Using Machine Learning." *International Journal of Interactive Multimedia and Artificial Intelligence* 1: 1. doi:10.9781/ijimai.2020.12.004.

Kwon, Joon-myoung, Kyung Hee Kim, Jose Medina-Inojosa, Ki Hyun Jeon, Jinsik Park, and Byung Hee Oh. 2020. "Artificial Intelligence for Early Prediction of Pulmonary Hypertension Using Electrocardiography." *Journal of Heart and Lung Transplantation* 39 (8): 805–14. doi:10.1016/j.healun.2020.04.009.

Laï, M. C., M. Brian, and M. F. Mamzer. 2020. "Perceptions of Artificial Intelligence in Healthcare: Findings from a Qualitative Survey Study among Actors in France." *Journal of Translational Medicine* 18 (1): 1–13. doi:10.1186/s12967-019-02204-y.

Lee, Hee, and S. N. Yoon 2021. "Application of Artificial Intelligence-Based Technologies in the Healthcare Industry: Opportunities and Challenges." *International Journal of Environmental Research and Public Health* 18 (1): 1–18. doi:10.3390/ijerph 18010271.

Macrae, Carl. 2019. "Governing the Safety of Artificial Intelligence in Healthcare." *BMJ Quality and Safety* 28 (6): 495–98. doi:10.1136/bmjqs-2019-009484.

Mahomed, S. 2020. "COVID-19: The Role of Artificial Intelligence in Empowering the Healthcare Sector and Enhancing Social Distancing Measures during a Pandemic." *South African Medical Journal* 110 (7): 610–13. doi:10.7196/SAMJ.2020.V110I7. 14841.

Mansour, Romany Fouad, Adnen El Amraoui, Issam Nouaouri, Vicente García, Vicente García Díaz, Deepak Gupta, and Sachin Kumar. 2021. "Artificial Intelligence and Internet of Things Enabled Disease Diagnosis Model for Smart Healthcare Systems." *IEEE Access* 9 (1): 45137–46. doi:10.1109/ACCESS.2021.3066365.

Mendels, David A., Laurent Dortet, Cécile Emeraud, Saoussen Oueslati, Delphine Girlich, Jean Baptiste Ronat, Sandrine Bernabeu, Silvestre Bahi, Gary J.H. Atkinson, and Thierry Naas. 2021. "Using Artificial Intelligence to Improve COVID-19 Rapid Diagnostic Test Result Interpretation." *Proceedings of the National Academy of Sciences of the United States of America* 118 (12): 3–5. doi:10.1073/pnas.2019893118.

Omoruan, A. I., A. P. Bamidele, and O. F. Phillips. 2009. "Social Health Insurance and Sustainable Healthcare Reform in Nigeria." *Studies on Ethno-Medicine* 3 (2): 105–10. doi:10.1080/09735070.2009.11886346.

Palanica, Adam, Michael J. Docktor, Michael Lieberman, and Yan Fossat. 2020. "The Need for Artificial Intelligence in Digital Therapeutics." *Digital Biomarkers* 4 (1): 21–25. doi:10.1159/000506861.

Patel, Urvish K., Arsalan Anwar, Sidra Saleem, Preeti Malik, Bakhtiar Rasul, Karan Patel, Robert Yao, Ashok Seshadri, Mohammed Yousufuddin, and Kogulavadanan Arumaithurai. 2021. "Artificial Intelligence as an Emerging Technology in the Current Care of Neurological Disorders." *Journal of Neurology* 268 (5): 1623–42. doi:10.1007/s00415-019-09518-3.

Peek, Niels, Mark Sujan, and Philip Scott. 2020. "Digital Health and Care in Pandemic Times: Impact of COVID-19." *BMJ Health and Care Informatics* 27 (1): 2–4. doi:10.1136/bmjhci-2020-100166.

Randhawa, Gurprit K., and Mary Jackson. 2020. "The Role of Artificial Intelligence in Learning and Professional Development for Healthcare Professionals." *Healthcare Management Forum* 33 (1): 19–24. doi:10.1177/0840470419869032.

Sarkar, Arindam, Mohammad Zubair Khan, Moirangthem Marjit Singh, Abdulfattah Noorwali, Chinmay Chakraborty, and Subhendu Kumar Pani. 2021. "Artificial Neural Synchronization Using Nature Inspired Whale Optimization." *IEEE Access* 9: 16435–47. doi:10.1109/ACCESS.2021.3052884.

Schwalbe, Nina, and Brian Wahl. 2020. "Artificial Intelligence and the Future of Global Health." *The Lancet* 395 (10236): 1579–86. doi:10.1016/S0140-6736(20)30226-9.

Subiksha, K. P., and M. Ramakrishnan. 2021. *Smart Healthcare Analytics Solutions Using Deep Learning AI. Advances in Intelligent Systems and Computing*. Vol. 1245. Springer, Singapore. doi:10.1007/978-981-15-7234-0_67.

Tanwar, Sudeep, Karan Parekh, and Richard Evans. 2020. "Blockchain-Based Electronic Healthcare Record System for Healthcare 4.0 Applications." *Journal of Information Security and Applications* 50: 102407. doi:10.1016/j.jisa.2019.102407.

Ullah, Mujib, Asma Akbar, and Gustavo Gabriel Yannarelli 2020. "Applications of Artificial Intelligence in, Early Detection of Cancer, Clinical Diagnosis and Personalized Medicine." *Artificial Intelligence in Cancer* 3228 (2): 39–44.

Vatandsoost, Mohsen, and Sanaz Litkouhi. 2019. "The Future of Healthcare Facilities: How Technology and Medical Advances May Shape Hospitals of the Future." *Hospital Practices and Research* 4 (1): 1–11. doi:10.15171/hpr.2019.01.

Veeramakali, T., R. Siva, B. Sivakumar, P. C. Senthil Mahesh, and N. Krishnaraj. 2021. "An Intelligent Internet of Things-Based Secure Healthcare Framework Using Blockchain Technology with an Optimal Deep Learning Model." *Journal of Supercomputing* 77 (9): 9576–96. doi:10.1007/s11227-021-03637-3.

Yaqoob, Ibrar, Khaled Salah, Raja Jayaraman, and Yousof Al-Hammadi. 2021. "Blockchain for Healthcare Data Management: Opportunities, Challenges, and Future Recommendations." *Neural Computing and Applications* 1–16. doi:10.1007/s00521-020-05519-w.

Zhang, Ran, Xin Tie, Zhihua Qi, Nicholas B. Bevins, Chengzhu Zhang, Dalton Griner, Thomas K. Song, et al. 2021. "Diagnosis of Coronavirus Disease 2019 Pneumonia by Using Chest Radiography: Value of Artificial Intelligence." *Radiology* 298 (2): E88–97. doi:10.1148/RADIOL.2020202944.

12 Parkinson's Disease Pre-Diagnosis Using Smart Technologies
A Review

Mohammad Yasser Chuttur and
Azina Nazurally
University of Mauritius, Mauritius

CONTENTS

12.1   INTRODUCTION

Parkinson's disease (PD) is a neurodegenerative movement disorder which affect millions worldwide [1]. The exact causes of PD are still unknown; however, it is believed that hereditary and environmental factors could be the origin of the illness [2]. To date, there is no corresponding treatment for the disease, and medical practitioners address the condition primarily through symptoms management. Because an early diagnosis of the disease can support long term management of

PD in patients, it is essential to detect early warning signs of PD. Medical practitioners, however, can miss those early signs, which can be very subtle to human eyes and traditional monitoring devices.

Digital healthcare transformation with AI uses smart technologies such as robots, IoT sensors, machine learning algorithms and blockchain, among others, for delivering impactful healthcare services [3]. AI techniques are helpful because they can easily process a large amount of data to assist in medical diagnosis and uncover disease-related patterns not discovered before. In fact, with the deployment of intelligent sensors in IoT networks and the application of blockchain in telemedicine, the transfer and analysis of medical data can be rapidly, safely, and conducted cost-effectively over long distances for medical diagnosis and saving lives [4–9]. From this perspective, it is necessary to develop medical diagnosis techniques that can be easily incorporated into a framework, such as telemedicine, to deliver better healthcare services especially for PD diagnosis.

To this end, many researchers have recently proposed several machine learning algorithms to distinguish PD patients from healthy patients. Different types of biomarkers data such as voice, drawing, keyboard tapping, and gait movements have been used and the classification performance scores reported indicate that machine learning algorithms are very promising technologies for supporting robust decision-making for PD diagnosis. However, despite the marked advancements in the field, AI application for PD diagnosis is still inexistent in current clinical settings. To better understand this gap, a review of some recent works that make use of machine learning techniques for PD diagnosis is essential. Such a review will not only help underscore the potential of machine learning techniques for PD diagnosis but also reveal important areas that need to be addressed for future research.

The rest of the chapter is organized as follows. Section 12.2 will introduce some popular types of motor symptoms markers commonly used for creating PD datasets. In Section 12.3, different types of PD diagnosis biomarkers, along with the corresponding machine learning algorithms applied, and the performance score reported in recent studies will be described. This is followed by a discussion about the relevance of the proposed techniques for real-world settings and useful recommendations for future research directions in Section 12.4. Finally, concluding remarks are given in Section 12.5.

12.2   PARKINSON'S DISEASE SYMPTOMS

PD symptoms appear and progress differently for each individual, and these are usually classified as either motor- or non-motor-related. Motor-related symptoms associated with PD are well known, easily distinguished, and more reliable indicators of the disease. Examples of common motor-related symptoms are listed in Table 12.1. In contrast, non-motor signs are less evident because they can be easily confused with other types of diseases and, therefore, cannot always be relied on for accurate diagnosis of the disease [11, 12]. Examples of non-motor-related symptoms include a disturbed sense of smell (hyposmia or even

TABLE 12.1
Motor Symptoms Associated with PD, According to Mortimer et al. [10]

Motor Symptom	Description
Tremor	Usually, a tremor starts in one side of the body and eventually affects the other. Some patients may also experience internal tremors.
Bradykinesia	Patients suffer from slow movements, motor coordination issues and micrographia.
Postural instability	The patient is unable to remain upright and stable.
Walking/gait difficulties	Caused by bradykinesia and postural instability.
Rigidity	In the initial stages, the limbs or torso experience muscle stiffness.
Dystonia	A movement disorder that causes involuntary and repetitive muscle movements. Not all PD disease patients are affected by dystonia.
Vocal symptoms	Changes in voice tone and emotion may occur because of bradykinesia. Patients often speak in a monotone manner or even stutter.

anosmia), sleep disorders, vision problems, depression, cognitive changes and personality disorders.

PD symptoms and their severity also vary from patient to patient. In the early and initial stages, patients may experience mild tremors, which occur only on one side of their body and minor posture and walking style changes. The tremors and other symptoms may then affect both sides of the body, causing the patient to encounter challenges in daily activities. In mid-stages, the pathological hallmarks comprise rigidity, loss of balance as well as slow movement. When the disease progresses, the patient no longer remains independent as s/he may not be able to walk. In addition, hallucinations and delusions may also start to become frequent.

To better determine the progression and the stage in which a patient is regarding the disease, researchers use a rating scale specifically developed for the purpose [13]. The 'Hoehn and Yahr Scale', for instance, was introduced in 1967 to rate motor symptoms severity on a scale of 1 to 5 [14]. The scale was subsequently used as a benchmark for developing the 'Unified Parkinson's disease Rating Scale' (UPDRS), which is often used nowadays in the medical diagnosis of PD. UPDRS also includes a scale rating for non-motor symptoms [13]. Over the years, the UPDRS has been further improved and updated to include scale ratings for additional symptoms not considered in previous scales [15].

Given the nature of the disease, PD diagnosis remains a challenging and complex task [16–18]. No standard test exists to diagnose PD accurately, and medical practitioners often rely on a minimum of two motor symptoms through physical examinations for PD diagnosis. However, the assessment of movements is sometimes subtle to the human eyes, error-prone, resulting in misdiagnosis. Hence, accurate and precise PD diagnosis approaches that complement existing techniques are needed [6].

12.3   DIAGNOSIS MARKERS

As cited in Cova et al. [19], the "NIH Biomarkers Definitions Working Group" defines a biomarker as "a characteristic that is objectively measured and evaluated as an indicator of normal biological processes, pathogenic processes or pharmacologic responses to a therapeutic intervention". There can be different types of biomarkers or markers, with each having a special purpose. For example, a diagnostic marker can be used to diagnose a specific condition in a patient. In contrast, a staging marker is used to evaluate the severity of a disease in a person. The prognostic markers are another type of biomarker that can forecast the risk or progression of a disease. When it comes to PD, diagnostic markers are essential to detect early signs of the disease before symptoms of the disease become more apparent in patients. The most reliable markers for PD are based on motors symptoms [19]. This section will describe common motor symptoms markers and recent works that have used those markers to develop PD pre-diagnosis models using machine learning.

12.3.1   Voice Markers

Patients at risk of developing PD or who are already affected by PD often have difficulty speaking. Related speech symptoms may comprise a lowered voice tone and problems to utter words correctly. Symptoms may progress over time, from subtle changes in speech capabilities to severe difficulty communicating using spoken words. For this reason, early degradation in voice or speech signals can be critical to the pre-diagnosis of PD. Individuals are asked to perform predefined speech exercises to obtain voice markers, which are recorded and later analyzed. The activities require individuals to read vowels, for example, vowel /a/or vowel /i/, complete words, short sentences, or numbers [20]. Acoustic analysis is performed on the recorded data with the primary goal of detecting any variations of features like voice tremor amplitude, jitter, and shimmer [21].

An example of using voice markers to pre-diagnose PD using machine learning can be found in the work of Wroge et al. [22]. The authors used the voice dataset created for the mPower study, which Sage Bionetworks conducted. The dataset contained 5,826 vocal recordings of the phonation *aa*, which lasted 10 seconds each. The recordings were preprocessed and cleaned using the Voice Activation Detection algorithm, and all background noises were removed. 'Audio-Visual Emotion recognition Challenge (AVEC)' 2013 and 'Geneva Minimalistic Acoustic Parameter Set (GeMAPS)' features were used to train Gradient Boosted Decision Tree, Extra Trees, Random Forest, SVM and ANN classifiers. The authors report that the ANN gave the highest recall rates of 0.82 and 0.79 when validated with the AVEC 2013 and GeMaps features, respectively. The highest accuracy of 86% was obtained when trained with the AVEC features by the ANN.

In another work, Grover et al. [23] predicted the severity of PD using a deep neural network (DNN) classifier. The classifier model had five layers which comprised one input, three middle (30 neurons) and one output layer and were trained with the PD Telemonitoring vocal data from the UCI repository. The dataset contained a total of 5,875 recordings collected from 42 people. The recordings were preprocessed and normalized. The preprocessed data were split into 80% and 20% for training and evaluation, respectively. The deep learning classifier categorized the output into either severe or non-severe based on UPDRS metrics with an accuracy of 81.7%.

Berus et al. [24] also trained and validated multiple Artificial Neural Networks (ANNs) on the UCI repository for classifying PD patients and control subjects. The dataset used contained vocal recordings from 20 PD patients and 20 control subjects. Noise removal was performed on the recordings. Features were extracted using Pearson's and Kendall's correlation coefficient, Principal Component Analysis and Self-Organising Map. The ANNs classified the features into 0 (PD Disease) and 1 (No PD Disease). An accuracy of 86.4% was obtained in this case.

Similarly, Patra et al. [25] tested various machine learning approaches on a vocal dataset obtained from the UCI repository. The latter contained data for 23 patients and 31 healthy people. Random Forest, Decision Tree, Logistic Regression and KNN were trained and validated through 10-fold cross-validation. The Random Forest Classifier attained the highest accuracy of 84.5%. The Decision Tree, Logistic Regression and KNN, in contrast, gave accuracies of 79.9%, 82.0% and 76.3%, respectively.

The vocal dataset from the UCI repository was further used by Gunduz [26]. Here, the author implemented a CNN for classification purposes, and the dataset contained data collected from 188 patients and 64 control individuals. The CNN was implemented with nine layers in total and SoftMax activation. Leave-one-person-out cross-validation was applied to the model. The author found that when combining vocal features, CNN can yield a classification accuracy of 91.7%.

Recently, Karan et al. [27] have used SVM and Random Forest (RF) classifiers on two voice marker datasets; one from the UCI repository and the other from a custom-built dataset, which contained voice data for 25 patients and 20 healthy individuals. The vocal recordings were composed of phonations of a and o. Acoustic, Mel frequency Cepstral Coefficient (MFCC) and IMF-based features such as energy, entropy, Intrinsic Mode Function Cepstral Coefficient, spectral entropy and statistical features were extracted from the dataset for training and testing two classifiers, namely SVM and RF. The authors reported that a maximum accuracy of 96% for SVM and RF could be achieved depending on the acoustic features used and the number of cross-fold validations conducted when training the classifiers.

Solana-Lavelle et al. [28] further considered reducing the number of features extracted from voice recordings to improve performance for PD pre-diagnosis. The authors used the UCI Machine Learning Repository PD datasets for 188 patients and 64 control individuals' vocal records. Although the authors extracted 754 features through feature analysis, only 8–20 features were considered for classification purposes. The classifiers tested were the KNN, Multi-Layer Perceptron, SVM and RF. The authors reported that the SVM attained the highest accuracy of 94.7% when 20 features were used.

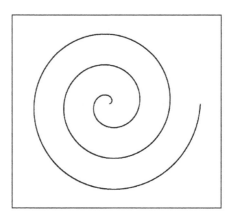

FIGURE 12.1   Spiral drawing template used in early PD detection.

12.3.2   DRAWING MARKERS

PD patients often experience early forms of tremors and bradykinesia. For this reason, drawing exercises can be used to detect the disease at an early stage. The activities are of two types: static or dynamic, which consist of drawing spirals or meanders. An example of a spiral drawing template that is shown to subjects during static and dynamic drawing tests for the early detection of PD is shown in Figure 12.1.

In static drawing tests, the subjects follow an existing line to reproduce the sketch presented to them. In contrast, in dynamic drawing tests, subjects are asked to reproduce a sketch shown for a short lapse of time only. Through different drawing exercises, several features, such as the speed at which the drawings are reproduced, the smoothness of the drawings, pen pressures and kinematics, can be mapped to the bradykinesia and tremor symptoms to establish any early occurrence of PD [29, 30]. Given the ease of data capture and analysis, several studies have used drawing markers for classifying PD patients.

For instance, Drotár et al. [31] used the PaHaWh and writing dataset, which contained data from 37 PD patients and 38 control subjects. The authors extracted various features such as spiral drawings and handwriting pressure from the dataset, which were then fed to three machine learning classifiers, namely the SVM, Adaboost and K-Nearest Neighbour (KNN). The classifiers were all trained and validated using the stratified 10-fold cross-validation method. Finally, the authors reported that the SVM classifier gave the best results with an accuracy of 81.3%.

Gil-Martín et al. [29] further examined the usefulness of spiral drawings for PD diagnosis. However, the authors used a different dataset comprising drawings from 62 patients and 15 control subjects. Each person was asked to perform three tasks, and each task was recorded five times. The records were each sampled at 100 Hz and flagged as 1 (PD disease) and 0 (no PD disease). Fast Fourier Transform was applied to the recordings. A CNN which took spectrum points as input was used for classification purposes. Features were automatically extracted by the CNN. The latter was equipped with a dropout layer to prevent overfitting, and the subject-wise cross-validation technique was used. In this case, the authors reported a high classification accuracy of 96.5%.

Angelillo et al. [32] also analyzed the handwritings of 37 patients and 38 healthy people from the PaHaW dataset. The participants were asked to perform various tasks, which included drawing spirals, writing in cursive format and writing specific words. Features were then extracted and formatted into a feature vector, which was fed into three different classifiers, namely SVM, Linear Discriminant Analysis and Adaboost. These classifiers were trained and validated using stratified 10-fold cross-validation with the extracted features. A voting algorithm was then used to combine the results obtained from the classifiers. It was found that the SVM classifier performed better than the other classifiers, with an accuracy of 88.75%.

Díaz et al. [33] used a smaller drawing dataset comprising sine waves and spirals collected from 12 healthy subjects and 15 PD patients. The collected data were rescaled, cleaned and digitalized. The histogram of oriented gradients (HOG) technique was then used on the processed dataset for feature extraction. Those features were finally used as input to a RF classifier which achieved an accuracy of 83%.

Ali et al. [34] tried to increase the performance of PD data classifiers. The authors used the HandPD dataset, which consisted of drawing data from 74 PD subjects and 18 control subjects. To boost the accuracy, the authors proposed to use Chi2 along with the Adaboost model. Chi2 has been used for feature selection and extraction, while random under-sampling has been performed to reduce outliers in the dataset. The features were then ranked by Chi2 and fed to an Adaboost classifier which was trained and validated using the stratified K-fold validation technique. This approach, however, gave a classification accuracy of 76.4%, which turned out to be lower than previously reported results.

And recently, Kamble et al. [30] used the spiral drawing dataset from the UCI repository. The dataset considered contained static and dynamic spirals drawing collected for 25 PD and 15 healthy subjects. Kinematics and spatiotemporal features were extracted and were fed to four machine learning (ML) classifiers, namely Logistic Regression, C-Support Vector Classification (SVC), K-nearest neighbour (KNN) classifier and ensemble model Random Forest Classifier (RFC). The authors reported the best performance of 91.6% accuracy when using Logistic Regression and RFC.

12.3.3   KEYBOARD TAPPING MARKERS

Researchers have also used keyboard keystrokes dynamics to differentiate between PD individuals from healthy controls. This is because individuals suffering from PD may suffer from bradykinesia, which is a slowing down of physical movements, irregular motor coordination and micrographia. Consequently, PD affected individuals will not have the same keyboard tapping patterns as healthy individuals. In general, features from keystroke latency time, time a key is depressed, and time a key is held are extracted and fed into classifiers to determine whether an individual is suffering from PD or not [35].

Adams [36] conducted an experiment in which he analyzed keystrokes timing information collected from 103 subjects, of which 32 had PD, and the remainder were controls. The author determined that when exposed over an extended period, PD individuals would have hand and finger movements different from healthy subjects. The author was particularly interested in the hold and latency time observed for keystrokes, which were fed into an ensemble ML classifier comprising of eight ML models, namely SVM, Multi-Level Perceptron, Logistic Regression, RF, Nu-Support Vector Classification, Decision Trees, KNN and Quadratic Discriminant Analysis. Data preprocessing steps consisted in replacing missing values, data normalization, separation of the dataset into two groups (hold and latency) and dimension reduction. Using the mentioned approach, the author reported a high classification accuracy with an AUC of 0.98.

In another study conducted by Iakovakis et al. [37], the authors evaluated the performance of CNN for the early detection of PD when using typing data obtained from smartphones. Two datasets were used. One dataset consisted of keyboard typing keystrokes collected from 18 early PD patients and 15 healthy controls during regular clinic visits. The other dataset consisted of keyboard typing keystrokes obtained from 27 PD patients and 84 healthy controls who installed and used the iPrognosis application on their phones in their daily activities. The CNN was compiled using RMSprop and Adam optimizers and validated using LOSO (Leave-one-subject-out) cross-validation technique. The authors reported that their approach for the analysis of keyboard typing gave a good classification performance of 0.89 and 0.79 Area Under the Curve (AUC) for keystrokes data collected from in-clinic visits and the iPrognosis application, respectively.

Peachap et al. [35] recently proposed a novel approach to use wavelets and spectral features extracted from keyboard keystrokes data to distinguish between PD and control patients keystrokes datasets. The authors argue that their approach outperformed state of the art methods for classifying PD datasets with a reported classification accuracy ranging between 93.5% to 100% for Pattern recognition artificial neural network (PR-ANN), the SVM, the K-NN and the Logistic regression classifiers. The features of interest used in their research are the hold time, the latency and the flight time of keystrokes that were obtained from Tappy Keystroke Data. The dataset comprised keystrokes data from 286 PD and 203 control subjects. A 10-foldcross-validation technique was applied to the dataset prior to classification to avoid data overfitting.

Instead of using keystrokes data from a keyboard, Williams et al. [38] demonstrated that video recordings could also be used to assess bradykinesia in people. In their experiment, the authors observed the action of finger tapping in 70 people, 40 of them being PD disease patients and the remaining being control participants, in video recordings. Observations about finger tapping were fed to a CNN for segmentation, and once frame motion was captured, dimension reduction was performed. Selected features (tapping frequency, amplitude, and variability) were extracted and fed into Naïve Bayes, Logistic Regression and the (SVM) classifiers. The LOSO cross-validation technique was used. The best classification accuracy of 69% was obtained using the SVM classifier.

12.3.4   GAIT MARKERS

Gait is an individual's manner or style of walking. As mentioned earlier, one of the major symptoms of PD in patients is a decrease in or lack of control over physical motion ability. PD patients, therefore, may also have trouble walking and experience different forms of stress on their legs when walking. Researchers have exploited this characteristic in PD patients by using sensors that, when attached to the body of an individual, can collect motion data. When analyzed, motion data can yield patterns that can distinguish between healthy and PD individuals. Examples of motion data that are usually captured are motion speed, stiffness, reduced smoothness of locomotion, reduced step length, reduced balance, shuffling of steps, etc. [39–41].

An example of using gait markers in a ML classifier can be found in the work of Açıcı et al. [39]. The PhysioNet dataset and data from the Laboratory for Gait and Neuro dynamics, Movement Disorders Unit of the Tel Aviv Sourasky Medical Center were used in this study. The dataset contained data collected from ground reaction force sensors worn under the foot for a total of 93 patients and 73 healthy subjects. Features extracted from the sensor data fed to a RF classifier. The 10-fold cross-validation was applied to avoid overfitting the data to the classification model, and the authors reported a high classification accuracy of 98.0%.

Similarly, Cavallo et al. [42] assessed the performance of ML techniques when using gait information for PD classification. In their study, data were collected from sensors attached to the upper limbs for 30 healthy individuals, 30 Parkinson's patients and 30 idiopathic hyposmia patients. Although a total of 48 features were extracted from the collected data, only 39 features were retained and fed into four classifiers, namely RF, SVM and Naïve Bayes. In the end, the RF classifier gave the best result with an accuracy of 95.0%.

Recently, Xia et al. [43] investigated the performance of two deep neural networks models, i.e., CNN and LSTM, to classify PD patients based on gait analysis. The CNN was used to extract an abstract representation of the gait signals, which was fed to the LSTM for robust feature extraction. A 5-fold cross-validation was performed on the deep neural networks for data obtained from the PhysioNet dataset. The proposed model yielded the best accuracy of 99.0%, depending on the subset of the dataset used.

In another study, El Maachi et al. [44] also used neural networks and gait markers to detect PD. The authors used a DNN built from a 1 Direction CNN (1DCNN) to analyse vertical ground reaction force measurements signals obtained from a sensor placed on an individual's foot. The authors also used data obtained from the PhysioNet dataset. The DNN extracted the relevant features and fed them into a RF model for classification. The proposed method yielded a classification accuracy of 98.7%.

12.3.5   MULTI-MARKER APPROACHES

In some studies, researchers have evaluated the classification performance of ML models by using input data collected for more than one marker. Aghanavesi et al. [45] for instance, proposed an approach that made use of both tapping and spiral drawing markers in classifying the severity of PD. In their study, participants interactions were recorded while performing some tapping and spiral drawing exercises on their smartphones. A total of 37 spatiotemporal features were extracted through time series analysis of the recordings. After dimension reduction, the features of interest obtained from principal component analysis were fed into four classifiers: SVM, Logistic Regression, Regression Tree and Multi-Layer Perceptron. In their evaluation, the authors compared the performance of the classifiers with the rating assigned by three independent movement disorder specialists. Therefore, instead of calculating classification accuracy, the authors calculated the correlation of results obtained by each classifier with the PD severity assessment of the three specialists. The authors reported that the best correlation result of 0.57 was obtained with the SVM classifier.

Vasquez-Correa et al. [46] also tried to diagnose PD using a CNN deep learning model. The authors used a combination of voice, gait and drawing markers in a dataset containing recordings of 44 patients and 40 healthy individuals. Each recording was 60 minutes long, where 15 minutes was attributed to speech, 15 minutes to handwriting and the remaining to gait. The authors reported having achieved a classification accuracy of 97.6% with their proposed technique.

Pham et al. [47] further evaluated the performance of RF, KNN and SVM when using a combination of voice and drawing-based markers to distinguish between PD and healthy individuals. In their work, the authors used the 'Parkinson Speech Dataset with Multiple Types of Sound Recordings' and the 'Improved Spiral Test Using Digitized Graphics Tablet for Monitoring PD Disease' datasets available at the UCI Machine Learning Repository. Compared to the other classifiers, the SVM yielded the best accuracy of 95.8%.

In another study, Prince et al. [48] proposed a multi-source ensemble learning method that combined data from four markers: tapping, gait, voice and memory, for detecting PD. Data for each marker was collected from 1,513 subjects through different activities that involved the use of a smartphone. Features extracted from the collected data were fed to a classifier ensemble composed of Logistic Regression models, RF models, DNN and CNN. Each of these classifiers was initially separately trained using 10-fold cross-validation. When compared to the performance obtained for individual classifiers, the ensemble approach gave the highest accuracy of 82.0%.

12.4   DISCUSSIONS

As seen in Section 12.3, several ML techniques that use numerous motor symptoms biomarkers, namely voice, drawing, tapping and gait-based markers for PD pre-diagnosis, have already been proposed and experimentally tested. Similarly, in their comprehensive literature review, Mei et al. [18] report that researchers have extensively and successfully applied numerous ML algorithms for PD diagnosis. Therefore, the high classification accuracy observed in past studies makes it evident that ML techniques are promising technologies that can assist medical practitioners in the early detection of PD.

But before one can claim that AI-powered applications for PD diagnosis can offer robust decision-making solutions, empirical evidence on the effectiveness of ML applications in real-world settings is a prerequisite. Currently, no empirical evidence that shows the successful deployment and adoption of ML application for the diagnosis PD in real-world settings exist. Consequently, researchers are encouraged to consider future research strategies that can improve the relevance of ML for PD diagnosis in real-world environments. Some recommendations for future research are given further.

12.4.1 RECOMMENDATIONS FOR FUTURE WORKS

ML techniques used in past studies for PD diagnosis have been mostly trained and tested in laboratories on experimental datasets and not in real clinical settings. Thus, there is a high need for ML techniques, which have already passed the experimental phase, to be thoroughly and rigorously validated through clinical trials in the presence of experts in the field. Validation in a clinical setting should also consider real-world data with subjects from all demographics to avoid any bias emanating from an experimental dataset [49].

In addition, due consideration should be given to the sample size for validating any proposed solution. Past studies have used relatively small sample sizes that are not sufficient for translation into real-world application. It should be highlighted that developed solutions that are tested and validated under clinical trials, with the acknowledgement of medical experts, will also help establish trust in the technology for both patients and medical practitioners.

Furthermore, the fact that AI-powered medical solutions are often forsaken because of the associated ethical implications should not be overlooked. Medical staff and patients alike are reluctant to adopt any AI-based solutions unless issues related to trust, transparency and data privacy are addressed. AI-powered solutions are often questioned on their algorithmic fairness and reliability [50]. Hence, future studies on using smart technologies for PD diagnosis should also consider technology acceptance evaluation and address relevant ethical issues related to the adoption of such technology.

Machine learning applications are well known to be resource-intensive that may require a considerable amount of processing power and quality data to guarantee performance. Hence, further research is needed to evaluate the requirements for different telemedicine or telediagnosis frameworks that would ensure that biomarker data can be accurately captured and processed to produce a reliable diagnosis.

Finally, individuals do not all experience the same PD symptoms. In some individuals, symptoms are primarily non-motor-related, whereas, in others, symptoms may be more motor-related. In other cases, individuals may have a combination of motor and non-motor-related symptoms. In this case, future studies should also consider non-motor-related symptoms or combine different modalities to develop systems that can supply medical practitioners with reliable information to support their decision-making for an accurate diagnosis.

12.5 CONCLUSION

Many studies have already shown the effectiveness of ML techniques in accurately classifying different forms of PD motor symptoms markers. Therefore, there is a high potential for including ML algorithms in smart applications to support decision-making during PD pre-diagnosis. In this chapter, different ML algorithms to process some popular motor-related biomarkers along with the corresponding performance scores obtained have been described. It is found that although many studies have achieved good classification performance scores, there is a lack of consideration on the part of researchers to propose, implement, and test system architectures that can be used as proof of concept for real-world smart PD diagnosis applications. Researchers have also overlooked the importance of non-motor symptoms, ethical concerns and larger samples when developing PD pre-diagnosis models. In the future, instead of replicating research for testing the effectiveness of ML algorithms in PD pre-diagnosis, researchers are encouraged to consider assessing the implementation of smart PD pre-diagnosis technologies in real-world settings.

CONFLICT OF INTEREST

There is no conflict of interests.

FUNDING

There is no funding support.

DATA AVAILABILITY

Not applicable.

REFERENCES

1. R. Balestrino and A. H. V. Schapira, "Parkinson's disease," *European Journal of Neurology*, vol. 27, no. 1, pp. 27–42, 2020, doi: 10.1111/ene.14108.
2. L. V. Kalia, S. K. Kalia, and A. E. Lang, "Disease-modifying strategies for Parkinson's disease," *Movement Disorders*, vol. 30, no. 11, pp. 1442–1450, 2015.
3. M. Krishnan, C. Chinmay, S. Banerjee, C. Chakraborty, and A.K. Ray, "Statistical analysis of mammographic features and its classification using support vector machine," *Expert Systems with Applications*, 37, 470–478, 2009. ISSN: 0957-4174, doi:10.1016/j.eswa.2009.05.045

4. S. Dhawan, C. Chakraborty, J. Frnda, R. Gupta, A. K. Rana, and S. K. Pani, "SSII: Secured and high-quality Steganography using Intelligent hybrid optimization algorithms for IoT," *IEEE Access*, vol. 9, pp. 87563–87578, 2021.

5. A. K. Gupta, C. Chakraborty, and B. Gupta, "Secure transmission of EEG data using watermarking algorithm for the detection of epileptic seizures," *Traitement du Signal*, vol. 38, no. 2,pp. 473–479, 2021.

6. T. Kaur and T. K. Gandhi, "Deep convolutional neural networks with transfer learning for automated brain image classification," *Machine Vision and Applications*, vol. 31, no. 3, pp. 1–16, 2020.

7. A. Kishor, C. Chakraborty, and W. Jeberson, "A novel fog computing approach for minimization of latency in healthcare using machine learning," *International Journal Of Interactive Multimedia And Artificial Intelligence*, vol. 1, no. 1, pp. 1–11, 2020.

8. J.M. Díaz, A.B. Shariq, M.O. Edeh, C. Chinmay, S. Qaisar, D.L.H.F. Emiro, A.C. Paola, "Artificial intelligence-based kubernetes container for scheduling nodes of energy composition," *International Journal of System Assurance Engineering and Management*, 1–14, 2021 doi. 10.1007/s13198-021-01195-8

9. D. Sujata, C. Chinmay, K.G. Sourav, K.P. Subhendu, "Intelligent computing on time-series data analysis and prediction of Covid-19 pandemics," *Pattern Recognition Letters*, 151, 69–75, 2021, doi:10.1016/j.patrec.2021.07.027.

10. J. A. Mortimer, F. J. Pirozzolo, E. C. Hansch, and D. D. Webster, "Relationship of motor symptoms to intellectual deficits in Parkinson's disease," *Neurology*, vol. 32, no. 2, Art. no. 2, Feb. 1982, doi: 10.1212/WNL.32.2.133.

11. K. R. Chaudhuri, D. G. Healy, and A. H. Schapira, "Non-motor symptoms of Parkinson's disease: diagnosis and management," *The Lancet Neurology*, vol. 5, no. 3, pp. 235–245, 2006.

12. S. Muzerengi, S. Muzerengi, H. Lewis, M. Edwards, E. Kipps, A. Bahl, P. Martinez-Martin, and K.R. Chaudhuri, "Non-motor symptoms in Parkinson's disease: An underdiagnosed problem,"*Aging Health*, vol. 2, no. 6, pp. 967–982, 2006. doi:10.22 17/1745509X.2.6.967.

13. P. Martinez-Martin, C. Rodriguez-Blazquez, and M. J. Forjaz, "Rating Scales in Movement Disorders☆," in *Encyclopedia of Movement Disorders*, K. Kompoliti and L. V. Metman, Eds., Oxford: Academic Press, 2010, pp. 8–16. doi: 10.1016/ B978-0-12-374105-9.00068-X.

14. M. M. Hoehn and M. D. Yahr, "Parkinsonism: onset, progression, and mortality," *Neurology*, vol. 17, no. 5, Art. no. 5, May 1967, doi: 10.1212/WNL.17.5.427.

15. C. G. Goetz et al., "Movement disorder society-sponsored revision of the unified Parkinson's disease rating scale (mds-updrs): Process, format, and clinimetric testing plan," *Movement Disorders*, vol. 22, no. 1, Art. no. 1, 2007, doi: 10.1002/mds.21198.

16. M. Alissa, "Parkinson's disease diagnosis using deep learning," arXiv preprint arXiv:2101.05631, 2021.

17. R. W. de Souza et al., "Computer-assisted Parkinson's disease diagnosis using fuzzy optimum-path forest and restricted Boltzmann machines," *Computers in Biology and Medicine*, vol. 131, p. 104260, 2021.

18. J. Mei, C. Desrosiers, and J. Frasnelli, "Machine learning for the diagnosis of Parkinson's disease: A review of literature," *Frontiers in Aging Neuroscience*, vol. 13, p. 184, 2021.

19. I. Cova and A. Priori, "Diagnostic biomarkers for Parkinson's disease at a glance: Where are we?," *Journal of Neural Transmission*, vol. 125, no. 10, pp. 1417–1432, 2018, doi: 10.1007/s00702-018-1910-4.

20. Betul Erdogdu Sakar, Muhammed Erdem Isenkul, C. Okan Sakar, and Olcay Kursun, "Collection and analysis of a Parkinson speech dataset with multiple types of sound recordings," Jul. 2013. https://www.researchgate.net/publication/260662600_Collection_and_Analysis_of_a_Parkinson_Speech_Dataset_With_Multiple_Types_of_Sound_Recordings (accessed Jan. 26, 2021).

21. P. Gillivan-Murphy, N. Miller, and P. Carding, "Voice Tremor in Parkinson's Disease: An Acoustic Study," *Journal of Voice*, vol. 33, no. 4, pp. 526–535, Jul. 2019, doi: 10.1016/j.jvoice.2017.12.010.

22. T. J. Wroge, Y. Özkanca, C. Demiroglu, D. Si, D. C. Atkins, and R. H. Ghomi, "Parkinson's Disease Diagnosis Using Machine Learning and Voice," in *2018 IEEE Signal Processing in Medicine and Biology Symposium (SPMB)*, Dec. 2018, pp. 1–7. doi: 10.1109/SPMB.2018.8615607.

23. S. Grover, S. Bhartia, Akshama, A. Yadav, and K.R. Seeja, "Predicting severity of Parkinson's disease using deep learning," *Procedia Computer Science*, vol. 132, pp. 1788–1794, Jan. 2018, doi: 10.1016/j.procs.2018.05.154.

24. L. Berus, S. Klancnik, M. Brezocnik, and M. Ficko, "Classifying Parkinson's disease based on acoustic measures using artificial neural networks," *Sensors* (14248220), vol. 19, no. 1, Art. no. 1, Jan. 2019, doi: 10.3390/s19010016.

25. A. K. Patra, R. Ray, A. A. Abdullah, and S. Ranjan, "Prediction of Parkinson's disease using Ensemble Machine Learning classification from acoustic analysis," *Journal of Physics*, vol. 1372, no. 1, p. 8, Aug. 2019.

26. H. Gunduz, "Deep learning-based Parkinson's disease classification using vocal feature sets," *IEEE Access*, vol. 7, pp. 115540–115551, 2019, doi: 10.1109/ACCESS.2019.2936564.

27. B. Karan, S. S. Sahu, and K. Mahto, "Parkinson's disease prediction using intrinsic mode function based features from speech signal," *Biocybernetics and Biomedical Engineering*, vol. 40, no. 1, Art. no. 1, Jan. 2020, doi: 10.1016/j.bbe.2019.05.005.

28. G. Solana-Lavalle, J.-C. Galán-Hernández, and R. Rosas-Romero, "Automatic Parkinson's disease detection at early stages as a pre-diagnosis tool by using classifiers and a small set of vocal features," *Biocybernetics and Biomedical Engineering*, vol. 40, no. 1, Art. no. 1, Jan. 2020, doi: 10.1016/j.bbe.2020.01.003.

29. M. Gil-Martín, J. M. Montero, and R. San-Segundo, "(1) (PDF) Parkinson's disease detection from drawing movements using convolutional neural networks," Aug. 01, 2019. https://www.researchgate.net/publication/335235994_Parkinson's_Disease_Detection_from_Drawing_Movements_Using_Convolutional_Neural_Networks (accessed Nov. 15, 2020).

30. M. Kamble, P. Shrivastava, and M. Jain, "Digitized spiral drawing classification for Parkinson's disease diagnosis," *Measurement: Sensors*, vol. 16, p. 100047, Aug. 2021, doi: 10.1016/j.measen.2021.100047.

31. P. Drotár, J. Mekyska, I. Rektorová, L. Masarová, Z. Smékal, and M. Faundez-Zanuy, "Evaluation of handwriting kinematics and pressure for differential diagnosis of Parkinson's disease," *Artificial Intelligence in Medicine*, vol. 67, pp. 39–46, Feb. 2016, doi: 10.1016/j.artmed.2016.01.004.

32. M. Angelillo, D. Impedovo, G. Pirlo, and G. Vessio, "Performance-driven handwriting task selection for Parkinson's disease classification," 2019, pp. 281–293. doi: 10.1007/978-3-030-35166-3_20.

33. C. A. G. Díaz et al., VIII Latin American Conference on Biomedical Engineering and XLII National Conference on Biomedical Engineering, *Proceedings of CLAIB-CNIB 2019*, October 2–5, 2019, Cancún, México. Springer Nature, 2019.

34. L. Ali, C. Zhu, N. Amiri Golilarz, A. Javeed, M. Zhou, and Y. Liu, "Reliable Parkinson's disease detection by analyzing handwritten drawings: Construction of an unbiased cascaded learning system based on feature selection and adaptive boosting model," *IEEE Access*, pp. 1–1, Jul. 2019, doi: 10.1109/ACCESS.2019.2932037.

35. A. B. Peachap, D. Tchiotsop, V. Louis-Dorr, and D. Wolf, "Detection of early Parkinson's disease with wavelet features using finger typing movements on a keyboard," *SN Applied Science*, vol. 2, no. 10, p. 1634, Sep. 2020, doi: 10.1007/s42452-020-03473-9.

36. W. R. Adams, "High-accuracy detection of early Parkinson's Disease using multiple characteristics of finger movement while typing," *Plos One*, vol. 12, no. 11, Art. no. 11, Nov. 2017, doi: 10.1371/journal.pone.0188226.

37. D. Iakovakis et al., "Motor impairment estimates via touchscreen typing dynamics toward Parkinson's disease detection from data harvested in-the-wild," *Frontiers in ICT*, vol. 5, p. 28, Nov. 2018, doi: 10.3389/fict.2018.00028.

38. S. Williams et al., "Supervised classification of bradykinesia in Parkinson's disease from smartphone videos," *Artificial Intelligence in Medicine*, vol. 110, p. 101966, Nov. 2020, doi: 10.1016/j.artmed.2020.101966.

39. K. Açıcı, Ç. Erdaş, T. Aşuroğlu, M. Kılınç Toprak, H. Erdem, and H. Oğul, A Random Forest Method to Detect Parkinson's Disease Via Gait Analysis, *International Conference on Engineering Applications of Neural Networks* 2017, p. 619. doi: 10.1007/978-3-319-65172-9_51.

40. L. di Biase et al., "Gait analysis in Parkinson's disease: An overview of the most accurate markers for diagnosis and symptoms monitoring," *Sensors (Basel)*, vol. 20, no. 12, p. 3529, Jun. 2020, doi: 10.3390/s20123529.

41. L. Lonini et al., "Wearable sensors for Parkinson's disease: Which data are worth collecting for training symptom detection models," *npj Digital Medicine*, vol. 1, no. 1, Art. no. 1, Nov. 2018, doi: 10.1038/s41746-018-0071-z.

42. F. Cavallo, A. Moschetti, D. Esposito, C. Maremmani, and E. Rovini, "Upper limb motor pre-clinical assessment in Parkinson's disease using machine learning," *Parkinsonism & Related Disorders*, vol. 63, pp. 111–116, Jun. 2019, doi: 10.1016/j.parkreldis.2019.02.028.

43. Y. Xia, Z. Yao, Q. Ye, and N. Cheng, "A dual-modal attention-enhanced deep learning network for quantification of Parkinson's disease characteristics," *IEEE Transactions on Neural Systems and Rehabilitation Engineering*, vol. 28, no. 1, Art. no. 1, Jan. 2020, doi: 10.1109/TNSRE.2019.2946194.

44. I. El Maachi, G.-A. Bilodeau, and W. Bouachir, "Deep 1D-Convnet for accurate Parkinson's disease detection and severity prediction from gait," *Expert Systems with Applications*, vol. 143, p. 113075, 2020.

45. S. Aghanavesi, D. Nyholm, M. Senek, F. Bergquist, and M. Memedi, "A smartphone-based system to quantify dexterity in Parkinson's disease patients I Elsevier enhanced reader," Mar. 14, 2017. https://reader.elsevier.com/reader/sd/pii/S235291481730023 0?token=4293F07FC1675096C26718809FEE430C2EC73921B3A2E4045A7F2FD 0902765C83BCAFE1A32D6C164D7211A9871703083 (accessed Nov. 13, 2020).

46. J. C. Vasquez-Correa, T. Arias-Vergara, J. R. Orozco-Arroyave, B. Eskofier, J. Klucken, and E. Noth, "Multimodal assessment of Parkinson's disease: A deep learning approach," *IEEE Journal of Biomedical and Health Informatics*, vol. 23, no. 4, Art. no. 4, Jul. 2019, doi: 10.1109/JBHI.2018.2866873.

47. T. D. Pham and H. Yan, "Tensor decomposition of gait dynamics in Parkinson's disease," *IEEE Transactions on Biomedical Engineering*, vol. 65, no. 8, Art. no. 8, Aug. 2018, doi: 10.1109/TBME.2017.2779884.

48. J. Prince, F. Andreotti, and M. De Vos, "multi-source ensemble learning for the remote prediction of Parkinson's disease in the presence of source-wise missing data," *IEEE Transactions on Biomedical Engineering*, vol. 66, no. 5, Art. no. 5, May 2019, doi: 10.1109/TBME.2018.2873252.

49. G. Briganti and O. Le Moine, "Artificial intelligence in medicine: Today and tomorrow," *Frontiers in Medicine*, vol. 7, p. 27, Feb. 2020, doi: 10.3389/fmed.2020.00027.

50. S. Gerke, T. Minssen, and G. Cohen, "Ethical and legal challenges of artificial intelligence-driven healthcare," *Artificial Intelligence in Healthcare*, pp. 295–336, 2020, doi: 10.1016/B978-0-12-818438-7.00012-5.

13 Emerging Technologies to Combat the COVID-19 Pandemic

Leila Ennaceur
Gabes University, Tunisia

Soufiene Ben Othman
University of Sousse, Tunisia

Chinmay Chakraborty
Birla Institute of Technology, Mesra, Ranchi , Jharkhand, India

Faris A. Almalki
Taif University, Taif, Saudi Arabia

Hedi Sakli
EITA Consulting 5 Rue du Chant des Oiseaux,
Montesson, France

CONTENTS

DOI: 10.1201/9781003247128-13

13.1 INTRODUCTION

As the novel coronavirus diseases continue their assault across the globe, with the appearance of new virus variants even in the presence of vaccines, many peoples are still under varying threats of contamination. However, several technological approaches can limit the impact of the COVID-19 pandemic. In fact, the Internet of Things (IoT), blockchain, AI and new generation telecommunications networks, have been in the foreground (Chinmay et al. [1]). The World Health Organization (WHO), and the Center for Disease Control (CDC) consider that digital technologies may play an important role in the management of coronavirus disease. Various technological solutions have taken place-replacing humans to minimize contact and kerb the massive spread of the disease (Priyanka et al. [2]).

In health, like other sectors (energy, industry, banking), many objects already communicated, but at a basic level, and only within their own technical universe, with limited capacities. With the IoT, these objects can now communicate 'alone' and project directly into the Web for remote management and control. With the development of increasingly integrated technologies and increasingly miniaturized equipment, information that they carry is now accessible very quickly and easily.

Health is a tremendous opportunity for the IoT. Beyond the connection of biomedical devices in hospital wards, it is especially on parallel applications that the IoT can reveal its potential, by bringing a finesse of view and management unpublished. Whether for the care of the patient, examinations or treatments, hospitalization at home, or the preventive component, the quantity and quality of data collected by more sensors in addition to being smarter, can provide solutions, improve flows and transform practice. Various companies today offer hospitals a real-time geolocation solution for their patients, their personal and their medical devices. Thus, hospitals will resolve problems in their various flows and activities, and consequently they can optimize their management and improve patient care [3].

For more than a year now, with the pandemic caused by the coronavirus disease, the world has been moving towards a technological approach to cope with the spread of the disease. Finds its strength through groupings and human/human contact. The IoT is also interesting in terms of traceability of the drug circuit outside the hospital. Via connected drug packaging, the various players in the care pathway will be able to know whether a patient is following his prescribed treatment. The IoT then finds a major role, through its ability to manage the condition of a patient from a distance. The instructions required by the WHO are thus applied to control and limit the spread of the disease. Sensors are in high demand for the development and distribution of the COVID-19 vaccine. Through this article, we present the role of new technologies in improving the quality of care. Then technological innovations were designed specifically to deal with COVID-19.

This chapter is organized as follows. In the second section we discuss the COVID-19 preventive measures. Section 13.3 presents smart healthcare and new technologies in the field of health facing COVID-19. We end with a conclusion and discussion.

13.2 COVID-19 PREVENTIVE MEASURES

As part of the COVID-19 response, health workers may be exposed to occupational risks. Put them at risk of illness, injury and even death. To mitigate these dangers and protect the health, safety and wellbeing of health workers, it is necessary to put in place well-coordinated and comprehensive measures for infection prevention and control, occupational health and safety, management of health personnel, mental health and psychosocial support. Lack of adequate occupational health and safety measures can lead to an increase in the rate of work-related illnesses among health workers, a high rate of absenteeism, a decrease in productivity and a deterioration in quality of care.

To this issue, WHO presented an updated document on interim guidelines titled 'COVID-19: Occupational health and safety for health workers' published on 2nd February 2021. This version, based on recent data available, provides guidance on occupational health and safety measures for worker occupational health and health services in the context of the COVID-19 pandemic. In addition, it updates the occupational health and safety rights and responsibilities of healthcare workers in accordance with International Labor Organization (ILO) standards.

In the same approach, Sujata et al. [4] in their article give a complete review of the COVID-19 pandemic and the role of new technologies in managing its impact as they describe the main measures to be followed to protect oneself. These measures emphasize the need to maintain physical distance between people. To the same extent, direct contact with infected persons presents a great risk of contamination. From here, we interpret the role of new technologies to apply these measures. New communication technologies and mobile networks have greatly served people to keep continuous communication through the online social network. Robotics, Artificial Intelligence (AI), and the IoT have been further exploited in various coronavirus disease management solutions.

13.3 SMART HEALTHCARE AND NEW TECHNOLOGIES

In times of emergency such as during a pandemic, technological innovations often materialize. This is currently happening in various countries of the world where new technologies are experiencing unprecedented advances encouraged by governments. In the healthcare field, we are facing a profound change, which has given rise to new uses, for caregivers and patients. The actors in this market must react and develop their innovative products as quickly as possible to meet new needs (Othman et al. [5]).

In addition, research laboratories and companies in the health sector are faced with a dominant challenge: to fight against the virus responsible for the global crisis in the short term as well as to improve the quality of life and the wellbeing of the population on the long term. New advanced technologies, such as AI, Big Data, machine learning, robotization or even information and communication technologies are therefore the main components of the solution. Thousands of healthcare start-ups are springing up around the world today. Table 13.1 below regroups the main technologies used.

TABLE 13.1
Smart Healthcare Technologies to Fight COVID-19

No	Emerging Technology	How Technology is Used During the Pandemic
1	*Telemedicine* as the practice of medicine through telecommunications and technologies enables remote health benefits and the exchange of related medical information.	• Help caregivers for remote triage, evaluation, and care for patients. • Reduce the risk of viral infection for patients and healthcare providers. • Recommended in areas with limited medical resources during COVID-19.
2	*Internet of Things (IoT)*, which enables the interconnection between the Internet and objects, has largely proven its efficiency in supporting decision-making and preventing possible risks.	• Any object attached to a sensor is used to inform caregivers about the evolution of the clinical condition of patients. • Help in real-time monitoring of hospitalized people and in decision-making.
3	*Drone Technology* has become a key tool to support those operating on the front lines during the pandemic. At the same time, governments are discovering new uses to accomplish missions that require more safety and caution.	• Carry out awareness-raising tasks. • Monitor a well-defined area and control the crowd and respect for physical distancing and the wearing of masks. • Supply infected areas with food and medicine. • Disinfect public places.
4	*Robots* have the capacity to be very useful in difficult times, when the human being is forced to adapt. During the health crisis, they help reduce the pressure on health workers and offer isolated people greater access to the outside world.	• Heal the sick. • Take samples for suspicious people. • Deliver food and medicine to hospital patients and for infected people quarantine. • Disinfect parts and replace those responsible for cleaning. • Raise citizens' awareness in parks and in large, closed areas.
5	*Mobile Applications* have become a very useful tool in the fight against the coronavirus. They can help reduce human-human interaction and therefore limit the spread of disease	• Informatics tool for decision support and monitoring of the spread of viruses in health centres [15]. • Using a high-speed telecommunications network, it helps to track the locations of gents in targeted areas, to report infected patients and recording data in gigantic databases. It models the monitoring results, depending on the capabilities of the applications used, for specific needs.
6	**Artificial Intelligence (AI**) is in great demand to respond to the COVID-19 health crisis. It helps public authorities to better anticipate and manage the crisis linked to the pandemic. AI-based tools continue to multiply and deliver good results.	• Make people aware of COVID-19. • Monitor the mobility of people and draw up the complete itinerary of the areas concerned. • Detect suspected cases of COVID-19 and contact the people concerned. • Report the lack of personal protective equipment (PPE) and ensure their distribution. • Provide updated information regarding the COVID-19 disease in real time to ensure a preventive study to the concerned which clarifies the uncertainties.

In addition, digital health is one of the most powerful sectors in terms of investment. Governments must take full advantage of digital technologies to deal with the COVID-19 pandemic and address a wide range of issues related to the pandemic. The pandemic is forcing governments and societies to turn to digital technologies to respond to the crisis, and increasingly governments are adopting digital communication channels to provide reliable information on global and national COVID-19 developments.

Faced with this pandemic, total containment and other social distancing measures have been imposed in different countries. During this period, people are faced with a difficult psychological situation. They rely on the Internet for information and advice. Governments are urged to deploy effective digital technologies to contain the pandemic. The Internet and new communication technologies have helped to mitigate the effect of distancing and quarantine administered to some around the world. We have all felt the major role of Information and Telecommunications Technologies, ICTs, during the pandemic in bringing people together, sharing information, screening, distribution of medicines and food, for awareness-raising, concerning the disease, wearing a mask and respecting physical distancing, especially in public places and in various other cases (Othman et al. [6]).

13.3.1 TELEMEDICINE FACING COVID-19

Telemedicine can improve the quality of care provided to patients in a place where healthcare is not available. This review considers that in remote or locked-down locations, telemedicine offers a practical solution for patients. The telemedicine technology allows patients to make a consultation from their home without having to visit the doctor or hospital (Vinay et al. [7]). The main advantages of this technology during the COVID-19 pandemic are:

- Avoid face to face interactions and therefore reduce the risk of infection;
- Slow down the spread of the virus thanks to the limited movement of patients;
- Reduce the risk of contamination for the healthcare worker;
- Automatic appointment reminder for the patient;
- Remote management of health services;
- Reduction of healthcare costs; and
- Improve the quality of care and consequently patient satisfaction.

Telemedicine that employs the use of the Wearable Sensor Network (WSN), is one of the most beneficial methods for monitoring people's daily lives. It can monitor body temperature as well as heart rate and other vital clinical parameters in patients remotely. It then offers a digital solution that helps caregivers in the remote monitoring of suspected cases. To achieve this digital solution, he uses Lab VIEW software for monitoring medical parameters. Everyone involved in this system uses wireless communication to reduce contact with suspicious people. Patient medical parameters are retrieved from the sensors and saved to backup servers. The caregiver can retrieve data from their cell phone to avoid the use of common tools such as keyboard and mouse. It uses as materials:

- NodeMcu;
- DHT11 temperature sensor;
- Location sensor; and
- 2 workstations.

It uses the ThingSpeak platform that allows aggregating, visualizes and analyze data streams live in the cloud. This platform collects data from the sensors to visualize the temperature variation. Depending on the temperature changes, the subject may or may not be confirmed as a suspected case of COVID-19. Thanks to the WSN and ThingSpeak information processing, infection with the COVID-19 virus will be reduced. This solution allows:

- Remote monitoring of temperature and localization of suspected cases in real-time;
- Avoid direct contact with suspected cases;
- In case of detection of high-temperature values, notifications will be sent remotely to caregivers on their smartphones; and
- The server records the data necessary for the statistical study of the spread of the virus across the country.

13.3.2 INTERNET OF THINGS IN HEALTHCARE

The Internet of Medical Things (IoMT), also known as the healthcare IoT, is a coupling of medical devices and software applications providing extended health services, which are connected to health informatics systems. IoMT involves the application of IoT concepts and these benefits in the healthcare field. This requires specific sensors, medical equipment capable of connecting them, portable devices and the development of the necessary applications, which ensure the proper management of connected objects. This intelligent environment has a major role in improving health benefits (Faris et al. [8]).

The healthcare industry has adopted the IoMT solution for collecting, analyzing and transmitting medical data. This technology shows promise in reducing the load on the health systems. The applications of IoMT include:

- Remote patient monitoring;
- Tracking of drug orders;
- The use of portable devices; and
- Transmit health information to the relevant professional health services.

The architectural representation of an IoMT solution is based on a 3-layer model: perception layer, network layer and application layer. The lower perception layer is designed to collect the required data from patients. It brings together portable IoMT-based devices that allow remote clinical examination. The network layer is the backbone of an IoMT system for real-time telemedicine, and therefore of an intelligent healthcare platform. It brings together all the terminals allowing the transmission and reception of patient files. These are stored on cloud servers, which consolidate both medical records and additional patient information.

The application layer is the level with which the caregiver interacts. This layer is dedicated to the management of the intelligent medical platform. It is an easy-to-operate personalized interface with a dashboard, which shows the clinical status of a patient remotely. Caregivers rely on the information provided for decision-making, management of patient visits, for statistics, as they form a solid database. This database is used to better understand the evolution of coronavirus disease, and for future research.

By leveraging the benefits of the latest technologies, such as sensor networks and IoT, this study presents the investigation, results and applications of the use of IoT innovation. It describes the most recent uses of IoT in healthcare to alleviate the COVID-19 crisis. Much research has focused on the comfort of the elderly by avoiding going to the hospital for treatment and even longer waiting times for a role, which exposes them to the risk of contamination. To this end, Chinmay et al. [9] describe their solution 'A home hospitalization system based on the Internet of Things, fog computing and cloud computing' which is an intelligent health service. It will be a promising service, which aims to alleviate the suffering of patients. In this proposed system, an environmental detection unit and a mobile application, which acts as the fog server, monitor the sick room. This application allows real-time monitoring and control of environmental factors in the hospital room. The patient is monitored remotely through a mobile application that allows nurses to measure vital signs and prepare medical reports. Clinical data is stored in a NoSQL database, which is extensively used in real-time web applications. This cloud database is generally faster and used for Big Data use. It makes it possible to process a large amount of data.

The IoT consists of several functions including the collection, transfer, analysis and storage of data. IoT technology has the advantage of monitoring people infected with coronavirus disease. Kumar et al. in the article [10] presents the solution for detecting symptoms of COVID-19 at an early stage. It is a device worn on the wrist; a solution based on the IoMT. This solution, knowing the most common symptoms of the disease including fever, dry cough, fatigue, anorexia, anosmia and dyspnoea. It is possible, according to him, to detect the disease from such symptoms. Therefore, prevent the spread of the disease.

The system architecture is composed as follows; several sensors, a battery, a 32-bit ARM Cortex microcontroller, a Bluetooth module responsible for sending data to the smartphone. The user can manipulate some components like an LED and a push button. A system requires energy autonomy to be able to use the device effectively. For this reason, the device is equipped with an LED screen for displaying notifications.

Another IoT model (Faris et al. [11])can be adopted in each region to manage the current state of business, prevent new epidemics in geographic regions, resume economic activities and plan for adequate emergency measures. Infrastructure is made up of the following components:

- Examination based on machine learning of the most common symptoms of COVID-19, namely body temperature and cough for each person using the means of transport;
- Control social distancing in public places;
- Check the wearing of protective masks in public places;
- Remote medical monitoring of the elderly and people in quarantine and isolation; and
- Smart healthcare in hospitals during emergencies.

The paradigm helps manage COVID-19 and mitigate its impact. The architecture comprises three levels. The first relates to the diagnosis of infected people and the monitoring of common symptoms of COVID-19 as it explains the proposed method to ensure social distancing and the detection of masks in public places. The next level describes remote health monitoring of isolated, quarantined and elderly people. In addition, the last level shows the smart healthcare based on advanced IT in emergency hospitals to overcome the lack of human resources available to care for a population flow in a time of crisis.

Othman et al. [12], which is based on the blockchain, propose a solution in guarantees the confidentiality of the data, and research the suspicious contacts then warns the parties concerned. Solution helps track infected people who need to be quarantined. The information collected is recorded in the cloud. This solution uses a smartphone application that can check for COVID-19 cases after analyzing the symptoms and checking whether it is infected or not thanks to an Adaptive Neuro-Fuzzy Interference System (ANFIS) and a K-Nearest Neighbour (KNN). The solution is characterized by an accuracy rate of approximately 95.9%.

Shivam et al in their article [13] propose an intelligent "EdgeSDNI4COVID" contactless architecture applicable in industry which is strongly affected by the pandemic. We are talking about a risk-free industry 4.0 based on a network of sensors whose data will be monitored remotely. The architecture is based on two SDN layers for Software Defined Networking and the NFV layer for Network Function Virtualization to ensure the monitoring of data collected from IoT sensors.

13.3.3   DRONE TECHNOLOGY

Drones as autonomous remote-controlled machines represent a technological evolution that has been able to overlap in different fields. They are characterized by a crucial role during pandemics caused by coronavirus disease. It helps governments and people during the lockdown. We have already noticed the use of this technology to make people aware of the need to wear masks, physical distancing, again for screening by measuring the temperature in public places of citizens. As again for disinfection and replenishment with food and drugs for people in quarantine or those who occupy areas rather difficult to reach. Drones have also made it possible to control the movement of citizens to demand and force the application of curfews in various countries around the world. It ensures a minimum of human interaction. During the COVID-19 pandemic period, and especially during periods of containment, drones are used a lot (Chinmay et al. [14]).

The drone can cover several areas during its flight. Once equipped with thermal, position, and camera sensors, drones can be used for 24-hour monitoring of groups in public areas, for announcements, for screening, and again for medical supplies. They can be a real substitute for less expensive manpower. Kumar et al. have designed an intelligent surveillance system [15] for the control of social distancing. This system is based on a drone capable of identifying violations of the social distancing policy. The system is based on the YOLO-v3 tiny fast object detection algorithm. It actually uses a detector that adapts to systems with low computation. The drone detects people and identifies if there are two people or several that are close to each other at a certain distance. The drone can then be located in a well-defined area and integrate a global positioning system that locates the observed area and detects the road. It, therefore, follows a predefined navigation pattern while flying above. The drone is equipped with a system capable of detecting objects, locating them, and measuring the distance between objects (Saxena et al. [16]).

13.3.4 ROBOTICS TECHNOLOGY

Medical robots include technical devices and machines used in the medical field that perform or assist mechanical tasks. In addition to assisting surgeons, robots can have support functions in the daily lives of patients. Thus, the latter can have multiple applications to help the disabled or caregivers (Bhushan, et al. [17]).

Medical robots come to assist surgeons, interns or nursing staff in tasks that are beyond their human capacities or that simply cannot be performed by humans. Here, fatigue during long surgical operations is a major element. Contrary to some fiction, robotics in medicine is not intended to completely replace humans. Medical robots mainly play an assistant role and must instead give the doctor an augmented hand, capable of performing difficult movements with extraordinary finesse and precision. They offer a wide range of uses and processing possibilities and can, in specific configurations, simplify certain processes and perform them precisely. Medical robots are sometimes called manipulators because they do not act autonomously and must be piloted by a person. The technique in this sense, therefore, offers a positive manipulation or optimization of human capacities (Bhushan et al. [18]).

Driven by innovation and with the importance that this represents for society, authorized medical robots are increasingly popular around the world; medical technology is thus opening new application horizons. With the COVID-19 pandemic, robots provide the solution to provide healthcare centres with a secure environment for caregivers who are facing a major challenge; treat infected people and protect themselves against this disease. In addition, the robots are used for surface disinfection by ultraviolet (UV) radiation. It thus replaces cleaning personnel and consequently reduces the probability of contamination of the latter. Robotic technology once used has proven its potential in many acts. The application of robots in healthcare systems has shown encouraging solutions to prevent COVID-19 cases (Shen et al. [19]).

With the simultaneous integration of machine learning algorithms and AI, robots have proven to be more efficient in the treatment and diagnosis of infection. One of the marked uses of robots is for mass screening. This solution adopted in various countries around the world makes it possible to acquire data to interpret the health assessment of individuals and consequently prevent infected cases. During the situation caused by the coronavirus disease, the autonomous robot system provided substantial support to health workers by performing repetitive operations. Indeed, a tireless solution performs tasks with a low margin of error.

Knowing that the physical distancing required by the WHO is the best solution to prevent the spread of the disease, robots are used in hospitals to reduce the impacts of the COVID-19 pandemic. Robotics aims to increase the autonomy of machines by endowing them with perceptual, decision-making and action capacities. Kaye et al. [20] used a robot in several healthcare centres around the world even during the appearance of the COVID disease, in Germany, in France, in Italy, and some African countries such as Tunisia and Rwanda.

Awaisi et al. in their article [21] provide a comprehensive study of the robotic systems that emerged during the pandemic. They focused on the challenges presented in almost all industries with the increasing demand for robotic systems and hence robotic developers are opening many opportunities.

There are various types of robots with a certain type of applications:

- *Telerobot:* like re-habilitation robot and telerobot arm for ultrasound;
- *Collaborative robot:* for swabbing and manual swabbing robot;
- *Autonomous robot:* UV disinfecting and self-driven delivery robot;
- *Social robot:* robot guide and the robot dog in the park; and
- *Wearable robot:* smart helmet and temperature and face recognition helmet.

To conclude, the current state of technological development, forced by the global health situation, paves the way for the fusion of robotics, AI, Big Data, advanced imaging systems and nanotechnologies so to meet human needs.

13.3.5   MOBILE APPLICATIONS

Various applications have been developed to help limit or even stop the spread of COVID-19. Thus, several developers, each in their own way participate in this wrestling company. Many platforms have been developed with education or healthcare field for example. These Android applications help citizens, caregivers and governments to manage the crisis well.

Ijaz et al. [22] notably propose an Android data collection application, LISUNGIcovid19. This application is based on the Open Data Kit (ODK) platform, like open-source mobile data collection software. The solution is made up of two parts: a mobile platform and a data collection server. This application helps decision-making in containment planning, as it represents a means of evaluating the health crisis management strategy; it can be adopted by the governorate in that order. LISUNGIcovid19 is built around a Client-Server architecture at three levels:

- **Desktop clients:** these are the Web applications for creating forms. It uses Excel and ODK XLSForm. The form was created with Excel then, converted to XForms format recognized by ODK tools using ODK XLSForm;
- **ODK Aggregate v1.7.3 server:** after form creation, it is downloaded to a server instance created in advance.; and
- **Mobile Client:** the mobile application used to collect data using a form already created.

The solution invites the user to answer a questionnaire concerning his state of health, or if he has an infected loved one, his opinion concerning the confinement in his region, etc. These questions allow statistics of contamination and spread of the virus to be drawn up. Allowing the decision-maker to make a reliable decision and manage the crisis caused by this pandemic.

There are still other mobile applications in the voice analysis framework for asthma-COVID-19 for early diagnosis and prediction. It is a mobile application based on AI and cloud Computing proposed by Sachin et al. in [23]. Asthma patients have a higher risk potential than others. In fact, asthma and COVID-19 cause detectable voice changes. The proposed solution is based on voice monitoring and represents a precise tool for predicting early pulmonary disease. The proposed asthma–COVID-19 detection system is based on voice analysis. It is a diagnostic method for the detection of COVID-19 asthma, which causes significant voice changes. The app relies on AI for the detection of voice changes caused by asthma and COVID-19. Cloud computing technology enables the collection, analysis and storage of data. With a smartphone device with an integrated mic, the user can operate the mobile application. This allows the user to be monitored continuously. It runs in the background during a voice search or a phone call. All you need is a short voice recording to operate the app. When a voice recording is made, the collected data is sent to the cloud for analysis and extraction of characteristics.

13.3.6 Artificial Intelligence (AI)

AI is based on computers and programs capable of performing skills generally associated with human intelligence and amplified by technology, such as the ability to:

- Process large amounts of data;
- Discern patterns and models undetectable by a human;
- Understand and analyze these models;
- Interact with humans;
- Learn gradually; and

- Continuously improve its performance.

During the pandemic, with the digitization of healthcare, large quantities of data will be processed. However, researchers and decision-makers must deal with the sheer volume of data known as Big Data. This justifies how AI could be crucial in the development and improvement of health systems globally. AI here helps solve complex problems in different fields including medicine. Bouraoui et al. [24] propose a combined method derived from AI and statistics from alternative epidemiological models to estimate the speed of spread and develop scenarios and prevent confirmed cases of COVID-19 in Algeria.

Wang et al. in [25] took the case of Indonesia when on July 6, 2020, there were 64,958 infected people including 3,241 people declared dead. He pointed out that this number is due to congestion in various places, such as markets, train stations, terminals and places of worship. He considers that the new policy proposed by the government to combat the spread of covid-19 has negative effects on productivity. To this end, it offers an integrated COVID-19 early prevention solution. The solution is a Smart Gate based on AI and the integration of a website. It helps control the density of the community in various locations and reminds the population to follow the health protocols recommended by the government. The solution is called COVID-19 Early Prevention Devices (INCEPS).

The Smart Gate system developed based on artificial intelligence is designed to be integrated into the INCEPS website. The smart door is equipped with various features including mask recognition camera, temperature sensor, automatic gate, disinfectant with spray box and door disinfectant. The temperature sensor measures the temperature of the object according to the infrared (IR) waves emitted by the target without hitting. The system automatically checks whether the visitor has normal body temperature and that he is wearing a mask. Therefore, visitors will be able to enter when they pass the smart door check, and hence, the door will be automatically open. A disinfectant spray can be used to sterilize visitors and the objects they still carry in a place reserved for them. The system thus checks whether the clothes and bodies of visitors are sterilized, so that they enter a public place, carry out various activities and feel safe.

Several searches have been proposed in the literature to detect COVID-19 cases. AI based on the medical image was used to analyze and identify infected cases. The system measures and monitors disease and differentiates between affected and healthy patients.

Medical imaging such as x-rays and computed tomography (CT) are necessary diagnostic tools to judge whether the case has the virus or not. Emerging technologies, such as AI, further strengthen the power of medical imaging and help medical specialists. For confirmation of infected individuals, doctors require the Reverse Transcription Chain Reaction Polymerase (RT-PCR) test. At the same time, especially at the start of the disease outbreak, the RT-PCR test tends to be insufficient in many more affected areas. Specialists then adopt the technique of medical imaging, such as chest x-ray and thoracic CT. The technique was adopted particularly in China, to identify many cases as contaminated by COVID-19 if characteristic manifestations in CT were observed. Knowing that suspected patients are asked to be tested several times before arriving at a definite diagnosis, imaging results is used for detecting suspicious cases (Kamboj et al. [26]).

Chinmay et al. in [27] discussed the role of medical imaging coupled with AI. It describes the imaging platform and machine learning methods including segmentation, diagnosis and prognosis. During this period, surveillance cameras are adopted in the scanning rooms, on the CT machine with better access to patients. Thus, the digitization room and the control room are completely isolated. Each has its own entrance to avoid unnecessary contact between technicians and patients. The correction of the patient's position on the bed in the examination room is provided by visual and audible prompts from the video transmitted by the AI cameras. Following a motion analysis algorithm and the patient's position, the algorithm automatically recovers the 3D pose. The technician can adjust if necessary. Once everything is checked, the patient's bed will be moved into the CT.

Kuzlu et al. [28] present a document allowing classifications by areas of people affected or not by COVID-19. the identification is made thanks to the CNN neuron network. The system can detect areas infected with coronavirus disease from radiological images through deep learning based on YOLO. Another COVID-19 case prediction system for autoregressive integrated moving average (ARIMA) can serve the most countries affected by the COVID-19 virus including India.

Other research focuses on the quality of the data transmitted and takes advantage of the strength of the algorithms to resolve certain constraints linked to the transmission of data. Chinmay et al. in [29] attempt to minimize latency in online healthcare through fog computing. In fact, in the IoT, the multimedia data is widely used in the health sector. So, they consider that the transmission times must be revised and optimized to satisfy the maximum number of users. To achieve this goal, they propose a novel intelligent multimedia data segregation (IMDS) scheme based on machine learning (k-fold random forest) applied in the fog computing environment. The simulation results in about 95% reduction in latency compared to the existing model, this contributes to improving the quality of care.

13.4   CONCLUSION AND DISCUSSION

Even with the manufacture of vaccine, the COVID-19 virus continues its assault on the globe in the form of the new variants. Globally, the situation is not adequately improved, and billions of people are under an almost constant threat. This situation threatens the economy of countries and increases the number of victims. Faced with this situation, a multitude of technological solutions is participating to face the pandemic.

Various technologies have been used to provide intelligent systems that facilitate the work of caregivers and speed up the process of treating patients. Much research has focused on improving the quality of care during the pandemic as well as for contagious diseases in general. COVID-19 pandemic has accelerated the need for automation technologies that prevent the transmission of the virus.

To date, physical distancing is the only measure to control the spread of the coronavirus, even with the discovery of a specific vaccine, and vaccination campaigns have been launched in countries around the world. To this end, the world is preparing for technological innovations, which can support humans in certain tasks requiring direct contact with COVID-19 patients. This article began by describing the various efforts deployed to put an end to the pandemic and the preventive measures followed by the various countries around the world to bypass the virus and prevent its spread to the maximum.

These efforts are based on new technologies to manage the impacts of the coronavirus disease. The majority intelligent systems do not only have the advantage of remote monitoring of the patient, but also of having a database on the disease, the symptoms, the age group reached, the organs attacked in the patients, the rate of disease progression in each region. All this information help doctors and officials in making decisions about what treatment is needed for each patient, as well as how countries should act to avoid massive population attacks.

The monitoring system is equipped with a platform, which allows the medical staff to monitor the patients admitted in real time. In addition, all the data will obviously be recorded on cloud servers for real-time use, as well as for failing the statistics necessary for the good management of the disease. We recall that the major objective is to offer caregivers a healthy environment that promotes the speed of care and its effectiveness. In addition, the occupational health and safety of nursing staff is essential to enable them to perform their work in this time of crisis. Their protection must be a priority.

CONFLICT OF INTEREST

There is no conflict of interests.

FUNDING

There is no funding support.

DATA AVAILABILITY

Not applicable.

REFERENCES

1. Chinmay, C., and Arij, N.A., Intelligent Internet of Things and Advanced Machine Learning Techniques for COVID-19, *EAI Endorsed Transactions on Pervasive Health and Technology*, 7, 1–14, 2021, doi:10.4108/eai.28-1-2021.168505

2. Priyanka, D., and Chinmay, C., Application of AI on Post Pandemic Situation and Lesson Learn for Future Prospects, *Journal of Experimental & Theoretical Artificial Intelligence*, 1–24, 2021, doi:10.1080/0952813X.2021.1958063.

3. Othman, S.B., Bahattab, A.A., Trad, A., and Youssef, H., LSDA: Lightweight Secure Data Aggregation Scheme in Healthcare using IoT, in *10th International Conference on Information Systems and Technologies*, Lecce, Italy, Dec 28, 2019–Dec 30, 2019, doi:10.1145/3447568.3448530.

4. Sujata, D., Chinmay, C., Sourav, K.G., Subhendu, K.P., and Jaroslav, F., BIFM: Big Data-Driven Intelligent Forecasting Model for COVID-19, *IEEE Access*, 1–13, 2021, doi:10.1109/ACCESS.2021.3094658.

5. Othman, S.B., Bahattab, A.A., Trad, A., et al., Confidentiality and Integrity for Data Aggregation in WSN Using Homomorphic Encryption, *Wireless Pers Commun*, 80, 867–889, 2015, doi:10.1007/s11277-014-2061-z.

6. Soufiene, B.O., Bahattab, A.A., Trad, A., and Youssef, H., RESDA: Robust and Efficient Secure Data Aggregation Scheme in Healthcare using the IoT, in *2019 International Conference on Internet of Things, Embedded Systems and Communications (IINTEC)*, Tunis, Tunisia, 2019, pp. 209–213, doi:10.1109/IINTEC48298.2019.9112125.

7. Chamola, V., Hassija, V., Gupta, V., and Guizani, M., A Comprehensive Review of the COVID-19 Pandemic and the Role of IoT, Drones, AI, Blockchain, and 5G in Managing Its Impact, *IEEE Access*, 8, 90225–90265, May 26, 2020.

8. Almalki, F.A., and Soufiene, B.O., EPPDA: An Efficient and Privacy-Preserving Data Aggregation Scheme with Authentication and Authorization for IoT-Based Healthcare Applications, *Wireless Communications and Mobile Computing*, 2021, 18, 2021, Article ID 5594159, doi:10.1155/2021/5594159.

9. Chinmay, C., Performance Analysis of Compression Techniques for Chronic Wound Image Transmission under Smartphone-Enabled Tele-wound Network, *International Journal of E-Health and Medical Communications (IJEHMC), IGI Global*, 10(2), 1–20, April 2019.

10. Kumar, M., and Chand, S., A Secure and Efficient Cloud-Centric Internet-of-Medical-Things-Enabled Smart Healthcare System With Public Verifiability, *IEEE Internet of Things Journal*, 7(10), 10650–10659, Oct. 2020, doi:10.1109/JIOT.2020.3006523.

11. Almalki, F.A., Ben Othman, S., A Almalki, F., and Sakli, H., EERP-DPM: Energy-Efficient Routing Protocol Using Dual Prediction Model for Healthcare Using IoT, *Journal of Healthcare Engineering*, 2021, 15, 2021, Article ID 9988038, doi:10.1155/2021/9988038.

12. Bahattab, A.A., Trad, A., and Youssef, H., PEERP: An Priority-Based Energy-Efficient Routing Protocol for Reliable Data Transmission in Healthcare using the IoT, *Procedia Computer Science*, 175, 373–378, 2020, doi:10.1016/j.procs.2020.07.053.

13. Saxena, S., and Bhushan, B., Mohd Abdul Ahad, Blockchain Based Solutions to Secure IoT: Background, Integration Trends and a Way Forward, *Journal of Network and Computer Applications*, 181, 103050, 2021, doi:10.1016/j.jnca.2021.103050.

14. Chinmay, C., Computational Approach for Chronic Wound Tissue Characterization, *Elsevier: Informatics in Medicine Unlocked*, 17, 1–10, 2019, doi:10.1016/j.imu.2019. 100162.

15. Kumar, A., Abhishek, K., Bhushan, B., and Chakraborty, C., Secure Access Control for Manufacturing Sector with Application of Ethereum Blockchain, *Peer-to-Peer Networking and Applications*, 1–17, 2021, doi:10.1007/s12083-021-01108-3.

16. Saxena, S., Bhushan, B., and Ahad, M. A., Blockchain Based Solutions to Secure IoT: Background, Integration Trends and a Way Forward, *Journal of Network and Computer Applications*, 103050, 2021, doi:10.1016/j.jnca.2021.10305.

17. Bhushan, B., Sahoo, C., Sinha, P., and Khamparia, A., Unification of Blockchain and Internet of Things (BIoT): Requirements, Working Model, Challenges and Future Directions, *Wireless Networks*, 27(1), 55–90, 2020, doi:10.1007/s11276-020-02445-6

18. Bhushan, B., Sinha, P., Sagayam, K. M., and Andrew, J., Untangling Blockchain Technology: A Survey on State of the Art, Security Threats, Privacy Services, Applications and Future Research Directions, *Computers & Electrical Engineering*, 90, 106897, 2021, doi:10.1016/j.compeleceng.2020.106897.

19. Shen, Y. et al., Robots under Covid-19 Pandemic: A Comprehensive Survey, *IEEE Access*, 9, 1590–1615, 2021.

20. Kaye, R., Chang, C.W.D., Kazahaya, K., Brereton, J., and Denneny, J.C., COVID-19 Anosmia Reporting Tool: Initial Findings, *Otolaryngol.–Head Neck Surgery*, 163, 132–134, 2020.

21. Awaisi, K.S., Hussain, S., Ahmed, M., Khan, A.A., and Ahmed, G., Leveraging IoT and Fog Computing in Healthcare Systems, *IEEE Internet of Things Magazine*, 3(2), 52–56, June 2020, doi:10.1109/IOTM.0001.1900096.

22. Ijaz, M., Li, G., Lin, L., Cheikhrouhou, O., Hamam, H., and Noor, A., Integration and Applications of Fog Computing and Cloud Computing Based on the Internet of Things for Provision of Healthcare Services at Home, *Electronics*, 10, 1077, 2021, doi:10.3390/electronics10091077

23. Sachin, D., Chinmay, C., Jaroslav, F., Rashmi, G., Arun, K.R., Subhendu, K.P., SSII: Secured and High-Quality Steganography Using Intelligent Hybrid Optimization Algorithms for IoT, *IEEE Access*, 9, 1–16, 2021, doi:10.1109/ACCESS.2021.3089357.

24. Fu, J., Liu, Y., Chao, H., Bhargava, B.K., and Zhang, Z., Secure Data Storage and Searching for Industrial IoT by Integrating Fog Computing and Cloud Computing, *IEEE Transactions on Industrial Informatics*, 14(10), 4519–4528, Oct. 2018, doi:10.1109/TII.2018.2793350.

25. Wang, T., and Chen, H., A Lightweight SDN Fingerprint Attack Defense Mechanism Based on Probabilistic Scrambling and Controller Dynamic Scheduling Strategies, *Security and Communication Networks*, 2021, 23, 2021, Article ID 6688489. doi:10.1155/2021/6688489.

26. Kamboj, P., Khare, S., and Pal, S., User Authentication Using Blockchain Based Smart Contract in Role-Based Access Control. *Peer-to-Peer Netw. Appl.*, 1–16, 2021, doi:10.1007/s12083-021-01150-1.

27. Chinmay, C., Joel JPC Rodrigues, A Comprehensive Review on Device-to-Device Communication Paradigm: Trends, Challenges and Applications, *Journal of Wireless Personal Communications*, 114, 185–207, 2020, doi:10.1007/s11277-020-07358-3.

28. Kuzlu, M., Fair, C., and Guler, O., Role of Artificial Intelligence in the Internet of Things (IoT) Cybersecurity, *Discov Internet Things*, 1, 7, 2021, doi:10.1007/s43926-020-00001-4.
29. Sachin, D., Chinmay, C., Jaroslav, F., Rashmi, G., Arun, K.R., Subhendu, K.P., SSII: Secured and High-Quality Steganography Using Intelligent Hybrid Optimization Algorithms for IoT, *IEEE Access*, 9, 1–16, 2021, doi:10.1109/ACCESS.2021.3089357.

14 The Role of Machine Learning and Internet of Things in Digital Health Transformation

Arij Naser Abougreen
University of Tripoli, Libya

Chinmay Chakraborty
Birla Institute of Technology, Mesra, Ranchi , Jharkhand, India

CONTENTS

14.1 INTRODUCTION

In the last 50 years, the population of cities has increased dramatically (S. Bhattacharya et al., 2020 [1]). In the future, cities around the world will be transformed to be smart cities (M. Al-Emran et al., 2020 [2]). Smart cities aim to effectively manage the energy consumption, maintaining a green environment and increasing the individuals' abilities to effectively utilize the modern ICT (Z. Ullah et al., 2020 [3]). The development in information technologies have affected most

DOI: 10.1201/9781003247128-14

sectors (A. C. Martín et al., 2019 [4]). The importance of IoT was recently appreciated by all academicians and researchers (D. N. Le et al., 2019 [5]). In IoT, every object can connect to the internet and objects can exchange data between each other. Through IoT large amounts of data are sent every second (S. Dhawan et al., 2021 [6]). IoT applications can assist in achieving smart city (SC) concept and provide enhanced services (F. Righetti et al., 2018 [7], A. Zanella et al., 2014 [8]). So, there is an urgent need to teach IoT technology for engineers (M. Al-Emran et al., 2020 [2]). In addition, AI is a significant tool which has a great impact on various sectors (L. Chen et al., 2020 [9]). ML is an emerging concept which is a branch of AI. ML enables computers to perform several tasks such as classification, clustering, predictions and pattern recognition (F. Zantalis et al., 2019 [10]). ML can support smart cities concept and it had remarkable contribution to several sectors with superb results (S. Nosratabadi et al., 2020 [11]). The most common IoT and ML applications for smart cities are environmental monitoring, smart parking, traffic monitoring, smart education, smart health and smart buildings and smart agriculture (F. Righetti et al., 2018 [7], W. M. Septiawan et al., 2019 [12], J. Barker et al., 2019 [13], S. Sasi Priya et al., 2020 [14], S. Hussain et al., 2019 [15], R. Ben Ammar et al., 2019 [16]). IoT can solve several issues such as congestion and limited car parking facilities (A. Khanna et al., 2016 [17]). Traffic congestion is a common issue in cities especially in developing countries. This issue leads to energy consumption and air pollution. So, many systems have been proposed for monitoring traffic and overcome this issue (S. P. Biswas et al., 2015 [18], G. Ali et al., 2020 [19]). Also, unavailable free parking slots will cause traffic congestion. Congestion and parking are related to each other. Thus, there is an urgent need to develop effective smart parking systems (G. Ali et al., 2020 [19]). Smart monitoring traffic is an active research topic owing to the emerging technologies of ML and IoT (M. Sarrab et al., 2020 [20]). Furthermore, employing advanced technologies can enable students to learn effectively and digital resources can be accessed via a wireless network (Z.-T. Zhu et al., 2016 [21]). Smart education environment is recommended. Employing IoT in education will enhance the quality of education (M. Abdel-Basset et al., 2019 [22]). The objective of smart classroom is to enhance teaching and learning (P. K, 2020 [23]). Also, the concept of smart farming relates to utilizing technologies in agriculture in order to increase production (H. Kaur et al., 2019 [24]). Figure 14.1 demonstrates the applications of IoT and ML for SC. Smart health is used to improve healthcare via providing several services such as accurate early diagnosis, diseases prediction and health monitoring. Thus, it has a positive impact on healthcare industry (Z. Rayanal., 2018 [25]).

[Alt Text: diagram demonstrates the applications of IoT and ML in SC. In this diagram, there are seven oval shapes which indicates these applications which are: Smart Education, smart health, Smart Buildings, Traffic Monitoring, Smart Agriculture, Environmental Monitoring and Smart Parking].

The main contributions of this chapter are:

- A review of IoT and ML approaches that have been used for various smart cities applications is presented;

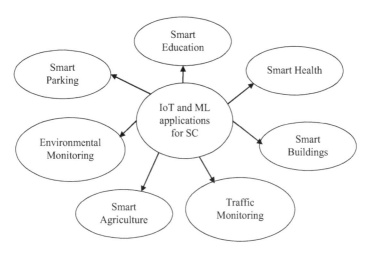

FIGURE 14.1 IoT and ML applications for SC.

- Discussion on the role of AI, IoT and blockchain in the development of the healthcare sector in the era of digital health transformation;
- Discussion on the challenges of IoT in SC; and
- Empowering researchers for further work on applications of ML and IoT in SC.

The chapter is organized as follows: in section 14.2 IoT and ML applications for SC is presented. Sections 14.2.1–14.2.7 review IoT and ML applications for environmental monitoring, smart parking, traffic monitoring, smart education, smart health, smart buildings and smart agriculture respectively. Section 14.3 presents the IoT challenges in SC. Secured SCs is discussed in section 14.4. Sections 14.5 and 14.6 present conclusion and future work respectively.

14.2 IOT AND ML APPLICATIONS FOR SC

14.2.1 ENVIRONMENTAL MONITORING

Poor air quality has a negative impact on individual's health and crops (F. Righetti et al., 2018 [7]). In (W. M. Septiawan et al., 2019 [12]), a new deep learning (DL) has been presented to analyze IoT data. Long Short-Term Memory (LSTM) networks were utilized for forecasting the future values of air quality in a SC. The findings demonstrated that the proposed LSTM-based model is an effective model due to its high obtained prediction accuracy.

It is required to develop smart environmental monitoring which can monitor the natural resources remotely (S. Abraham et al., 2017 [26], S. L. Ullo et al., 2020 [27]). In (S. Abraham et al., 2017 [26]), IoT system was designed for monitoring both of air and soil quality. Graphical user interface (GUI) was utilized for displaying the real-time data. Thus, abnormalities can be detected, and users notified via email.

In (D. E. N. Ganesh et al., 2017 [28]), Wireless sensor networks (WSN) platform was designed for environmental monitoring purpose. This approach is cost-effective, reliable and suitable for long term environmental data acquisition.

IoT is commonly used as platform in smart campus. In (N. P. Sastra et al., 2017 [29]), a WSN in IoT was designed for environmental monitoring for building smart campus. Sensors were employed to gather information. Then this information was delivered to a web server via 802.11 standards. Thus, the collected information was available on internet. This network can operate only when WiFi service is available.

Air pollution is one of the issues that need to be controlled (M. S. Jamil et al., 2015 [30]). In (M. S. Jamil et al., 2015 [30]), WSN nodes were deployed around the city and on public transport and cars for gathering data about the air polluting. This method is an efficient approach for monitoring the environment.

In (C. Toma et al., 2019 [31]), a real-time pollution monitoring system was proposed. This system involves sensors and IoT telecommunication protocols. Data was acquired and transmitted via telecommunication channels.

Many disasters happen annually, such as floods and earthquakes. Thus, early warning systems (EWS) are needed (A. L. Pyayt et al., 2011 [32]). In (A. L. Pyayt et al., 2011 [32]), ML was employed for detecting abnormal behaviour.

In (R. J. Kuo et al., 2019 [33]), a recurrent neural network (RNN) was employed for forecasting the air quality. Data has been gathered from Taiwanese government. Gaussian process algorithm was utilized for choosing the best parameters in the model. The results have demonstrated that this approach outperformed back-propagation neural network and basic RNN.

In (T. Malche et al., 2019 [34]), a secure and reliable IoT-based environmental monitoring system has been proposed. This system was utilized for monitoring a wide spectrum of gases. The stored and transmitted data were authenticated and encrypted.

14.2.2 SMART PARKING

Recently, people face a real issue of parking their vehicles owing to the increased number of vehicles. So, it is significant to provide smart parking systems to enable drivers to find available parking slots (S. Begade et al., 2019 [35], R. Kumar et al., 2020 [36]). In (S. Begade et al., 2019 [35]), a real-time parking system using IoT was proposed. Through this system, data about parking spaces can be accessed by users. Moreover, booking of parking spaces can be performed using smartphone app. There are many benefits of this system such as reducing fuel consumption, time and pollution.

Advanced smart parking systems can inform users about the existence of vacant nearby parking spaces (R. Salpietro et al., 2015 [37]). In (R. Salpietro et al., 2015 [37]), an approach for automatic detection of parking actions via the analysis of smartphone embedded sensors and Bluetooth connectivity was proposed. In addition, the parking action is disseminated via a combination of Internet connection to a remote server, and Device-to-Device (D2D) connections over Wi-Fi Direct links. Thus, other potential interested users will be notified.

In (A. Khanna et al., 2016 [17]), IoT-based smart parking system was proposed. This system can monitor the availability of parking spaces. So, every user can search for the available parking spaces via a mobile application. This mobile application is connected to the cloud. Through this application, the user can select any parking slot.

In (R. Kumar et al., 2020 [36]), a real-time parking system was proposed based on ML and IoT. This system has employed smart sensors, cloud computing, ML algorithms and cyber-physical system. The advantage of this system is the ability to indicate the usage of reserved and unreserved parking slots, unauthorized parking and detecting objects in parking slots.

In (R. Lookmuang et al., 2018 [38]), IoT-based smart parking system has been proposed to provide information about vacant space and determine the location of available parking slot for reducing traffic issue in the parking area. This system is capable of detecting a vehicle plate number and informing the driver of a parking place for his car. This system was designed using hardware and software based on the concept of IoT and mobile application. The driver can also pay the parking fee using their mobile phone.

Most smart parking systems around the world gather and share real-time data with their users through mobile phone apps. However, ML algorithms can be utilized for predicting the future availability which may leads to reducing traffic congestion (J. Barker et al., 2019 [13]). In (J. Barker et al., 2019, [13], ML algorithms were employed for future car parking availability rates prediction. Various ML algorithms have been tested which are K Nearest Neighbour (KNN), KStar, Linear Regression model, Multi-Layer Perceptron model and Random Forest. It was found that KStar algorithm has produced the best results during highly variable conditions.

In (G. Ali et al., 2020 [19]), a deep LSTM network framework was proposed for predicting the availability of a parking slot. This framework was integrated with IoT. This system can forecast the availability of parking space with considering the parking location, days of the week and hours.

In (S. Yamin Siddiqui et al., 2020 [39]), a car parking location forecasting using Deep Extreme Machine Learning (DEML) was proposed. The obtained precision rate was 91.25% which demonstrates the effectiveness of this approach.

In (S. Saharan et al., 2020 [40]), ML was employed for predicting the occupancy of parking lots and determining the parking prices for the next arriving cars. Four ML models have been used and compared which are Linear (LIN), Decision Tree (DT), Neural Network (NN), and Random Forest (RF). RF has achieved the highest accuracy which was 99.01%. The findings exhibit the effectiveness of this approach over other exiting methods. Table 14.1 demonstrates a summary of ML and IoT approaches that has been used for smart parking

14.2.3 TRAFFIC MONITORING

In (I. M. O. Widyantara et al., 2015 [41]), an IoT-based traffic monitoring system (TMS) was proposed to monitor the traffic in Denpasar city. In this system, GPS tracker devices have been employed as embedded sensors. Also, general

TABLE 14.1
Summary of ML and IoT Approaches That Have been Used for Smart Parking

Author	Proposed Technique	Contributions
R. Salpietro et al. [37]	IoT	Smart parking system has been proposed.
A. Khanna et al. [17]	IoT	a smart parking system for monitoring the availability of parking space was proposed.
R. Kumar et al. [36]	ML+ IoT	a real-time parking system was proposed.
R. Lookmuang et al. [38]	IoT	A smart parking system has been proposed.
J. Barker et al. [13]	ML	ML algorithms were employed for future car parking availability rates prediction.
G. Ali et al. [19]	ML+ IoT	A framework was proposed for predicting the availability of parking slot.
S. Yamin Siddiqui et al. [39]	DEML	A car parking location forecasting system was proposed.
S. Saharan et al. [40]	ML	An effective smart parking pricing system has been proposed.

packet radio service (GPRS) technology was utilized for transporting data to the server. Moreover, the visualization of road density category is viewed to the users through Web-GIS (Geographic Information Systems) media. So, users can know information about the traffic accurately.

Heavy traffic congestion leads to different kinds of pollution. This pollution will have a negative impact on people's health. To address this issue, a smart system which can monitor and control the traffic congestion is needed (A. K. M. Masum et al., 2018 [42]). In (A. K. M. Masum et al., 2018 [42]), an IoT-based real-time TMS was proposed. In this system, ultrasonic sensors are employed for measuring the traffic density. Then, the sensor data is analyzed, and the traffic signal time is set via traffic management algorithm. Moreover, the controller delivers the data to a cloud server via a Wi-Fi module. The advantages of this system are easy maintenance, simplicity of installation and cost-effective. However, security aspect should be considered.

In (J. Zaucha et al., 2019 [43]), an IoT-based-road TMS was proposed. A traffic monitoring algorithm has been deployed to Raspberry Pi. Also, analysis and visualizing of the traffic patterns were performed via ThingSpeak platform. Furthermore, an automatic setting of green times is permitted based on road intersections traffic.

In (G. M. Lingani et al., 2019 [44]), DL-based TMS was proposed. The approach was employed for still images, recorded-videos, real-time live videos for detecting, classifying, tracking and computing moving object velocity and direction in an intersection via convolution neural network (CNN).

Road traffic data involves huge volumes, and it is difficult to monitor these data manually (S. Sasi Priya et al., 2020 [14]). In (S. Sasi Priya et al., 2020 [14]), CNN was utilized for traffic monitoring and control. The model classifies the input images into fire accident, accident, heavy traffic and low traffic. The accuracy of the model was 80%.

Management of traffic signal is one of the main current issues (S. K. Janahan et al., 2018 [45]). In (S. K. Janahan et al., 2018 [45]), IoT-based Traffic Monitoring Signal timing was developed. In this model, the timing of traffic signal depends on number of cars on the specific roadside. Data analysis was done using KNN algorithm. This system has the capability for reducing the waiting time of the drivers.

14.2.4 SMART EDUCATION

Smart education term is a significant concept. Recently, this concept has gained a great attention. This concept refers to utilizing advanced technologies to develop the education. Smart classroom transforms the traditional way of education to a digital way in order to provide a smart learning environment (K. Palanivel, 2019 [46], H. EL Mrabet et al., 2017 [47], A. C. Martín et al., 2019 [4], W. Shi et al., 2019 [48]). ICTs can enhance learning (H. EL Mrabet et al., 2017 [47]). IoT has a positive impact on education since IoT can enable the education system to be more effective (K. Palanivel, 2019 [46], H. EL Mrabet et al., 2017 [47]).

In (J. Britto et al., 2019 [49]), an IoT-based smart classroom was proposed. This system is composed of many wireless nodes, a middleware and user interface. All wireless nodes communicate with the middleware via Message Queue Telemetry Transport (MQTT) protocol. Also, the user can interact with the middleware through speech in order to control the electrical devices such as light, fan and projector from anywhere. The benefit of this approach is that it is a cost-effective method.

In (M. Ur Rahman et al., 2016 [50]), a model for providing a smart learning environment at Indian institutes was proposed. It was found that IoT is a powerful tool which can enhance the learning process.

In (S. Liu et al., 2019 [51]), a ML-based system for smart classroom was designed. Sensors were employed for measuring the students' physiological responses for every learning part. Moreover, reinforcement learning has been utilized for selecting the suitable learning activities. The findings have exhibited that the proposed system can enhance the performance of students.

In (A. Pacheco et al., 2018 [52]), an on-device DL inference was implemented for smart classroom prototype. Also, object recognition was performed for controlling various classroom devices such as lights and projector using smartphone camera. Three DNNs have been used which are Inception v3, MobileNet and SqueezeNet. It was found that the prototype has performed control and recognition tasks effectively. Also, the findings demonstrate that Inception V3 model has achieved the best accuracy. However, it was the slowest.

In (S. K. Gupta et al., 2019 [53]), a student's affective content analysis approach was proposed for calculating the students' engagement score to be as feedback to the faculty member and therefore assists in enhancing the students' learning process. The students' moods have been forecasted via analyzing their facial expressions in the classroom environment. Modified-Inception-V3 model was employed

TABLE 14.2
Summary of ML and IoT Approaches That Have been Used for Smart Education

Author	Proposed technique	Contributions
J. Britto et al. [49]	IoT	Smart classroom for controlling various electrical devices remotely has been proposed.
M. Ur Rahman et al. [50]	IoT	A smart learning environment at Indian institutes was proposed.
S. Liu et al. [51]	ML	A smart classroom was designed to enhance the performance of students.
A. Pacheco et al. [52]	DL	A Smart classroom was proposed. It can control various classroom devices effectively.
S. K. Gupta et al. [53]	DL	DL-based system was proposed for calculating the students' engagement score to enhance students' learning process.
S. Hussain et al. [15]	DL	A model has been proposed to predict students' performance.
H. M. R. Hasan et al. [54]	ML	ML was used to predict the student's performance.

for recognizing students' moods. This work was performed in India. The achieved test accuracy for mood classification was 87.65%.

Students is the very crucial part of educational organizations. Finding out students' current status and predicting their future performance is very crucial process to avoid the poor predicted findings (H. M. R. Hasan et al., 2019 [54]). DL plays a significant role in recognizing academically weak students so that it can assist them improve their performance (S. Hussain et al., 2019 [15]), In (S. Hussain et al., 2019 [15]), a DL-based model has been proposed to predict students' performance in Assam colleges, India. A dataset of 10,140 student records was employed in this work. The obtained accuracy was 95.34%. This model enables teachers to assist students of poor predicted performance in improving their final exam marks.

In (H. M. R. Hasan et al., 2019 [54]), ML was used to predict the student's performance in the final exam. Two models were employed which are KNN and DT Classifier model and a data 1,170 students were utilized to train the models. The highest accuracy was achieved by DT Classifier model which was 94.88%. This work will be useful for students and teachers. Table 14.2 exhibits a summary of ML and IoT approaches that has been used for smart education

14.2.5 SMART HEALTH

The smart healthcare system has lately gained popularity and is becoming increasingly necessary as a result of substantial advances in current technology, particularly in AI and ML (M. Nasr et al., 2020 [55]). In the era of digital health transformation, ML and IoT play significant roles in the development of healthcare sector. In addition, blockchain has a great influence on healthcare sector via solving the data management issue and providing encryption and immutable storage ([56]; A. Banotra et al., 2021 [57]). Blockchain has been gaining importance in recent years owing to its powerful features (M. Kaur et al., 2021 [58]). Blockchain can provide an effective solution to overcome IoT challenges. Security is one of the essential challenges of using IoT in medical field. Although Blockchain can solve security issue, it suffers from some issues such as complexity and scalability especially when utilized by IoT devices (N. Chendeb et al., 2020 [59]). Researchers have been developed several effective systems which can utilize these great technologies to assist doctors in diagnosis and monitoring for patients.

Diagnosis and monitoring individual's health are crucial tasks. So, there is an urgent need to employing advanced technologies to assist patients and doctors in monitoring and tracking the sensitive medical data (D. A. M. Budida et al., 2018 [60]). In (D. A. M. Budida et al., 2018 [60]), an IoT-based healthcare system was proposed in order to enhance the healthcare industry. This system has the ability to measure the real-time patients body parameters via sensors. Then, the measured data is transferred to Microcontroller which deliver the data to MySQL database server. These data can be viewed to the patients via smartphone app. Also, abnormal data can be detected via decision-making algorithms. Thus, patients and care takers are notified in case of any emergency.

In (H. Pandey et al., 2020 [61]), Health Monitoring System using ML and IoT was proposed in order to predict heart diseases in an early stage. In this system, sensor was utilized to collect data. Also, IFTTT enables sensor's data to be observed in google sheet and further employed in ML algorithms. Several ML algorithms were used and compared. KNN, support vector machine (SVM), random forest classifier and DT. It was found that SVM has achieved the highest accuracy which was 86%.

In (G. An et al., 2019 [62]), ML was used for glaucoma diagnosis. This approach has achieved an AUC of 0.963. It was found that this classification model can effectively distinguish between healthy and glaucomatous eyes.

In (R. Ben Ammar et al., 2019 [16]), ML-based method was employed for Alzheimer's disease (AD) diagnosis in an early stage.

The results exhibited that this model classifies Alzheimer's patients from healthy people with an accuracy of 79%.

In (A. Rghioui et al., 2020 [63]), ML algorithms were employed for monitoring Diabetic Patients. Sensors have been utilized for gathering several measurements from patients' bodies. Different ML algorithms were utilized which are naïve Bayes, sequential minimal optimization (SMO), J48, ZeroR, OneR, simple logistic and random forest. The findings have demonstrated that SMO algorithm has outperformed the other algorithm and it has achieved an accuracy of 99.66%.

In (I. Machorro-Cano et al., 2019 [64]), a smart health platform for controlling overweight and obesity via IoT and ML was proposed. Weka API and the J48 ML algorithms have been utilized for identifying the critical variables and classifying patients. However, Apache Mahout and RuleML have been employed for generating medical recommendations.

Healthcare monitoring systems have become a great concern around the globe (M. M. Islam et al., 2020 [65]). In (M. M. Islam et al., 2020 [65]), IoT-based health monitoring system was proposed. Sensors were utilized to gather data about heartbeat, body and room temperature. Thus, the medical staff can process and analyze the situation of the patient.

Coronavirus disease 2019 (COVID-19) is a contagious disease that spreads rapidly around the world. Rapid detection of people infected with COVID-19 is a critical challenge. Thus, there is a great challenge for research community to develop effective AI systems which can assist in diagnosis the disease (Y. E. Almalki et al., 2021 [66], C. Chakraborty et al., 2021 [67]). In (Y. E. Almalki et al., 2021 [66]), COVID Inception-ResNet model was proposed for diagnose the COVID-19 patients rapidly using chest X-rays. The achieved accuracy of this model was 95.7%.

Over the last few decades, the prevalence of skin cancer has increased. Detecting skin cancer at an early stage helps patients to recover faster (A. Khamparia, 2020 [68]). In (A. Khamparia, 2020, [68], a novel approach for detecting and classification of skin cancer using IoT and DL was proposed. It was found that this system can assist specialists effectively in the diagnosis and treatment of skin cancer.

In (J. Feng et al., 2021 [69]), DL was employed for lung cancer detection from CT images. In this work, the denoizing and detection tasks has been integrated. Via this approach, competitive findings have been achieved.

In (A. K. Gupta et al., 2021 [70]), an effective cloud-enabled Health IoT system was proposed for monitoring epileptic seizures in real time. In this system, Short Time Fourier Transform was employed for obtaining two-dimensional Electroencephalogram (EEG) data from one dimensional EEG. This process was followed by digital watermarking technique for secure transmission of EEG data.

In (N. Chendeb et al., 2020 [59]), a Secure Healthcare Digital System was proposed. In this system, Blockchain technology has been integrated with IoT and high scalability, security and low latency were achieved.

In (A. Kishor et al., 2020 [71]), fog computing technology was utilized to minimize the latency of e-healthcare. Fog computing can process, store and analyze the data nearer to IoT and end-users to reduce the latency issue. In this work, k-fold random forest has been proposed in the fog computing environment and total latency (transmission delay, computation delay, and network delay) was calculated. Using this approach, 95% minimization in latency was achieved. Thus, this method can assist in enhancing the quality of services in e-healthcare and it is suitable for heterogeneous networks.

In (C. Chakraborty, 2019 [72]), a computational method for chronic wound tissue characterization has been proposed. Fuzzy c-means clustering was utilized for wound image segmentation task. Moreover, various computational learning schemes: Naïve Bayes, Linear discriminant analysis, DT and Random Forest were utilized for classifying the percent of wounded tissue in a segmented region. The overall accuracy of the system was 93.75%.

There is an urgent need for secure and effective remote patient monitoring systems (G. Srivastava et al., 2019 [73]). In (G. Srivastava et al., 2019 [73]), a secure healthcare model was presented. In this system, a blockchain was integrated with IoT. This system has solved the challenges of integrating blockchain with IoT such as low scalability and data storage. The system consists of overlay network, cloud storage, healthcare providers, smart contracts and IoT devices for patients. In addition, a double encryption scheme has been employed.

In (A. Banotra et al., 2021 [57]), a model for healthcare sector using blockchain and IoT was presented. In this model, IoT devices was utilized for collecting real-time data. However, these data were stored in blockchain. It was found that this system needs to be improved to reduce the processing time. Table 14.3 demonstrates a summary of ML and IoT approaches that has been used for smart health.

TABLE 14.3

Summary of ML and IoT Approaches That Have been Used for Smart Health

Author	Proposed Technique	Contributions
D. A. M. Budida et al. [60]	IoT	Smart healthcare system proposed.
H. Pandey et al. [61]	ML+IoT	A health monitoring system for predicting heart diseases in an early stage.
G. An et al. [62]	ML	An approach for glaucoma diagnosis proposed.
R. Ben Ammar et al. [16]	ML	An approach for Alzheimer's disease (AD) diagnosis in an early stage proposed.
A. Rghioui et al. [63]	ML	A system for monitoring Diabetic Patients.
I. Machorro-Cano et al. [64]	ML+IoT	A platform for controlling obesity and being overweight proposed.
M. M. Islam et al. [65]	IoT	Health monitoring system was proposed.
Y. E. Almalki [66]	ML	An effective system for COVID-19 diagnosis was proposed.
A. Khamparia [68]	DL+IoT	A novel system for detection and classification skin cancer was proposed.
J. Feng et al. [69]	DL	Two path CNN was utilized for lung cancer detection.
A. K. Gupta et al. [70]	IoT	An effective real-time cloud-enabled Health IoT system was proposed for monitoring epileptic seizures.
N. Chendeb et al. [59]	IoT + Blockchain	A Secure Healthcare Digital System was proposed.
A. Kishor et al. [71]	IoT+ML+Fog Computing technology	A New Fog Computing method for Reduction of Latency in Healthcare using ML has been proposed.
C. Chakraborty [72]	ML	A computational method for chronic wound tissue characterization has been proposed.
G. Srivastava et al. [73]	IoT+Blockchain	A secure healthcare model was presented.
A. Banotra et al. [57]	IoT+Blockchain	A healthcare model was introduced.

14.2.6 SMART BUILDINGS

Smart building is an essential element to improve cities and infrastructures (A. Daissaoui et al., 2020 [74]). Building energy management (BEM) system is needed to identify devices that consume a lot of energy and to monitor energy usage (W. Tushar et al., 2016 [75]). It is also useful to control energy wastage. In (W. Tushar et al., 2016 [75]), an IoT-based BEM was proposed for performing analysis on energy usage pattern and the wastage. This system was performed in an office using wireless sensor network. It was found that IoT can assist in reducing energy wastage.

In (H. Park et al., 2018, [76], an IoT platform for smart building was prepared. Health profiles of the occupants has been accumulated. Also, a dynamic thermal model of occupants has been proposed to guarantee thermal comfort of the occupants.

The aim of smart buildings is to guarantee that the resources are effectively utilized and for providing comfortable living for individuals. In (I. Sülo et al., 2019 [77]), LSTM was utilized for predicting the energy consumption values of the buildings.

forecasting energy consumption in smart Buildings is very significant (S. Bourhnane et al., 2020 [78]). In (S. Bourhnane et al., 2020 [78]), Artificial Neural Networks (ANN) was employed for energy consumption forecasting and scheduling. The resulted accuracy was modest owing to the small size of the dataset.

14.2.7 SMART AGRICULTURE

In (T. A. A. Ali et al., 2018 [79]), a real-time IoT monitoring system for precision agriculture was proposed. This system can monitor the variation in several parameters such as weather, water, soil and fire detection. Farmers is notified via an email in order to take the appropriate action. This system is affordable and low power consumption.

In (R. Dagar et al., 2018 [80]), IoT was utilized for smart agriculture. Sensors was used for aggregating information. This information was delivered to the server via WiFi network. Based on the delivered information, suitable action can be taken.

There is an increasing demand for food production owing to the rapid increasing of the global population (Doshi et al., 2019 [81]). It is expected that the global population will be about nine billion by 2050. Thus, agriculture is a significant sector which has a great impact on the economy of the developing countries (T. Talaviya et al., 2020 [82], J. Doshi et al., 2019 [81]). Traditional agriculture relies on farmers. This method is inefficient due to its drawback of wasting a lot of time in the field (T. Dindigul et al., 2020 [83]). So, innovation of new technologies is the need of the hour. Smart farming concept is utilizing of technology in agriculture to increase the quality and quantity of the production (H. Kaur et al., 2019 [24]). Smart farming can assist in handling the climate change and epidemics such as draught (A. Vij, S. Vijendra et al., 2020 [84]). ML is a branch of AI which can used in several fields. One of the most challenging tasks in agriculture is crop yield prediction owing to the dependency of the crop yield on various factors such as climate, weather and soil. ML is an efficient tool which can support crop yield prediction (T. van Klompenburg et al., 2020 [85]). CNN is commonly utilized in agriculture due to its strong ability of image processing (H. Kaur et al., 2019 [24]).

In (D. Elavarasan et al., 2020, [86], Deep Recurrent Q-Network has been proposed for yield prediction. The obtained accuracy was 93.7%.

In (P. Sharma et al., 2019, [87], segmented images have been employed to train CNN models on detection of plant diseases. Compared to the models that trains on full images, this approach has obtained higher performance with 98.6%.

14.3 IOT CHALLENGES IN SC

Security is one the main challenges of deploying IoT in SC. This aspect should be taken in the account to avoid any malicious attacks such as data stealing and privacy violations (F. Righetti et al., 2018 [7], B. Hammi et al., 2018 [88]). Due to process of gathering all data in the same IoT platform, the system may subject to vulnerabilities. Thus, serious measures are needed to guarantee the privacy and security of data and IoT systems must be resistant to cyberattacks (S. Talari et al., 2017 [89]). In addition, heterogeneity is a challenging issue due to the different format of gathered data which is gathered by various ways via various protocols. So, these data cannot be analyzed, processed and stored owing to the lack of standard format. Also, it is difficult to integrate data which is obtained from heterogeneous sources (B. Hammi et al., 2018 [88]). Moreover, Big Data is another IoT challenge owing to large number of connected devices. So, it is difficult to transfer, store and analyze the gathered data by this huge number of devices (S. Talari et al., 2017 [89], E. Ahmed et al. [90]). In addition, one of the most significant challenges related with enabling IoT for smart building is improving energy efficiency of the smart building (A. Totonchi et al., 2018 [91]). There are several challenges related to smart parking using IoT such as the unsuitable current infrastructure, the high cost of installed equipment and high cost of maintenance (S. Rupanr et al., 2019 [92]). In smart education using IoT, student's data is collected and stored in the network. So, protecting the privacy of student's data is a challenging task. Also, the high cost of implementing IoT in the educational organizations is a big challenge (M. Abdel-Basset et al., 2019 [22]). In addition, teachers should be trained on using technological tools. Furthermore, excellent internet connectivity is needed (M. Ur Rahman et al., 2016 [50]). Reliability is another challenge in designing IoT system for SCs. Unreliable systems may lead to data loss, delays and wrong decision. For example, failures in IoT health systems may cause patient death (I. Khajenasiri et al., 2016 [93]).

14.4 SECURED SCS

Owing to the heterogeneity and dynamic features of SCs, conventional cyber-security protecting approaches can't be applied directly to smart SC applications. Moreover, security threats should be taken into account when designing new systems. Real-time authentication is one of the essential requirements of intelligent systems. Thus, it is necessary to guarantee that services of a heterogeneous system can be accessed by authorized clients only. Also, encryption is mostly utilized to provide reliable communication. Smart systems must be capable of maintaining efficient functioning even under attacks. In addition, intrusion detection is very significant. However, developing smart intrusion prediction systems (IPS) is better than detection after attacks (L. Cui et al., 2018 [94]). In (S. Chakrabarty et al., 2016 [95]), a secure IoT architecture for SCs has been proposed. This architecture composes of four blocks which are Black Network for adding privacy, Trusted Software Defined Networking Controller for secure routing, Unified Registry for identity authentication and Key Management System. In (I. Alrashdi et al., 2019 [96]), Random Forest ML algorithm was employed for anomaly detection of IoT cyberattacks in SC. The results have demonstrated that this approach has achieved highest classification accuracy of 99.34%.

14.5 CONCLUSION

The populations of cities are growing rapidly. So, smart solutions are needed to enhance the quality of life. Advanced technologies such as ML and IoT can enable implementing SC concept. In this chapter, a review on the applications of ML and IoT in smart cities is presented. The recent research studies of IoT and ML systems for environmental monitoring, smart parking, traffic monitoring, smart education, smart health, smart buildings and smart agriculture have been studied. The results demonstrated that ML and IoT approaches had remarkable contribution to the development of smart cities. IoT can assist teachers in performing their work effectively. It also can enhance the learning process of students. ML is a very effective tool in predicting student's performance. Also, ML and IoT play significant roles in the development of healthcare sector. Moreover, the challenges of IoT in SCs have been discussed. The findings demonstrate that blockchain can provide an effective solution to overcome the security challenge of IoT. Thus, secure healthcare digital systems can be achieved via integrating IoT with Blockchain. Also, fog computing technology can be integrated with IoT systems to minimize the latency of e-healthcare

14.5.1 FUTURE SCOPE

Several research opportunities have been detected, such as designing reliable and secure IoT systems for SC and improving energy efficiency of the smart building. Also, implementing IoT systems in developing countries is highly recommended. Future work on smart parking systems for predicting the availability of parking space which can consider the weather conditions and social events information is needed. Furthermore, investigation of the roadside parking space availability and traffic congestion information should be conducted. Several ML approaches should be compared in order to provide efficient utilization of energy. In addition, novel IoT systems which can overcome the challenges of IoT are needed. Also, more secure healthcare digital systems are required.

REFERENCES

1. S. Bhattacharya, S. R. K. Somayaji, T. R. Gadekallu, M. Alazab, and P. K. R. Maddikunta, "A review on deep learning for future smart cities," *Internet Technol. Lett.*, 1–6, e187, 2020.
2. M. Al-Emran, S. I. Malik, and M. N. Al-Kabi, A Survey of Internet of Things (IoT) in Education: Opportunities and Challenges, vol. 846. Springer International Publishing, Switzerland, 2020.
3. Z. Ullah, F. Al-Turjman, L. Mostarda, and R. Gagliardi, "Applications of Artificial Intelligence and Machine learning in smart cities," *Comput. Commun.*, vol. 154, no. February, pp. 313–323, 2020.
4. A. C. Martín, C. Alario-Hoyos, and C. D. Kloos, "Smart education: A review and future research directions," *Proceedings*, vol. 31, no. 1, p. 57, 2019.
5. D. N. Le, L. Le Tuan, and M. N. Dang Tuan, "Smart building management system: An Internet of Things (IoT) application business model in Vietnam," *Technol. Forecast. Soc. Change*, vol. 141, no. December 2018, pp. 22–35, 2019.
6. S. Dhawan, C. Chakraborty, J. Frnda, R. Gupta, A. K. Rana, and S. K. Pani, "SSII: Secured and high-quality Steganography using Intelligent hybrid optimization algorithms for IoT," *IEEE Access*, vol. PP, no. June, p. 1, 2021.
7. F. Righetti, C. Vallati, and G. Anastasi, "IoT applications in smart cities: A perspective into social and ethical issues," *Proc. - 2018 IEEE Int. Conf. Smart Comput. SMARTCOMP 2018*, pp. 387–392, 2018.
8. A. Zanella, N. Bui, A. Castellani, L. Vangelista, and M. Zorzi, "Internet of things for smart cities," *IEEE Internet Things J.*, vol. 1, no. 1, pp. 22–32, 2014.
9. L. Chen, P. Chen, and Z. Lin, "Artificial Intelligence in Education: A Review," *IEEE Access*, vol. 8, pp. 75264–75278, 2020.
10. F. Zantalis, G. Koulouras, S. Karabetsos, and D. Kandris, "A review of machine learning and IoT in smart transportation," *Future Internet*, vol. 11, no. 4. pp. 1–23, 2019.
11. S. Nosratabadi, A. Mosavi, R. Keivani, S. Ardabili, and F. Aram, "State-of-the-art survey of deep learning and machine learning models for smart cities and urban sustainability," *Lect. Notes Networks Syst.*, vol. 101, no. Ml, 2020, pp. 228–238.
12. W. M. Septiawan and S. N. Endah, "Suitable Recurrent Neural Network for Air Quality Prediction with Backpropagation Through Time," *2018 2nd International Conference on Informatics and Computational Sciences (ICICoS)*, pp. 196–201, 2019.
13. J. Barker and S. U. Rehman, "Investigating the use of machine learning for smart parking applications," *Proc. 2019 11th Int. Conf. Knowl. Syst. Eng. KSE 2019*, 2019.
14. S. Sasi Priya, Rajarajeshwari, K. Sowmiya, and P. Vinesha, "Road Traffic Condition Monitoring using Deep Learning," *Proc. 5th Int. Conf. Inven. Comput. Technol. ICICT 2020*, pp. 330–335, 2020.
15. S. Hussain, Z. F. Muhsin, Y. K. Salal, P. Theodorou, F. Kurtoğlu, and G. C. Hazarika, "Prediction model on student performance based on internal assessment using deep learning," *Int. J. Emerg. Technol. Learn.*, vol. 14, no. 8, pp. 4–22, 2019.
16. R. Ben Ammar and Y. Ben Ayed, "Speech Processing for Early Alzheimer's Disease Diagnosis: Machine Learning Based Approach," *Proc. IEEE/ACS Int. Conf. Comput. Syst. Appl. AICCSA*, vol. 2018, pp. 1–8, 2019.

17. A. Khanna and R. Anand, "IoT-based smart parking system," in *2016 International Conference on Internet of Things and Applications, IOTA 2016*, pp. 266–270, 2016.

18. S.P. Biswas, P. Roy, N. Patra, A. Mukherjee and N. Dey, "Intelligent traffic monitoring system". *In Proceedings of the Second International Conference on Computer and Communication Technologies*, vol. 380, pp. 535–545, 2015.

19. G. Ali et al., "IoT-based smart parking system using deep long short memory network," *Electronics*, vol. 9, pp. 1–17, 2020.

20. M. Sarrab, S. Pulparambil, and M. Awadalla, "Development of an IoT-based real-time traffic monitoring system for city governance," *Glob. Transitions*, vol. 2, pp. 230–245, 2020.

21. Z.-T. Zhu, M.-H. Yu, and P. Riezebos, "A research framework of smart education," Smart Learn. Environ., vol. 3, no. 1, pp. 1–17 2016.

22. M. Abdel-Basset, G. Manogaran, M. Mohamed, and E. Rushdy, "Internet of things in smart education environment: Supportive framework in the decision-making process," *Concurr. Comput.*, vol. 31, no. 10, pp. 1–12, 2019.

23. P. K, "Emerging technologies to smart education," *Int. J. Comput. Trends Technol.*, vol. 68, no. 2, pp. 5–16, 2020.

24. H. Kaur, "Deep learning in smart farming – concepts, applications and techniques," no. 16, pp. 3359–3371, 2019.

25. Z. Rayanal, M. Alfonse, and A. B. M. Salem, "Machine learning approaches in smart health," *Procedia Comput. Sci.*, vol. 154, no. 1985, pp. 361–368, 2018.

26. S. Abraham, J. Beard, and R. Manijacob, "Remote environmental monitoring using Internet of Things (IoT)," *GHTC 2017 – IEEE Glob. Humanit. Technol. Conf. Proc.*, vol. 2017-Janua, pp. 1–6, 2017.

27. S. L. Ullo and G. R. Sinha, "Advances in smart environment monitoring systems using iot and sensors," *Sensors (Switzerland)*, vol. 20, no. 11, 2020.

28. D. E. N. Ganesh, "IOT-based environment monitoring using wireless sensor network.," *Int. J. Adv. Res.*, vol. 5, no. 2, pp. 964–970, 2017.

29. N. P. Sastra and D. M. Wiharta, "Environmental monitoring as an IoT application in building smart campus of universitas udayana," no. December, pp. 1–5, 2017.

30. M. S. Jamil, M. A. Jamil, A. Mazhar, A. Ikram, A. Ahmed, and U. Munawar, "Smart environment monitoring system by employing wireless sensor networks on vehicles for pollution free smart cities," *Procedia Eng.*, vol. 107, pp. 480–484, 2015.

31. C. Toma, A. Alexandru, M. Popa, and A. Zamfiroiu, "IoT solution for smart cities' pollution monitoring and the security challenges," *Sensors (Switzerland)*, vol. 19, no. 15, 2019.

32. A. L. Pyayt, I. I. Mokhov, B. Lang, V. V. Krzhizhanovskaya, and R. J. Meijer, "Machine learning methods for environmental monitoring and flood protection," *World Acad. Sci. Eng. Technol.*, vol. 78, no. June, pp. 118–123, 2011.

33. R. J. Kuo, B. Prasetyo, and B. S. Wibowo, "Deep Learning-Based Approach for Air Quality Forecasting by Using Recurrent Neural Network with Gaussian Process in Taiwan," *2019 IEEE 6th Int. Conf. Ind. Eng. Appl. ICIEA 2019*, pp. 471–474, 2019.

34. T. Malche, P. Maheshwary, and R. Kumar, "Environmental monitoring system for smart city based on secure Internet of Things (IoT) architecture," *Wirel. Pers. Commun.*, vol. 107, no. 4, pp. 2143–2172, 2019.

35. S. Begade and V. B. Dharmadhikari, "Cloud Based Smart Car Parking System Using Internet of Things," in *Proceedings of the 2nd International Conference on Intelligent Computing and Control Systems, ICICCS 2018*, vol. 8, no. 1, pp. 1100–1105, 2019.

36. R. Kumar and G. Rani, "Machine Learning and IoT-based Real-Time Parking System: Challenges and Implementation," no. May, 2020.

37. R. Salpietro, L. Bedogni, M. Di Felice, and L. Bononi, "Park Here! a smart parking system based on smartphones' embedded sensors and short-range Communication Technologies," in *IEEE World Forum on Internet of Things, WF-IoT 2015 - Proceedings*, pp. 18–23, 2015.

38. R. Lookmuang, K. Nambut, and S. Usanavasin, "Smart parking using IoT technology," in *Proc. 2018 5th Int. Conf. Bus. Ind. Res. Smart Technol. Next Gener. Information, Eng. Bus. Soc. Sci. ICBIR 2018*, vol. 2017, pp. 1–6, 2018.

39. S. Yamin Siddiqui, M. Adnan Khan, S. Abbas, and F. Khan, "Smart occupancy detection for road traffic parking using deep extreme learning machine," *J. King Saud Univ. - Comput. Inf. Sci.*, no. xxxx, pp. 1–7, 2020.

40. S. Saharan, N. Kumar, and S. Bawa, "An efficient smart parking pricing system for smart city environment: A machine learning-based approach," *Futur. Gener. Comput. Syst.*, vol. 106, pp. 622–640, 2020.

41. I. M. O. Widyantara and N. P. Sastra, "Internet of Things for intelligent traffic monitoring system: A case study in denpasar," *Int. J. Comput. Trends Technol.*, vol. 30, no. 3, pp. 169–173, 2015.

42. A. K. M. Masum, M. Kalim Amzad Chy, I. Rahman, M. N. Uddin, and K. I. Azam, "An Internet of Things (IoT) based Smart Traffic Management System: A Context of Bangladesh," in *2018 International Conference on Innovations in Science, Engineering and Technology, ICISET 2018*, pp. 418–422, 2018.

43. J. Zaucha, M. Matczak, C. Rus, R. Marcuș, and O. Stoicuța, "Retractation note: Road traffic monitoring system with self-learning function using the raspberry Pi platform," *MATEC Web Conf.*, vol. 290, p. 06011, 2019.

44. G. M. Lingani, D. B. Rawat, and M. Garuba, "Smart traffic management system using deep learning for smart city applications," in *2019 IEEE 9th Annual Computing and Communication Workshop and Conference, CCWC 2019*, pp. 101–106, 2019.

45. S. K. Janahan, M. R. M. Veeramanickam, S. Arun, K. Narayanan, R. Anandan, and S. J. Parvez, "IoT-based smart traffic signal monitoring system using vehicles counts," *Int. J. Eng. Technol.*, vol. 7, pp. 309–312, 2018.

46. K. Palanivel, "Smart education architecture using the internet of things (IOT) technology," *Int. J. Manag. Edu.*, vol. 9, no. 2, pp. 46–70, 2019.

47. H. E.L. Mrabet and A. Ait Moussa, "Smart classroom environment via IoT in basic and secondary education," *Trans. Mach. Learn. Artif. Intell.*, vol. 5, no. 4, pp. 274–279, 2017.

48. W. Shi et al., "Review on Development of Smart Education," in *Proceedings - IEEE International Conference on Service Operations and Logistics, and Informatics 2019, SOLI 2019*, pp. 157–162, 2019.

49. J. Britto, V. Chaudhari, D. Mehta, A. Kale, and J. Ramteke, A Sixth Sense Door using Internet of Things. in *International Conference on Computer Networks and Communication Technologies*, vol. 15. Springer, Singapore, 2019.

50. M. Ur Rahman, V. Deep, and S. Rahman, "ICT and internet of things for creating smart learning environment for students at education institutes in India," *2016 6th International Conference-Cloud System and Big Data Engineering (Confluence)*, pp. 701–704, 2016.

51. S. Liu, Y. Chen, H. Huang, L. Xiao, and X. Hei, "Towards Smart Educational Recommendations with Reinforcement Learning in Classroom," in *Proceedings of 2018 IEEE International Conference on Teaching, Assessment, and Learning for Engineering, TALE 2018*, pp. 1079–1084, 2019.

52. A. Pacheco, E. Flores, R. Sanchez, and S. Almanza-Garcia, "Smart Classrooms Aided by Deep Neural Networks Inference on Mobile Devices," in *IEEE International Conference on Electro Information Technology*, vol. 2018, pp. 605–609, 2018.

53. S. K. Gupta, T. S. Ashwin, and R. M. R. Guddeti, "Students' affective content analysis in smart classroom environment using deep learning techniques," *Multimed. Tools Appl.*, vol. 78, no. 18, pp. 25321–25348, 2019.

54. H. M. R. Hasan, "Machine Learning A lgorithm for Student' s Performance Prediction," *2019 10th International Conference on Computing, Communication and Networking Technologies (ICCCNT)*, pp. 1–7, 2019.

55. M. Nasr, M. Islam, S. Shehata, F. K. Fellow, and Y. Quintana, "Smart healthcare in the age of AI: Recent advances, challenges, and future prospects," vol. 1, pp. 1–24, 2020.

56. https://health.economictimes.indiatimes.com/news/health-it/how-digital-health-and-ai-are-driving-intelligent-healthcare/83942999

57. A. Banotra, J. S. Sharma, S. Gupta, S. K. Gupta, and M. Rashid, "Use of blockchain and Internet of Things for securing data in healthcare systems," pp. 255–267, 2021.

58. M. Kaur, M. Z. Khan, and S. Gupta, "MBCP: Performance analysis of large scale mainstream blockchain consensus protocols," pp. 80931–80944, 2021.

59. N. Chendeb et al., "Integrating blockchain with IoT for a secure healthcare digital system to cite this version: HAL Id: hal-02495262 Integrating Blockchain with IoT for a Secure Healthcare Digital System," 2020.

60. D. A. M. Budida and R. S. Mangrulkar, "Design and implementation of smart Healthcare system using IoT," in *Proceedings of 2017 International Conference on Innovations in Information, Embedded and Communication Systems, ICIIECS 2017*, vol. 2018, pp. 1–7, 2018.

61. H. Pandey and S. Prabha, "Smart Health Monitoring System using IOT and Machine Learning Techniques," *2020 6th Int. Conf. Bio Signals, Images, Instrumentation, ICBSII 2020*, 2020.

62. G. An et al., "Glaucoma diagnosis with machine learning based on optical coherence tomography and color fundus images," *J. Healthc. Eng.*, vol. 2019, 2019.

63. A. Rghioui, J. Lloret, S. Sendra, and A. Oumnad, "A smart architecture for diabetic patient monitoring using machine learning algorithms," *Healthcare*, vol. 8, no. 3, p. 348, 2020.

64. I. Machorro-Cano, G. Alor-Hernández, M. A. Paredes-Valverde, U. Ramos-Deonati, J. L. Sánchez-Cervantes, and L. Rodríguez-Mazahua, "PISIoT: A machine learning and IoT-based smart health platform for overweight and obesity control," *Appl. Sci.*, vol. 9, no. 15, 2019.

65. M. M. Islam, A. Rahaman, and M. R. Islam, "Development of smart healthcare monitoring system in IoT environment," *SN Comput. Sci.*, vol. 1, no. 3, pp. 1–11, 2020.

66. Y. E. Almalki et al., "A novel method for COVID-19 diagnosis using artificial intelligence in chest x-ray images," *Healthc.*, vol. 9, no. 5, pp. 1–23, 2021.

67. C. Chakraborty and A. N. Abougreen, "Intelligent internet of things and advanced machine learning techniques for covid-19," *EAI Endorsed Trans. Pervasive Heal. Technol.*, vol. 7, no. 26, pp. 1–14, 2021.

68. A. Khamparia, "An internet of health things-driven deep learning framework for detection and classification of skin cancer using transfer learning," no. December 2019, pp. 1–11, 2020.

69. J. Feng, A. W. Godana, S. Liu, and D. J. Gelmecha, "DFD-Net: lung cancer detection from denoised CT scan image using deep learning," vol. 15, no. 2, 2021.

70. A. K. Gupta, C. Chakraborty, and B. Gupta, "Traitement du signal secure transmission of EEG data using watermarking algorithm for the detection of epileptic seizures," vol. 38, no. 2, pp. 473–479, 2021.

71. A. Kishor, C. Chakraborty, and W. Jeberson, "A novel fog computing approach for minimization of latency in healthcare using machine learning," no. March 2021, 2020.

72. C. Chakraborty, "Computational approach for chronic wound tissue characterization Informatics in Medicine Unlocked Computational approach for chronic wound tissue characterization," *Informatics Med. Unlocked*, vol. 17, no. December, p. 100162, 2019.

73. G. Srivastava, J. Crichigno, and S. Dhar, "A Light and Secure Healthcare Blockchain for IoT Medical Devices," *2019 IEEE Can. Conf. Electr. Comput. Eng.*, pp. 1–5, 2019.

74. A. Daissaoui, A. Boulmakoul, L. Karim, and A. Lbath, "IoT and big data analytics for smart buildings: A SURVEY," *Procedia Comp. Sci.*, vol. 170, pp. 161–168, 2020.

75. W. Tushar, C. Yuen, K. Li, K. L. Wood, Z. Wei, and L. Xiang, "Design of cloud-connected IoT system for smart buildings on energy management (invited paper)," *EAI Endorsed Trans. Ind. Networks Intell. Syst.*, vol. 3, no. 6, p. 150813, 2016.

76. H. Park and S. B. Rhee, "IoT-based smart building environment service for occupants' thermal comfort," *J. Sensors*, vol. 2018, 2018.

77. I. Sülo, Ş. R. Keskin, G. Doğan, and T. Brown, "Energy Efficient Smart Buildings: LSTM Neural Networks for Time Series Prediction," in *Proc. - 2019 Int. Conf. Deep Learn. Mach. Learn. Emerg. Appl. Deep. 2019*, pp. 18–22, 2019.

78. S. Bourhnane, M. R. Abid, R. Lghoul, K. Zine-Dine, N. Elkamoun, and D. Benhaddou, "Machine learning for energy consumption prediction and scheduling in smart buildings," *SN Appl. Sci.*, vol. 2, no. 2, 2020.

79. T. A. A. Ali, "Precision agriculture monitoring system using Internet of Things (IoT)," *Int. J. Res. Appl. Sci. Eng. Technol.*, vol. 6, no. 4, pp. 2961–2970, 2018.

80. R. Dagar, S. Som, and S. K. Khatri, "Smart Farming - IoT in Agriculture," in *Proceedings of the International Conference on Inventive Research in Computing Applications, ICIRCA 2018*, no. Icirca, pp. 1052–1056, 2018.

81. J. Doshi, T. Patel, and S. K. Bharti, "Smart Fanning using IoT, a solution for optimally monitoring fanning conditions," in *Procedia Comp. Sci.*, vol. 160, pp. 746–751, 2019.

82. T. Talaviya, D. Shah, N. Patel, H. Yagnik, and M. Shah, "Implementation of artificial intelligence in agriculture for optimisation of irrigation and application of pesticides and herbicides," *Artif. Intell. Agric.*, vol. 4, pp. 58–73, 2020.

83. T. Dindigul, "Smart irrigation system with monitoring and controlling using IoT," *Int. J. Eng. Adv. Technol.*, vol. 9, no. 4, pp. 1373–1376, 2020.

84. A. Vij, S. Vijendra, A. Jain, S. Bajaj, A. Bassi, and A. Sharma, "IoT and machine learning approaches for automation of farm irrigation system," in *Procedia Comp. Sci.*, vol. 167, pp. 1250–1257, 2020.

85. T. van Klompenburg, A. Kassahun, and C. Catal, "Crop yield prediction using machine learning: A systematic literature review," *Comp. Electron. Agric.*, vol. 177, no. January. Elsevier, p. 105709, 2020.

86. D. Elavarasan and P. M. Durairaj Vincent, "Crop yield prediction using deep reinforcement learning model for sustainable agrarian applications," *IEEE Access*, vol. 8, pp. 86886–86901, 2020.

87. P. Sharma, Y. P. S. Berwal, and W. Ghai, "Performance analysis of deep learning CNN models for disease detection in plants using image segmentation," *Inf. Process. Agric.*, vol. 7, no. 4, pp. 566–574, 2019.

88. B. Hammi, R. Khatoun, S. Zeadally, A. Fayad, and L. Khoukhi, "IoT technologies for smart cities," *IET Networks*, vol. 7, no. 1. pp. 1–13, 2018.

89. S. Talari, M. Shafie-Khah, P. Siano, V. Loia, A. Tommasetti, and J. P. S. Catalão, "A review of smart cities based on the internet of things concept," *Energies*, vol. 10, no. 4. pp. 1–23, 2017.

90. E. Ahmed, S. Member, I. Yaqoob, S. Member, and M. Guizani, "Internet of Things based smart environments: State-of-the-art, taxonomy, and open research challenges," pp. 1–11.

91. A. Totonchi, "Smart buildings based on Internet of Things: A systematic review," *Dep. Inf. Commun. Technol.*, 2018.

92. S. Rupanr and N. Doshi, "A review of smart parking using internet of things (IoT)," in *Procedia Comp. Sci.*, vol. 160, pp. 706–711, 2019.

93. I. Khajenasiri, A. Estebsari, M. Verhelst, and G. Gielen, "A review on internet of things solutions for intelligent energy control in buildings for smart city applications," in *Energy Procedia*, 2017, vol. 111, no. September 2016, pp. 770–779.

94. L. Cui, G. Xie, Y. Qu, L. Gao, and Y. Yang, "Security and privacy in smart cities: Challenges and opportunities," *IEEE Access*, vol. 6, no. March 2020, pp. 46134–46145, 2018.

95. S. Chakrabarty and D. W. Engels, "A secure IoT architecture for Smart Cities," *2016 13th IEEE Annu. Consum. Commun. Netw. Conf. CCNC 2016*, pp. 812–813, 2016.

96. I. Alrashdi, A. Alqazzaz, E. Aloufi, R. Alharthi, M. Zohdy, and H. Ming, "AD-IoT: Anomaly detection of IoT cyberattacks in smart city using machine learning," in *2019 IEEE 9th Annu. Comput. Commun. Work. Conf. CCWC 2019*, pp. 305–310, 2019.

15 Effective Remote Healthcare and Telemedicine Approaches for Improving Digital Healthcare Systems

Anubha Dubey
Independent researcher and analyst, Noida, Uttar Pradesh, India

Apurva Saxena Verma
Researcher computer science, Bhopal, MP, India

CONTENTS

DOI: 10.1201/9781003247128-15

15.1   INTRODUCTION

Telemedicine is the electronic form of communication to give healthcare support while at distance apart. In Greek, the word "*tele*" means "distance", and "*mederi*" is a Latin word meaning "to heal" (WHO, 1998 [1]). Previously, it was called "future treatment" or "experimental". But in today's world, telemedicine is a reality, and plays an important role in delivering healthcare and in other sectors like education, research, administration, etc. as proposed by Ajami S and Lamoodi P. 2014 [2]. In healthcare, telemedicine is an important way to help patients in maintaining proper care [3]. Most people in the world living in rural areas find difficulty in accessing good quality medical care, hence telemedicine comes into existence to call specialist physicians (Mc Lean S et al. 2011 [4]). The fast-moving world is becoming less healthy. In every four citizens, one is suffering from a disease. So, looking into the importance of cutting-edge technologies, the authors attempt to present a model which is flexible and dynamic in providing complete healthcare through telemedicine approaches.

Contributions discussed:

1. A set of techniques is adopted for making data accessible, reachable, viewed by doctors, to improve patient's health.
2. Most important, the payment mode is secure and transparent through blockchain. Personalized care is made through AI bots and blockchain ensures privacy and security.
3. Patient and doctor treatment satisfaction for providing tele-support is very important, and patient feedback is also a great criterion to improve the quality of services.
4. The present model is well organized for patient data management, medical health providers suggestions, reports, pharmacy are all interlinked and used only when needed. Any data breaching could be avoided as it is developed under the blockchain.

Practicing telemedicine is a good choice and will be the best way to acquire consultations over mobile in any of the places.

15.1.1 Chapter Organization

The chapter is organized thus: Introduction (15.1) with major contributions, telemedicine and AI and digital health transformations (15.1.2); telemedicine and cloud computing (15.1.3); telemedicine in blockchain with their utilities and advantages (15.1.4). This work is followed by motivation (15.1.7). Section 15.2 discusses method improvements and telemedicine approaches. Section 15.3 presents the working of the IAISTM model, including challenges, benefits, and advantages in the present scenario followed by remote monitoring through IAISTM (15.4) and the sustainability of work is covered in Section 15.5. Finally, the conclusion and future scopes are discussed in Section 15.6.

15.1.2 Telemedicine History

As the growth of telecommunication industry to 5G, telemedicine is also the part of interest during these 5 years showing as the new use of telecommunication industry. The National Aeronautics and Space administration distinctively showed a crucial role in the early expansion of telemedicine given by Wilson LS and Macder AJ 2015 [5]. NASA began working with telemedicine in the 1960s. The physical or biological parameters were transmitted from the spacecraft and the spacesuits during missions by Wilson LS and Macder AJ 2015 [5]. The story begins usually in 1971 when 26 sites in Alaska were chosen by the National Library of Medicine's Lister Hill National Center for Biomedical Communications to observe whether authentic communication would improve distant village healthcare. Satellite video consultations are used to upgrade the quality of rural healthcare in Alaska by Pacis DM et al. 2018 [6] and Peterson MC et al. 1992 [7]. Hence from 1977, the telemedicine centre at the Memorial University of Newfoundland has worked with regard to developing interactive audio systems for educational applications and the transmission of medical details (including the history of pain, treatment, etc.).

15.1.3 Telehealth and Telemedicine Consultation Centre

Telehealth is the system wherein technology uses electronic information, and telecommunications are made possible to effect remote clinical wellness of patients, and for professional health-related training for academics, as well as communal health management. The consultation site is the place where the patient presence is required, and all the types of equipment for scanning/converting, all kinds of medical treatment information are available was given by Roshan M.R. 2000 [8].

15.1.3.1 Components

As usual in a telemedicine system, hardware and software is required. The machinery includes a computer, printer, scanner and videoconferencing peripherals. Nowadays, the mobile phone network is sufficient to fulfil all the requirements. Only a printer is required when the reports are needed to send.

15.1.3.2 Benefits of Telemedicine

(a) Accessible in remote areas.
(b) Reduces the time and price of sufferer transportation/relocation.
(c) Always keep an eye on home care.
(d) The communication between health providers and patients is improved.
(e) Monitoring through sensors where transfer of the patient is not possible.
(f) Telecommunication industry made it possible to continue medical education and clinical research.
(g) The public will be more aware.
(h) Second opinions can more easily be taken if the patient is not satisfied initially.
(i) Medical practices could deliver more timely treatment and other services.
(j) Telementored plans – surgery employs hand robots.
(k) Surveillance of disease and tracking of those affected is possible.

15.1.4 TELEMEDICINE AND USE OF ARTIFICIAL INTELLIGENCE

During the pandemic of COVID-19, researchers and healthcare providers perform their duty to support all humans while at home, and their research continues. Jabarullah and Lee 2021 [9] highlighted the importance of AI and blockchain with the patient-centric model. Including challenges and overcomes of COVID-19.The paper is well written, and explains all dimensions of telemedicine approaches.

AI is advantageous to telemedicine (Reddy S. et al., 2019 [10]). AI helps in solving the problems of high volume demand of data, patient relocation and data transfer; and clinical demand is necessary when specialized expertise is needed. Hence sometimes person-to-person clinical interconnection is needed. In telehealth, AI tools could also improve the balance of order versus supply in healthcare facilities. AI can solve telecommunication link failures, manage the busy schedules of clinicians, and provide time to needy patients on demand. For this, AI innovation and working on the latest technology, the information and communication technology (ICT) people developed programs to match the accessibility of care providers with expertise. The understanding of clinical procedures requires recognition of new discoveries in remedies and procedures. These AI-based algorithms or chatbots will help medical practices to understand the patient's needs. This support will maintain and manage all these data in a secure manner through cloud computing. According to Russell and Norvig in 1995 [11], the scope of AI-based smart devices improves planning, research, learning, decision-making, communication, etc. Now, robotics will also help in AI-based telecommunication.

The computers are the intelligent partners that would mimic humans and solve their queries through cognitive performance.

Pacis D.M. et al. 2018 [6] describe the prospective influence of AI in telehealth in five basic ways: patient observation, healthcare information technology, intelligent assistance, proper diagnosis and collaborates information analysis. This will improve the quality of existing clinical practices, service delivery and utmost important models for secure AI for delivering care.

In recent years, there has been a fast improvement observed in the exponential increase in virtual data created by patients and healthcare systems. This will enhance the possibility of telehealth, AI, and maintain standards in all these systems.

Gors et al 2015 [12] proposed a system for medical care in remote areas. A case study of chronic obstructive pulmonary disease is well presented and used in a telemedical system with mobile and communication technologies.

Roshan M Rao in 2000 [8] observed that the role of examination is as low as 7.7%. The procedure of history taken by the HC provider and examination and clinical diagnosis will take time which affects the patient. Examinations make telecare quicker and trouble-free as such data is easy to store and transmit. The diagnosis of ultrasonography, CT scan, MRI, etc. towards making a resultant detection has been important for clinical examination, which improves the diagnosis and quality enhancement, leading to more timely diagnosis of diseases. This feature saves the physician time and is feasible.

15.1.5 DIGITAL HEALTH TRANSFORMATION USING AI

The world is growing quickly due to technological advancement, and now the digital transformation affects all our lives. The COVID-19 pandemic has changed the way of thinking, and healthcare is now the top priority. Digital health leads to the advancement of telemedicine, as all the work involves computer networks. This telecommunication and computer proficiency has reached the next generation of care and possible outcomes.

The safety of patients and data is the utmost priority. These new innovations have opened the path of value-chain in healthcare. The ecosystem of healthcare is developed with IoT-AI devices that include e-pharmacy, e-diagnostics, consultations through mobile phone and other healthcare solutions such as personal health and online delivery of healthcare.

The adoption of telemedicine approaches like IoT, robotics, automation, cloud, analytics and blockchain are needed to improve access and quality of their assistance.

AI and ML have improved patient monitoring and disease diagnosis. Now, the Internet of medical things (IoMT) has come into existence, which has the complete infrastructure of software applications, medical electronics devices, health systems and services. These tech services provide real-time monitoring and personalized notifications. This is the benefit of telemedicine approaches over digital health systems.

Importance of Telemedicine approaches:

A) Due to COVID-19, the uncertainty of treatment leads to the development of digital and remote consultations for timely treatment. This virtual care fills the gap in patient-doctor relations. Hence, telemedicine is well used and is projected for a good future technology.

B) AI programs improve the accessibility of clinical practices like diagnoses, monitoring patient health, developing care needs. This assistance automates the administrative work and lessens the costs. These telemedicine approaches are the next-generation operative technology that reaches everywhere in less time. There are certain opportunities like interpretability, privacy, and data standardization but there are health tech providers which use certain algorithms of AI ML to improve the drawbacks. Using chatbots, patients can access information about beds in hospitals. Here machine learning plays an important job by maintaining all the required documents, storing records for health and assist hospitals improving the resources. AI and ML collect all the correct information related to patient, doctor and hospitals for making healthcare system efficient, as given by Abdul RJ et al. 2021 [13].

C) Development of telemedicine will lead to the improvement in personalized healthcare. AI is developing day by day with hardcore algorithms and computer applications. This improves the way of thinking and provides solutions for personalized treatments. AI has reached drug discovery to clinical trials. It can also predict a patient's disease according to the symptoms were given or genetic and environmental markers. The preliminary diagnosis will affect good and correct treatment. Patient evaluation for risk of any disease can be diagnosed illustrated in Chinmay C. et al 2016 [14].

D) As the treatment is available virtual, it can reach remote areas. COVID-19 has shown the importance of telemedicine with digital media to reach remote areas and doctor approaches to common people. This intelligent healthcare model will make treatment possible through any geographical location. To improve the quality of telemedicine, four things need to be focused on: strong digital health infrastructure, skilled people, e-governance and awareness among people. There would be a telemedicine app or on-demand treatment websites where any of the patients can reach his/her doctor.

Virtual reality is one of the best possible solutions to fulfil the patient's need and take part in services.

E) Wearable devices are the devices that provide monitoring to high-risk patients. Many of the health tech giants work on wearable devices as they save money and are very helpful in pricing and gamification opportunities.

F) Big Data and other sources of information about patients provide systematic ways of predictive analysis of patient disease and health monitoring.

15.1.5.1   Digital Health Transformation through Blockchain

Blockchain is one of the preferred technologies used for data security. Healthcare has also touched this facility to gain advantages. A huge amount of health data is generated by digital means needs to be properly satisfied and secured; moreover knowledge extraction is vital for researchers to improve the disease diagnosis and treatment. Two frameworks like digital and virtual need to be protected from frauds and maintaining the data confidential. So from data release to data share to the data store, all are in one stage and processed step by step without any disturbance. There is a need to provide e-health solutions [15].

15.1.6   TELEMEDICINE THROUGH CLOUD COMPUTING

In 1961, John McCarthy said that "computation may someday be organized as a public utility" [16]. According to Ian Foster and his colleagues, cloud computing is a joint working of engrossed, practically realistic, scalable, and managed to compute, and a storage platform that provides assistance as and when required over the Internet. Cloud-enabled techniques are the topmost revolutionary change in the business prototype. Electronic health records (EHRs) are now executed in a client-server manner in a physician's office or a centralized server nest in a hospital data centre. Smart mobiles are presently used by many Indians, so all these (if patient) are interconnected.

Software is installed that is able to access, manage and share all the records of health as per authorization and authentication achieved. All this data is privately managed efficiently and effectively. To make more secure payments and digital health records, blockchain comes into play [17].

15.1.7   TELEMEDICINE AND BLOCKCHAIN

Patient information reliability and identity solitude for doctors/users are considerable challenges in contact tracing since they are kept in a centralized cloud. This may lead to the loss of users' possession of their respective data. Therefore, blockchain technology plays an essential role in providing security and privacy to users' data as it works on a decentralized network where users can have full control over their private data.

On the other hand, it is also essential to split patient applicable data with the healthcare associates nationally and internationally to avail well-built datasets for any disease study and to provide better medication, treatments for the health of the patient. It is vital to ensure that patient's peace is taken care of, and sharing methods do not violate data sharing rules worldwide. Complete information about the patient's health record like blood oxygen level and medication are stored securely in the database. Blockchain can be used here as on-time data handling and it also makes data sharing possible between hospitals and medical practitioners. Implementing blockchain can be used to eradicate the difficulties related to data faking, hacking and alterations. Blockchain provides distributed depositories.

Hence, the security, integrity and privacy of health-associated data can be enhanced and protected [18].

Blockchain has marked a good entry in bringing digital records and payment security. Its adoption in telehealth successfully demonstrates the state of clinical and research information, manage identifications of different appliances which could be used for remote patient tracking of diseases, protect health seeker identity and the deposit settlements. Hence blockchain has played a vital role in healthcare shown by Stowe S. and Harding 2010 [19].

In today's world, Internet-based technology is prevalent. Each one of us is using smartphones and smart devices according to our daily necessities. It is therefore easy to introduce telemedicine to people by the use of smartphones. Telemedicine services are affordable as compared to consulting the doctors personally in this pandemic situation. The Internet provides cloud storage, which is handy for the doctor and the patient at any time from anywhere in the world through the use of the cloud platform. Test reports of patients and their treatments are done by doctors and saved in libraries in well-ordered form through the cloud. The main reason for cloud computing in telemedicine is to supply information about the patient and make it accessible when required by the patient or the doctor. The data can be entered in the cloud database from the medical centres or designated data centres over the Internet through proper security. Tele-psychiatrist was the first benefit of cloud computing in the medical field. Psychiatrists generally connect with a patient on the Internet using video conferencing; it reduces costs and time.

Telemedicine services using the client–server architecture. The cloud platform is the best way to handle all the telemedicine records and provide full security to the patient record from unauthorized users. Cloud computing plays a key role in telemedicine services because any cloud platform has very easily accessible software provided, for use by doctors and patients. In India, 560 million people are using the Internet, so nowadays other than the cloud no technology is present.

15.1.8 MOTIVATION

During the COVID-19 pandemic, many people have suffered due lack of awareness and as a result not taking proper health precautions. To that end, the authors have tried to present a system which can reach everyone for maintaining proper health.

15.2 METHOD

15.2.1 AI-BASED BOT

In the age of AI, chatbots, also known as "conversational bots", have played a crucial role in maintaining virtual assistants that could use voice queries or message queries to get answers from doctors. This manages a conversation between physician/doctor and patient. This chatbot performs all the necessary actions and recommendations as needed. The AI interface is adaptable to user languages and preferences. This conversational bot cloud plays a crucial role in overcoming the present hurdles in healthcare. Fundamental healthcare is easy to afford, within reach and becomes feasible in this electronic era. This service is instant and personalized which makes telehealth a good start. Physicians use these applications to record, access and store the patient data. It is cheaper for patients. An AI-enabled chatbot assistant will work 24×7 and can care for a wide range of patients. Persons suffering from diseases, and weakened or handicapped people,

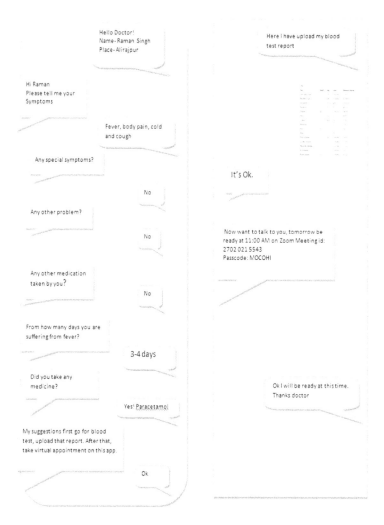

FIGURE 15.1 Aapka swasthay salahkar chatbot: this chatbot is made on the A1 algorithm, is easy to maintain, works as per the requirement, and is connected to the cloud platform.

and including people from remote areas, can access this bot efficiently and effectively. It is an easy way to reach a doctor for primary treatment.

This saves medical practices time and improves data security; on-demand healthcare is available, which is reassuring to patients. This chapter describes the "aapka swasthaya salahkar" chatbot, which is AI-enabled and offers promising results to patients [20].

Here, an example is taken of a patient who is suffering from a high fever and had a conversation using "aapka swasthaya salahkar" with the desired physician.

15.2.2 Cloud-Enabled Interface

Hybrid cloud interface is used because data as a service, software as a service (SaaS), platform as a service (PaaS) and infrastructure as a service (IaaS) are the most familiar and extensively trusted service models, but other templates consist of communication as a service (CaaS), database as a service (DbaaS), security as a service (SECaaS), identity management as a service (ImaaS) and desktop as a service (DaaS) are used as per the need. This enables data storage in a cloud given in Basu S. 2012 [21] and will be available on demand with specific requirements because security is a must. Cloud is used for telemedicine to both patients and doctors (Figure 15.2). Telemedicine and cloud computing services are combined to develop an adaptable method for patients and doctors, reducing the gap between them. Any application that is easily adjustable with cloud computing and smart devices is valuable in this era. Doctors can easily follow patients' health with its records by clicking in a particular application [22].

15.2.3 Blockchain Interface

The blockchain information is sensitive and personal, requiring secured sharing among peers, hospitals, medical practices, pharmacies, and health-related authorities to maintain patient records on time (Dubouitskaya et al., 2017 [23]; Saweros E 2019 [24]). Blockchain technology enforces trust because it does not involve any mediator. The consent management system is protected by different authorities/organizations [25, 26]. Blockchain features of immutability, traceability, and transparency make it suitable for healthcare data [27]. The IAISTM model (Figure 15.3) is well-suited to deliver all such services on time. Hence blockchain helps in maintaining all the sensitive and knowledgeable data in storage form in the cloud or in local systems.

15.3 WORKING OF IAISTM MODEL

Remote healthcare practicing makes telehealth and telemedicine an effective method. This technology requires electronic in-person encounters of medical seekers and medical specialists for making the right decision in treatment for remotely located patients. This is a kind of direct-to-consumer or business-to-business model. Here, patients can directly contact their preferred doctor to discuss health

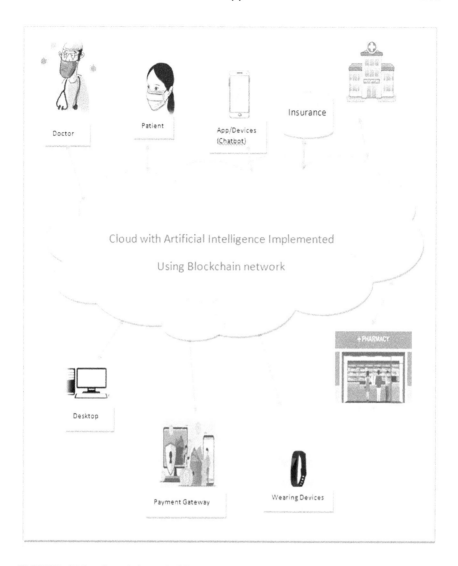

FIGURE 15.2 Correlation of different stakeholders, interconnection with cloud, and blockchain infrastructure that will be used in telemedicine.

status. In virtual appointments, patients contact doctors through video conferencing, which can be managed and maintained by AI bot "aapka sawasthya salahkar". All the required images are added to that. In this example (Figure 15.1), if a patient's test reports the malaria parasite is detected, this should be added to the link provided by the chatbot, and a virtual meeting with the doctor is assigned.

The existing telemedicine system has the issue of managing the health records of the patient. But in this above-mentioned IAISTM model, data sharing is not limited. This model provides single or multiple uses of data sharing among health

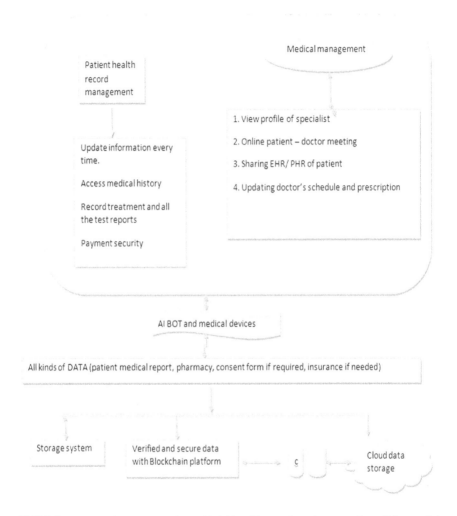

FIGURE 15.3   IAISTM: Innovative artificial intelligence-based secure telemedicine model has updated features of AI and cloud-blockchain for data handling, storage, and security.

parties. This system manages all the health records of patients, including previous medical history, blood tests, or any other images in past, present or future. If the patent needs pharmacy support or insurance, all these records are added and updated on time. If the patient uses a medical kit (from reputed manufacturers) or wearable devices for his disease monitoring and medication taken on time, all are recorded [28, 29]. In wearable devices, there is a system of alarm that makes patients remember to eat their medicines on time in critical situations or normal daily timely medicines. This centralized telehealth system consists of m-health, e-health based devices. Blockchain technology made transparency in medical kits or testing aids on the dispersed records. The smart tele system made all these for

TABLE 15.1

Comparison between Traditional Ways of Treatment and Modern Ways of Treatment (IAISTM)

Traditional system	IAISTM
Cost is high.	Cost is low.
Patient waiting time is high.	Patient waiting time is low.
Cloud based system is not involved.	Cloud based system is involved.
Health records can be manipulated.	No manipulation of health records.
Documentation is difficult to carry and maintain.	No need to carry documents, AI-enabled cloud has the system to manage and maintain health records.
All the data records are difficult to secure.	Data security and privacy is easy to maintain.
There is no transparency.	Transparency is maintained.
Reliability and integrity are low.	Reliability and integrity are high.

homecare devices with their performance evaluations. Patients can use it under doctor advice. Now the personal health record (PHR) system is also developed in the IAISTM model. It is an individual's health records of the present, past treatments as in our malaria case. This PHR is generated, maintained and properly managed to provide proper supervision to the patient. This system has the power to store extensive records of many patients.

All the contacts like the patient and his medical facilities are registered and authorized, and it allows the owner to share data with verified users (Daghar et al. 2018 [30]). The automated payment system is also decentralized with cryptocurrency tokens. Therefore, direct payment transfer and all settlements are done in a secure manner. The blockchain-based IAISTM model provides an option for cash on delivery, which is in the user's interest, as it can reduce payment frauds.

In remote areas, the IAI system is well maintained to provide medicines to given addresses, and the system is programmed so that the pharmacist will get money only when the particular drugs reach the patient. In our example, if the patient is ordered Quinone, a malarial drug, it will reach the patient by the authorized pharmacist with cash on delivery or digital secure payment mode.

If patients use any biomedical sensors or wearable devices, continuous monitoring of health is recorded, such as blood pressure and body temperature. Table 15.1 shows the comparison of traditional systems and new telemedicine models like IAISTM (as discussed above).

15.3.1 Dataset

Here, the example of malaria is used. If symptoms of the malaria parasite are diagnosed, the IATSTM model will work as classification machine learning (see Chinmay C. et al 2016 [31]). This is supervised in action. Machine learning performs better in good datasets, and outcomes are good for proper diagnosis and treatment. In ML there are many algorithms; the best possible algorithm for the data is a decision tree. This algorithm allows the computer to think like a human as the data is fed in, and it has the power to make a good decision which is easy to understand. It thinks like a tree, where "yes" and "no" are branches. Finally, it reaches the point which is helpful in decision-making.

Workplace for doctors: A distinctive place is designed for physicians to work with the proposed system. The system provides the AI bot data and a detailed overview of machine learning-based identification of disease based on the parameters (see Figure 15.4) and they can understand the present status of the patient. This information is useful for physicians to provide teleservices for the medical seeker. This workplace is a web-based application that provides worldwide access, so any patient or physician can use this service. The data is transmitted through sensors too if required.

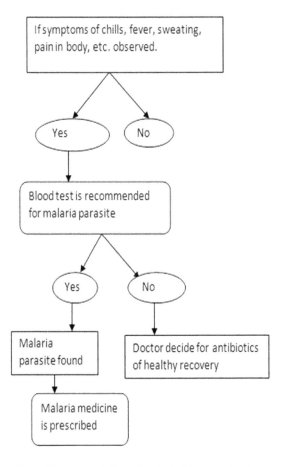

FIGURE 15.4 Schematic representation of malaria identification in any person through decision tree classification.

Communication service: the communication services include database connection with hardware which provides secure and robust transmission of information. There would be a central database for storing the data. Programming libraries and web services are commonly used [32].

Every service is connected to the Internet. High-speed Internet connectivity is very important for teleservices to come into existence and success. With these physicians could keep an eye on patient data and daily routine of medicine intake and position of fever or any health issue.

A decision tree helps to clearly diagnose any disease based on the symptoms identified and reports generated [33]. Patients will take the appointment through the AI bot "aapka sawasthay salahkar" and as per the questionnaire, he or she goes for a blood test and submits a report to the doctor, and then, accordingly, the doctor provides medication if the malaria parasite is found. Later, a person can check again to see if they have a fever, and if need be seek treatment. In any case, if any other symptom develops or they do not recover within seven days, or whatever is stated by the doctor, the patient and doctor talk again by the same app/chabot, and further treatment may be prescribed. The chatbot with IoT and machine learning transforms the thinking and treatment process. It looks like "tum mujhe symptoms do Hum tumhe sahi chikatsak denge". This is now a slogan for telemedicine-based therapies.

Analysis: the following three goals are achieved:

(a) The physician's workload is reduced.
(b) New knowledge is gained, and proper prediction of disease is done.
(c) Diseases could be monitored by physicians whenever they wanted.

This rule, or decision tree interpretation framework (Figure 15.4), allows the physicians to better understand the disease. Above all, patient–doctor and doctor–patient communication must be effective and offline too, so that there would be no problem if the network failed. The mobile client also gets a feedback form to share the views about how they feel the treatment went.

Figures 15.1–15.3 are interrelated. This must be patient-centric approach and provides full support to each patient. Expected diseases patients and outcomes and management of all the data are stored and used effectively. The technique to use is redesigned and cultivated as per the need. This model is used for other disease diagnosis also. All kinds of data, patients treated, untreated and left or died due to an outbreak is monitored through AI. This will help in exposed areas of diseases, and in development of medicines or vaccines. Although drug repurposing is possible with the use of bioinformatics approaches, decentralization is done for the use of data and databases.

AI models needs to be standardized and have training for hospital staff to enable proper usage, and shared every time a new step is added. Blockchain technology helps in this to distribute all the AI parameters with standards. Data sharing is done securely by blockchain, as data is transferred through blocks every time, without any breaching of patient privacy. The rules of AI are satisfied with machine learning algorithms for proper functioning of the IAISTM framework.

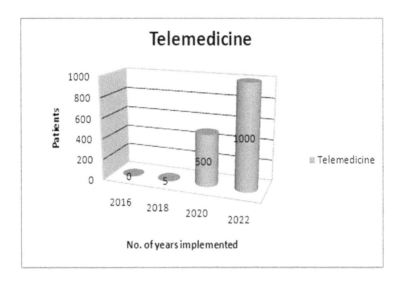

FIGURE 15.5   Increased use of telemedicine year by year.

Clinical trials can also be done as per the need, and their facts shared with medical practitioners with utmost utility to provide quick diagnosis and treatment with these decision rules (Figure 15.5).

Due to COVID-19, use of telemedicine is increasing, and it is expected that it will progress rapidly in the coming years. The graph in Figure 15.5 also shows that telemedicine will be the needed by everyone in the near future. It is feasible for all, and will save time. Markets will increase in this area. Smart phones with voice assistance have reached every locality, so people living in remote areas are also taking the advantage of telemedicine.

15.3.2   EFFECTIVENESS OF TELEMEDICINE IN PRESENT CONTEXT

Working together for health is the report given by WHO. At present more trained and skilled persons are required for effectiveness. Awareness and understanding of telehealth are a big decision to take. Having faith in such technologies is an important criterion to get better treatment or results. Eldercare is one of the future uses of telemedicine. This needs attention. The main thing is that telemedicine is here to stay with the existing healthcare system, to provide better treatment on time, reducing suffering. Presently, few countries are using this technology, but still it does a lot of work to reach developing countries. The advantage of this technique is that it can address deficiencies. Technology efficiency is one of the most important parameters to make telemedicine a success. In the near future, there may be apps available for illiterate people, and also to perform activities on telemedicine networks through Government awareness programmes and advertisements shown on the Internet/Facebook/television. It will focus on more veracious health needs.

In case of another disease, if the sensor is used, a mobile/smartphone [14] is available to fill the entire questionnaire about their disease progress. The activity of sensors is also captured and monitored. This would be available for a long time too. The collected data is automatically transmitted to the servers. In the telemedical workplace, nurses are sometimes there also for follow-up, and provide suitable support when required. If the nurse finds an abnormality, she can provide support, and if there is a technical error or issue, IT support is always available. Centres for telemedicine in hospitals provide all the necessary support and track all activities day and night.

15.3.3   DECISION-MAKING SYSTEM

Patients involved in the treatment are the ones to whom diagnostic and treatments are based on their communications with the doctors/nurses whilst using chatbots, or questionnaire-filling or video conferencing. The process and results obtained during consultations are crucial. Patient and healthcare provider satisfaction is necessary. In this telemedicine framework, interaction between any two is organized with technological capabilities. Practice makes it possible and leads to success. Here, patients and health professionals make use of their knowledge for better treatment possibilities. Decision-making policy is also shared for patient betterment. As it is very different from face-to-face consultations, skills and experience of improving and using this technology are essential. An AI-based system having inbuilt machine learning algorithms like decision trees is helpful to understand the disease cause and disease diagnosis. Patient disease management and treatment decision is also taking place with its help which saves the medical practices time [34].

15.3.4   SUMMARY OF TELEMEDICINE MODEL FOR MALARIA

The system developed and shown here is flexible and gives full support to patients. This furnishes a novel way of treatment at the doorstep and improves quality of life, reducing costs. The results found are encouraging.

Any of the health services need trustable data to provide accurate information about the protozoa/malaria parasite or any other disease predictions. There is a need to develop a patient-centric society with applications of digital technologies [9]. Bluetooth, mobile, tablets and laptops are all connected through IoT devices. They track the disease outcome, m-health, e-health, and are the basis of today's disease diagnosis and prediction. These data will help in the future spread of disease outcomes and pandemics [12]. With an AI-enabled bot, the patient fills in the form and learns about suffering, and informs the doctor about the disease. The doctor, having observed the symptoms through AI and previous data, learns about the particular disease. Figure 15.4 shows a person suffering from malaria, with the help of a decision tree. The physician then provides treatment for malaria. After 5–7 days, the patient receives the link to update their disease situation. This reaches physicians, and then, if necessary, a doctor or nurse will call and explain about medicines to continue or stop. They will also provide all the necessary measures for complete recovery.

This model provides automated supervision of each and every step so no data breaching. Data management is possible, which is helpful in diagnosis infections. The possibility of patient information sharing keeps the data as no further duplication. Formulation of raw data sets, AI, web-based toolkits and wearable devices is all handled with care as per government rules.

This infrastructure provides contact-free treatment and all medical help including the pharmacy. Drones and robots are used to find out about disease outbreaks, or to monitor patient health over time. Medical supplies and pharmaceuticals are also managed properly. This whole process is time-consuming, but well organized. This is also helpful in disaster management and insurance claims in cases of cancer-like disease.

15.3.5 BENEFITS OF CLOUD IN TELEMEDICINE

Cloud computing offers many advantages in tele-network for healthcare. It includes economic, commercial, operational and functional tasks under one umbrella. Better integration and privacy with security draw a lot of attention from health providers and researchers. Pharmacists and pharma companies are also using cloud for providing support to medicines and vaccine development. The cloud providers take care of secure payments too. Live video is possible if a doctor wants to check a patient, or needs consultations, diagnostics and treatment services. The data is stored and transmitted whenever necessary; m-health or m-care are part of medicine nowadays in the form of smartphone apps. Additional benefits of using cloud techniques in telemedicines include:

(i) Telemedicine gained rapid recognition by patients who are suffering from persistent health conditions, which must be frequently monitored. It is advantageous for both doctor and patient.

(ii) It is beneficial or discovered for those patients who live in remote areas and doctors can track the patient's health regularly.

(iii) Bandwidth of emailing larger files is accessible across the network.

(iv) Authorized access is maintained every time.

(v) Flexibility is there in that patient data can be accessed by doctors and shared by senior doctors for further treatment and tests.

(vi) Accessibility is one of the features of the cloud which is used beneficially here by uploading patient's data onto the cloud, which can then be accessed from anywhere in the world by authorized users.

(vii) It saves them time and travelling expenditure of the patient, and saves the time of the doctor too.

(viii) Disaster recovery: here, data is secured and can be recovered as data gets stored in the cloud.

(ix) Patient connectivity, health management and distribution of data are also part of cloud computing in telemedicine.

(x)   The whole tele-model is secured through encryption techniques, and blockchain plays a crucial role.

(xi) Cloud storage is possible for all kinds of past, present data, which can be migrated whenever needed.

15.4   REMOTE MONITORING THROUGH IAISTM

Monitoring the disease condition of a patient using a relevant sensor, data transfer from patient to a medical health provider, data integration with other data, patient care with decision support, and data storage is done with the cloud computing techniques. AI bot with the advancement of ICT components performs various functions. These AI bots are built through mathematical functions of machine learning with logic. This will enable handling of large volumes of data and data-sets. AI approaches have been applied to conducting and supervision of patients with chronic health conditions immediately finds data from GPS, motion sensors, etc. Classification and regression method of machine learning for the early iden-tification of disease like in our example, if a patient is diagnosed with the malaria parasite then they need to take the medicine recommended. And patient records its fever severity after taking medicine in the app linked with AI bot "aapka saw-asthaya salahker". This will feel like the doctor at home. That doctor also updates with a particular patient's day-to-day health and recovery. Medical practitioners recommend other medicines also to improve health by the same bot. These tele-health tools need to be improved for further assessment. Telehealth will lead to the development of medical informatics in near future.

The key participants in this feature are:

(i)   Patient: Any person who requires medical care is a patient. The data given by them may be helpful in understanding the disease better.

(ii)   Healthcare providers: This huge group includes physicians, specialists, hos-pitals, dispensaries, laboratories, repositories, researchers and pharmacies.

(iii) Payers: In case of tough diseases like cancer, etc. an insurance company plays an important role in paying.

(iv)   Pharmacy: Without these vital entities, healthcare wouldn't be possible. They are also updated with new techniques and have full records of med-icines distribution and stock of medicines, injections.

(v)   Pharma companies: The drug makers are the companies that work day and night to provide healthcare as prescribed. Their supply chain is so strong that it reaches every pharmacy and manages medication.

(vi)   Scholars and researchers: They are the ones who conduct pharmaceuti-cal and biomedical research. Nowadays, research is also digitally trans-formed. Big Data and machine learning develop such algorithms that can analyze data and give good predictions [9].

(vii) Government: People safety and handling emergencies are the big respon-sibilities of the Government. As they are policymakers for industry standards, they enforce and ensure regulations [9].

15.4.1   Benefits of IAISTM

(a) This model helps in decentralization. All the EHRs are stored, accessed and managed at multiple locations.
(b) The data is immutable: All the records stored are not changed. Due to the use of cryptography used in blockchain, it is possible to maintain data integrity.
(c) All the entries/records are transparently providing remote patient-centred data control.
(d) Patients can access physicians' profiles and talk with the AI BOT (like "aapka sawasthay salahkar") and confirm their schedule.
(e) By this model, drug province can be tracked.
(f) Anonymous identity of a patient can be maintained and tracked.

15.4.2   Wonders of AI and Blockchain

AI-based bots and other applications allow organizations to understand the data as an individual or population-based. In this COVID-19 pandemic, the trend of telemedicine reaches its top position because persons prefer remote treatment, as it is easy and timely. Blockchain plays a vital role in the metamorphose of health information exchange and making a secure payment gateway. Blockchain in healthcare has revolutionized the IT era with its moves of sharing, dispersal and encryption. Still, AI and blockchain are in their infancy, and will bring a lot more to the healthcare industry in the future. These technologies have the power to communicate in remote areas where doctors are also avoiding going personally. Blockchain has worked on mechanisms like proof-of-work (PoW), Byzantine fault-tolerant (BFT), zero-knowledge proof, and proof-of-stake (PoS) [26].

These intelligent contracts are utilized to increase the liquidity and faith between two people, doctor-patient relations, patient-hospital (any of the two parties). Blockchain provides the opportunity to handle the data in reality as discussed in Jabarulla and Lee, 2019 [10]. It is certain that the amalgamation of AI, IoT and blockchain will solve all the technical and other issues of healthcare in the future and every one of us will get better treatment and sustainable life. The most important points are:

 (i)   Patients have the authority to access and control their data.
 (ii) Any risk of data leakage can be identified within a time limit.
(iii) Any hindrance blockchain network can track and trace the information directly from the origin which is based on cryptography technology. All things are always in backup in a centralized server.
(iv) The data is audited from time to time if needed.
 (v) AI-based decision-making makes the process run smoothly.

The telemedicine approach surrounds the services of remote consultations basically through audio/video calls with tablets, mobile phones or computer availability. This will maintain contact-free discussion of disease and availability of treatment on time. Now, healthcare is becoming patient-centric, and there is no room for compromising in treatment (Chinmay C. 2016; 2019 [14, 33]).

15.5 SUSTAINABILITY OF THE WORK

Telehealth requires all the facts and figures with communication techniques to transmit health data for clinical and scholastic purposes. This model provides superior services in time, distance and difficult territories, economical, and a better approach is developed and reaches to progressing countries. Telehealth support in remote areas with the help of AI and blockchain is a must in today's fast-developing technology. This model also helps in remote monitoring of the health issues which involves data collection, distribution as per demand and need. This is also called e-health or electronic health, and m-health or mobile health are interrelated. These will help in teleradiology, telepathology, teledermatology, etc.

All the examination reports of imaging techniques like an ultrasound for gall stones or severe pain in the bladder, CT scan (tumour), MRI, etc. makes conclusive investigations in the clinical examinations of one or more patients.AI and blockchain made telemedicine reachable to remote areas in a low cost.

15.6 APPLICATION

(i) Telemedicine in public health: Telemedicine utilization for epidemiological surveillance is slowly approaching new steps with the evolution of technology as observed in geographic information systems (GISs). This not only works well in disease prevalence also shows valuable insights towards community wellbeing assessment. Risk factors are studied well for disease epidemiology. This will help in planning, assessing different intermediate policies for early diagnosis of disease, and monitoring health in an effective way.

(ii) Anticipating epidemics: Plays a central role in forecasting outbreaks. This is crucial to make the public aware of the symptoms of an outbreak in a community. This real-time monitoring of diseases on the local and global level will help people to maintain their health and necessary precautions for any epidemics.

(iii) Disease transmission: If GIS is used in this tele-model this will help to know spatial-temporal modelling of weather conditions which will help to understand disease transmission in remote areas. The spread of a disease facilitates and integrates different data from diverse sources so that this will make the public health programmes and make proper decisions on time (as observed in the COVID-19 outbreak).

(iv) Disease prevention: Revolution in information technology led to the development of telemedicine improves the way to adopt a healthy lifestyle, aware of health-related issues.

(v) Easily accessible: This is user-friendly, and if a person is unable to type, they can use a virtual assistant for medical treatment.

(vi) Promotes self-care: Telemedicine approaches promote self-care and all the self approaches to care for themselves. One person can evaluate their own health.

(vii) Quality improvement in services: Telehealth approaches are improving day by day for better connections in telecommunication by AI and blockchain services which require an IoT platform to fulfil all the safe health delivery need.

(viii) Awareness among medical care providers: For using telehealth services efficiently, computer literacy is important and adaptable to use all the features for AI and blockchain use. This telemedicine is a new avatar to provide good infrastructure for easy access and use. Every time when the new feature is added its demonstration is showed to healthcare providers and makes them efficient to use AI-based telehealth effectively.

15.7 CONCLUSION

This chapter signifies the importance of cutting-edge technology of AI and blockchain in health, which makes telehealth. It is the journey of tele-caller to telehealth (4T), happily utilizing telecommunication methods. The 4T is defined as tele-assessment, tele-diagnosis, tele-interactions and telemonitoring. This closed unity among healthcare participants to keep up all the health records up to date. Nowadays, an enormous amount of data is involved, requiring security and storage, so the cloud with blockchain minimizes the risk of data leakage. The current cloud–blockchain platform confirms the secured payments by cryptocurrency such as Ethereum, or having the option of pay on delivery. This information sharing in a network is fast, secure and has a shield of privacy maintenance to users. This work assisted physicians to check and communicate with patients in remote areas. This chapter also discussed the identification of a doctor, or how to contact the doctor of interest. Key features:

(a) Monitoring patients in remote areas to minimize error in treatment.
(b) Manage secure patient consent form.
(c) Minimize transaction time for payments.
(d) Drug delivery is transparent.
(e) Home-based diagnosis is safe as it can be used under physician direction.

The high impact of blockchain technology in the financial sector proves better in telehealth and telemedicine platforms. This AI–IoT–blockchain-based platform makes telemedicine systems error-prone. The challenges of telemedicine in this era are identified and managed every time with the help of an AI-blockchain system. Hence it is said that telemedicine fully destroys the utility of blockchain in its betterment. Last but not least, the fast-growing world in the telecommunication era makes a better environment in the medicine/health sector, as it also fastens the research in the medical field. The data available through telemedicine are also huge and require proper arrangement and further research for improving the algorithms to work more accurately and provide knowledge about the diseases and their treatments.

15.7.1 FUTURE SCOPE

With the advancement of technology, the future of these technologies is bright.

a) Telemedicine gives quality assistance to patients.
b) Patients have a choice of their physician based on comfortability.
c) It would become a well-organized possibility for preventative care.
d) Cost-effective and time-efficient ways make telemedicine a boon to medical care.
e) Specialist assistance will be more effective in the near future.
f) It develops more ways to personalized health planning.

The rich source of IoT–AI brings all the dreams to come true, now virtual assistance of doctors made feel "at home services". The connection with any of the doctors is possible. This new technology has improved the methods of patient treatment.

REFERENCES

1. World Health Organisation, 1998. A health telematics policy in support of WHO's Health-For-All strategy for global health development: Report of the WHO group consultation on health telematics, 11–16 December, Geneva, 1997. Geneva: World Health Organization.
2. Ajami S., Lamoochi P., 2014, Use of telemedicine in disaster and remote places. *Journal of Education Health Promotion*, 3, 26. And Communication, Springer, Phuket, Thailand, 2019, pp. 858–869. App. 10/904, 818.
3. World Health Organization, 2010, Telemedicine: Opportunities and developments in member states. Report on the second global survey on eHealth. Geneva: World Health Organization.
4. McLean S., Protti D., Sheikh A., 2017, Telehealthcare for long term conditions. *BMJ* 2011 Feb 3; 342: d120.nugget for privacy and security challenges. *The Journal of the International Society for Telemedicine and eHealth*, 5.
5. Wilson L.S., Maeder A.J., 2015, Recent directions in telemedicine: Review of trends in research and practice. *Health Information Research*, October 1, 21(4), 213–222.
6. Pacis D.M., Subido Jr E.D., Bugtai N.T., 2018, Trends in telemedicine utilizing artificial intelligence. *AIP Conference Proceedings*, February 13; 1933(1), 040009.
7. Peterson M.C., Holbrook J.H., Von Hales D., Smith N.L., Staker L.V., 1992, Contributions of the history, physical examination, and laboratory investigation in making medical diagnoses. *The Western Journal of Medicine*, February, 156(2), 163–5.
8. Roshan M., Rao A., 2000, A study on relative contributions of the history, physical examination and investigations in making medical diagnosis. *The Journal of the Association of Physicians of India* 48(8), 771–775.
9. Jabarullah Y.M., Lee H., 2021, A blockchain and artificial intelligence-based patient-centric Healthcare system for combating the COVID-19 pendemic: Opportunities and applications. *Healthcare*, 9, 1019.

10. Reddy S., Fox J., Purohit M.P. 2019, Artificial intelligence-enabled healthcare delivery. *Journal of the Royal Society of Medicine*, 112, 22–28.

11. Russell S., Norvig P., 1995, *Artificial Intelligence – A Modern Approach*. Prentice-Hall.

12. Gors M., Albert Michael, Schwedhelm Kai, Christian Herrmann, Schilling Klaus, 2015, Design of an advanced telemedicine system for remote supervision. *IEEE Systems Journal*.

13. Abdul R.J., Chinmay C., Celestine W., 2021, Exploratory data analysis, classification, comparative analysis, case severity detection, and Internet of things in COVID-19 telemonitoring for smart hospitals. *Journal of Experimental & Theoretical Artificial Intelligence*, 1–24. doi: 10.1080/0952813X.2021.1960634.

14. Chinmay C., Gupta B., Ghosh S.K., 2016, Mobile telemedicine systems for remote patient's chronic wound monitoring. *IGI: M-Health Innovations for Patient-Centered Care*, Ch. 11, 217–243, ISBN: 9781466698611.

15. Prokofieva M., Miah S.J., 2019, Blockchain in healthcare, Australas. *Journal of Information Systems* 23.

16. Rajaram V., 2014, John Mc Carthy-father of artificial intelligence. *Resonance*, 198–207.

17. Jin Zhanpeng, Chen Yu, 2015, Telemedicine in the cloud era: Prospects and challenges. *IEEE Pervasive Computing*.

18. Khatoon A., 2020, A blockchain-based smart contract system for healthcare management. *Electronics*, 9(1), 94. doi: 10.3390/electronics9010094.

19. Stowe S., Harding S., 2018, Telecare, telehealth and telemedicine, Eur. Geriatr. Med. 1 telemedicine program in a community setting. *Journal of Genetic Counseling*, 27(2), U.D. of Health, H. Services, et al., Personal Health Records and the HIPAA Privacyusing tangle. International Conference on Ubiquitous Information Management.

20. Bharti U., Bajaj D., Batra H., et al., 2018, Medbot: Conventional artificial intelligence powered chatbot for delivering tele-health after COVID-19. Proceedings of the fifth International Conference on Communication and Electronic System (ICCES 2020). Blockchain Technology. *Sustainable Cities and Society* 39, 283–297.

21. Basu, S. et al., 2012 Fusion: Managing healthcare records at cloud scale. *Computer*, 45(11), 42–49.

22. Ahmed S., Abdullah A., 2011, Telemedicine in a cloud—a review. *Proc. IEEE Symp. Computers & Informatics*, pp. 776–781.

23. Dubovitskaya A., Xu Z., Ryu S., Schumacher M., Wang F., 2020, Secure and trustableelectronic medical records sharing using blockchain, 2017. *American Medical Electronics*, 9(1), 94.

24. Saweros E., Song Y.-T., 2019, Connecting heterogeneous electronic health record systems using Tangle. *International Conference on Ubiquitous Information Management and Communication IMCOM 2019: Proceedings of the 13th International Conference on Ubiquitous Information Management and Communication (IMCOM) 2019*, pp. 858–869.

25. Genestier P., Zouarhi S., Limeux P., Excoffier D., Prola A., Sandon S., 2017, J.-GKR-e24. health records using blockchain technology, arXiv preprint arXiv: 1804.10078. *Informatics Association, AMIA Annual Symposium Proceedings*, vol. 650.

26. Zhang R., Xue R., Liu, L. 2019, Security and privacy on blockchain. *ACM Computing Surveys* 52, 1–34.

27. Verma A.S., Dubey A., 2021, *Computing Techniques for Securing Healthcare Data with Blockchain Technology*, Blockchain for Healthcare Systems, Issue 1, CRC Press, doi: 10.1201/97810031.

28. Li R., 2005 Multifunctional self-diagnostic device for in-home health-checkup, US Patent.
29. Weissman S.M., Zellmer K., Gill N., Wham D., 2018, Implementing a virtual health telemedicine program in a community setting. *Journal of Genetic Counseling*, April, 27(2), 323–325.
30. Dagher G. G., Mohler J., Milojkovic M, Marella P.B., 2018, Ancile: Privacy-preserving framework for access control and interoperability of electronic health records using Blockchain Technology, February. *Sustainable Cities and Society*, 39(1). doi: 10.1016/j.scs.2018.02.014.
31. Chinmay C., Gupta B., Ghosh S.K., Das D, Chakraborty C., 2016, Telemedicine supported chronic wound tissue prediction using different classification approach. *Journal of Medical Systems*, 40(3), 1–12. doi: 10.1007/s10916-015-0424-y.
32. Mielcarz T., Winiecki W. 2005, The use of web-services for development of distributed measurement systems. *Proc. IEEE IDAACS: Technol. Appl.*, pp. 320–324.
33. Chinmay C., 2019, Mobile health (m-Health) for tele-wound monitoring. *IGI: Mobile Health Applications for Quality Healthcare Delivery*, Ch. 5, 98–116, ISBN: 9781522580218. doi: 10.4018/978-1-5225-8021-8.ch005.
34. Kelvin K., Tsoi F., 2019, Application of artificial intelligence on a symptom diagnostic platform for telemedicine – a pilot case study. *IEEE International Conference on Systems, Man and Cybernetics*, Italy, October 6–9.

16 Legal Implication of Blockchain Technology in Public Health

Jayanta Ghosh
West Bengal National University of Juridical Sciences,
Kolkata, India

Ardhendu Sekhar Nanda
National Institute of Securities Markets and Maharashtra
National Law University, Mumbai, India

CONTENTS

DOI: 10.1201/9781003247128-16

16.1 INTRODUCTION

Genetics point towards worldly solace only to be nourished according to the adequate available standards of goods and services. Technologies act in a good way with the future goals of adding comfort in our everyday lives, prioritizing it to be the best intangible asset in the present-day scenario. Racing in the avenue of technologies, blockchain leads the game due to its features and easy access. Classy, encrypted representation at every step guides a customer towards minimalist life management inclusive of an advanced economy and beneficiary relationships [1]. To make life easier, people are drawn to vehicles that are faster and more efficient, meeting individual, community and regional needs. Technological indulgence would support the human efforts and would serve as a more successful way to layout living entities, moving forward in development [2].

Health is wealth and no less a person's primary goal for life. Maintenance is entirely worthy of living, and life span depends on the energy of the youth. Daily focus on lifestyle activities commemorates one's dedication towards the best of objectives. Some nations provide breath-taking compulsory insurance schemes, whereas some don't undertake an individual's health. Hassle-free healthcare is maintained only if the technology pushes us active to take care of ourselves at level one. The importance of healthcare and the necessity of self-care programmes are both represented in sociological theory. Healthcare institutions and treatment programmes both utilize advanced goods that conform with approved technology health solutions. Health insurance and life insurance protection look good when taking a glance at the finances [4].

Public health has become one of the most remarkable features of today's life, which is the primary responsibility of individual government. Health ministry has more significant roles than any other if they value the life of every citizen. WHO has multiple commissions and bodies to put a check on health and poverty. Challenging complexities arise with new diseases, new diagnosis methods, new treatments and the complexity goes up daily. With the scare of maintaining adequate principles of life perfectly, which are essential, multiple applications are available handy. Whether it is simple diet remainder or calculation of calories or how much water to drink per day, smaller connotations cater to lifestyle management. Ignorance of basics would lead to bodily patterns like the body mechanism, sleep patterns, and immunity cycles [3, 4].

Liabilities rise when mistakes occur via human work, but sooner or later, they will be replaced by "smart contracts" irreversibly. Pros and cons battle the league of excellence, but the indulgence of multiple technologies creates multiple bumps via the yonder of the corporate which cannot take care of their affairs. Technological singularity is the inconceivable solution among the maze of technologies always. Ultimately, it is the desire for technology to deliver the greatest service that motivates the pursuit of knowledge, and there is no guarantee that the pursuit will be fulfilled. The transaction method is increasing and seeming to be more organized on a blockchain network. All members of the government may see the advantages of a mutual demand-supply chain, which is supported by a range of economic viewpoints. Man to man (M2M) communication has been rendered obsolete, with technology still leading the way [9].

Individual care prioritizes the best efforts to maintain health on common grounds, irrespective of skilled doctors, additional help and paramedics. Whatever happens, happens for good in a way that would go divergent to various resources, clamped with checks and balances. In a country like India, the acute shortage of medical help shows the desperate ratio of doctors and patients, which succumbs to 1:1000. The gulf between satisfactory and good healthcare needs a palliative remedy, which technology may provide. The health-tech gadgets, which are creative, offer intellectual help, but this void is addressed by one-on-one reviews. If human compassion is traded for technical kindness, the two parties may agree on a compromise [10].

A rough drive arrives with the commercialization of the healthcare industry, where bioethics is challenged globally. One of the worst incidents lies with the ransomware attacking the NHS, the UK and some hospitals in Canada. Surprisingly, the cyber attacker demanded payments in cryptocurrency, which is claimed to be the best form of encrypted money to unlock systems. Due to the fragility of health IT infrastructure, the rise of social media has led to an increase in the severity of cyber-attacks. The health-tech industry also faces the problem of uneven treatment, as health-tech subscription is proportional to income. Human existence as a whole is damaged owing to classifying equality as a necessity. Unless there is rapid, widespread trust, terrorism or worse is possible: a bioterrorist event that no one can stop. If technology is not checked each second of service delivery, the healthcare business might be adversely affected, and vernacular decentralization may appear. The judicial system is severely skewed in favour of the rich, and the poor are especially hard hit [12].

16.2   EFFECTIVENESS OF BLOCKCHAIN TOWARDS PUBLIC HEALTH

Innovation is praised for its efficient role in today's life, on a par with digital contracts, and comfort is gestured to be needful. Law has become a public code in which the smart contract essentials percolate as per legal compliance. Blockchain is one of the leading innovations that run on a decentralized database and formulates data integrity and authenticity by encrypted measures. Blockchain stands upon four principles: a) Consensus; b) Provenance; c) Immutability; and d) Finality; transposing all these features into one successful application is the bitcoin network. Bitcoin, a decentralized payment system not controlled by any government or central bank, was the first to use blockchain technology. The state of a blockchain can only be altered by adding new data through consensus (i.e., with the consent of more than half of the network nodes). In this way, the blockchain can be thought of as a cryptographically secure append-only database that functions without the requirement for a central authority or clearinghouse. Drawing on the notion of lex informatica, we can connect law with information technology where the algorithms are legally enforceable, and the enforcement or applications go as per legal compliance. As per lex cryptography within the blockchain, data privacy is safe and secure with every transaction back and forth in the field of fintech [13]. Public health has grasped the fire of the hearts of many, especially in the developing and the underdeveloped ones.

16.2.1 BLOCKCHAIN INFLUX WITH TIME

One of our society's most significant economic and regulatory players is reduced with the help of blockchain technology. The approach of the market is also different from working hand in hand. To regulate the market and government aspects, it must comply with the legal mechanism while balancing power. An apt definition for the most successful blockchain to date is:

> A blockchain is a digitally distributed, decentralized, public ledger that anyone can upload programs to and leave the programs to self-execute, where the current and all previous states of every program are always publicly visible, and which carries a very strong crypto economically secured guarantee that programs running on the chain will continue to execute in exactly the way that the blockchain protocol.

Irreversible decentralized platforms are safer for any B2B or B2C transaction, where the customers feel secure on personal data privacy and the lack of government interventions. Citizens feel free when government interventions go minimal without any scrutiny unless taxes are paid on time. The future of the peer-to-peer(P2P) economy is blockchain technology. It implements a methodology for individuals to agree on a particular state of affairs and document that agreement by integrating P2P networks, cryptographic algorithms, distributed data storage and decentralized consensus processes. Individual actions before the blockchain development could not be coordinated via the Internet without the help of a centralized authority that verifies that the data hasn't been tampered with [14, 15].

Decentralized automated organizations (DAO) develop smart codes to simplify the legal language in any online application. Government banks and regulatory bodies have to create new end policies to have cross-checked on the transparency. Moreover, the corporations might have to get through multi-technology curvatures to keep data management intact with the strategies inflow. Individual decision-making as per source codes can be more accessible than the collective decision-making by a team as per the consensus. Review management can improvise the techniques in a short period, and everything goes on virtual [21].

Similar to the above can exist with the medical systems where individual patent details can be shared with a team of the doctors concerned only. Personal information is quite exclusive, and truthful information is supposed to be protected according to privacy policies. In biological research and therapeutic sectors, blockchain technology has shown significant promise. Even before starting a clinical trial or examination, it may be feasible to record all clinical consents, plans and procedures on a blockchain, thanks to the practical use of blockchain technology. Sensitive data requires to be updated, secure and available to the public. With the help of updated data can be possible to create a secure real-time database on patient healthcare setup. Therefore, blockchain can be the best possible means for this digital healthcare system which is dependable [22].

Because digitized medical records are accessible and shared and thus also facilitate better and faster decision-making, demand for the digitization of medical records has risen rapidly in the last decade. Today's most common use of blockchain technology is in the healthcare field, employed in medical records. Many doctors, radiologists, healthcare providers, pharmacists and researchers use medical records to diagnose and treat patients effectively. The safety of the patient's treatment while storing, transmitting and distributing such sensitive patient information can be jeopardized, putting the patient's health at risk. The incidence of these challenges may increase in patients with long-term diseases because of the pre-and post-treatment, monitoring and rehabilitation processes they've undergone before and after their treatment. To ensure effective treatment, keeping the patient's medical history updated is crucial.

Perhaps the growth of blockchain technology in medical applications worldwide is a strong guarantee for patients, that is, to use this blockchain technology to make their medical records unchangeable. Any interruption that comes in the technology can be quickly identifiable and adjustable. It is helpful for patients as well as for any activity related to criminal fraud or adulteration. Plus, it will be easier to share and review approved medical service records. When a patient sees a doctor, most providers of that patient tend to see a doctor quickly. With appropriate patient care algorithms, medication errors, allergies and medication solutions can be adapted to all blockchain registries reasonably quick, without the need for cumbersome medication commitment forms [24].

Therefore, blockchain will promote better access to care, medical record management, rapid confirmation of clinical information, expanded safety and more effective care treatment. Third-party involvement would be significantly less due to most minor indulgence, which may mark up the data privacy to the best possible scalability. Due to potential data integrity, medical services may remain behind other emerging ventures, but there is an incentive to grasp the blockchain in the medical field shortly. There are several focal points for managing electronic medical records. The adaptation of smart contracts discussed encourages us to handle all the trivial and significant exchanges in the medical industry. The smart contract provides an unbreakable blockchain looking for personalized treatments without breaking into the clinical framework. Through the integrated clinical system, blockchain smart contract resists making duplicate copies in higher centralized systems. For researchers, blockchain's potential support will provide a verified and timestamped version of scientific research. Just as smart contracts allow for patient data management, document blockchain records enable researchers to obtain a persistent form of their findings. Blockchain is an essential technology in the vast sector of the pharmaceutical industry [26].

16.2.2 SMART CONTRACT AND SMART CONSENT

A legitimate computer program with its architecture or code of functions and data would help to formulate an intelligent contract. The term "smart contracts" refers to computer code that automatically executes all or portions of a contract and is stored on a blockchain network, regardless of whether or not the code contains "real smartness." The code of blockchain technology guides smart contracts. This code has the agreement on a typical text-based contract that transfers information from one to another. Every code has duplicate nodes that support robust blockchain technology. This replication ensures that the code is effectively run as each new block is added to the network. In the end, a smart contract is neither smart nor a contract but an online agreement to assent a code to move forward with the blockchain-linked service. More or less, it is an automatic step to go ahead in any transaction with a simple click without any negotiation, and it's no less than an e-commerce click. Creating synergies with the fusion of IoT, AI and blockchain can deliver the best of goods and services.

Imagine a workplace that complies with blockchain applications like the smart dispute resolution system, smart conciliation, smart trust, smart finance, smart supply chain, smart analytics and what is not claimed to be smart! Every smart application is imbibed with a smart contract or the source code, formulated with the terms and conditions agreements act. Programming a code is like tailoring an attire as per the necessity of the event. A smart contract is a tailored code as per the services offered by a corporate. The replacement of computer to computer (C2C) has inflicted more excellent benefits via blockchain like a shared public ledger, multiple backups, immutability and convenience. Achieving the client goals would be the primary notion, followed by maintaining a "client block" in the distributed ledger [31].

Provision of equal access to healthcare benefits is a nation's zealous duty, inclusive of a qualitative healthcare system, efficient lifestyle, healthy connotations and updated insurance schemes. More or less, a human being's health data is locked up in a box or portfolio as a block of transactions which one would term necessary in the case of individual healthcare. Data infrastructure should be generous to handle fragmented data, consolidate heterogeneous data, maintain protocols and allow easy updates. Blockchain proves to be efficient in preserving the insurance of patients to subside their maintenance.

Many of the biggest roadblocks to effective healthcare are data related. Healthcare providers struggle to effectively use data due to the widespread dispersion of data across systems and substantial fragmentation. Data is gathered and kept in various locations for public health and planning reasons, including patient records, provider(s), and government archives. On the other hand, few places offer complete and longitudinal perspectives of the people in their systems. The inability to integrate data comprehensively, including risk factors, medical history and treatments, is a significant problem in moving forward.

Blockchain innovation could dispose of multiple obstructions by giving a distributed archive containing the entirety of this information, subsequently diminishing fragments. Conventions inside the chain can guarantee that information is consistently coded and steady throughout the framework, making a homogeneous climate helpful for liquid trade. At long last, this information can be stacked in a split second into the blockchain and be given to anybody with an entrance key using the conveyed record usefulness. Like monetary exchanges, trust is essential to information inside the medical services industry. Wellbeing data is constrained by medical clinics, wellbeing data trades; insurance agencies; and other go-betweens, who, while asserting reliability, are in a position to misuse that trust. Blockchain innovation lessens the job of these confided in go-betweens in getting and sharing people's wellbeing records, subsequently moving the force balance for specialists and patients [29].

The source code is effectively intellectual property once it becomes a true innovation, and there are potentials of malfunctioning or errors via the same designated IP. Protection of the IP goes at par with maintenance and control on the smart contracts, which is truly difficult to execute. As per the tokens and individual concerns, only the code can get into an experimental error to pause and check the significant error. But if there are no bugs, issues are untraceable, and remedies may go ineffective. Regulatory codes are equally playing a role in managing the governance of smart contracts. Interoperability and risk may exist colloquially, but sooner or later, the blocks are protected in a secure, private, and closed network [32].

16.3 BLOCKCHAIN LAWS AROUND THE GLOBE

"Trust Systems" are prone to easy damages and inefficiency, leading to bullish faults and violation of enforcing standards. Privacy blocks another pathway leading to complex transactions, and human mistakes synchronize to a mammoth task [33]. Single-handed technology, which consists of no third parties, encryption, trust, safety, and efficiency, provides a good solution in our economic background. Blockchain has adopted cryptographic solutions for critical data governance, confidence, and data management, proving to become an all-in-one finance solution. Laws have ethically adapted blockchain technologies with the fastest implication of the "Smart Dubai" initiative by UAE, where the city of Dubai is expected to be fully operational with blockchain technology. Initially pumped by bitcoin, many countries reacted to it under cryptocurrency and initial coin offerings (ICO) as a financial venture. Later on, Internet laws fastened hard with technology laws to give rise to "blockchain laws" or lex cryptographic.

Primary legislation runs parallel to the substitute and new legislations made for the public good, with some jurisprudence attached. The blockchain environment is relatively new and optimistic as per its growth and applications across the continents. Significant legislations created are Internet laws and developments concerning security exchanges. The total market capitalization of blockchain technologies goes up to $6.6 billion (USD), which forms the efficiency and visibility in organizations later. The economy needs regulation, and a regulatory body needs smart laws to prevent cybercrimes, money laundering and mis-finance. As the technology blooms, so are the bottlenecks for the rise and growth of the block-chain. A significant digital heist took place in 2017, in which the hacker stole around \$55 million of Ether, a digital currency. Despite the security, the hacker had the anti-engineering of blockchain, and specific blocks coded in action. Limitations are pretty substantial as the convenience and safety protruding from any technology to maintain the legal sanctity [36].

Quality assessment bodies surge up with crypto news withstanding the market position of legal trading, policy-making and analysis. Due to poor quality ICO, fintech solutions have been a degradation. Alternative currency ideas have hovered for a long time, but there have been multiple delicacies in conversion, storage, regulation, simplicity and records. Healthcare is unaffected by blockchain usage due to its "organizing power" in health-tech and electronic health records. Blocks are easier to maintain and process, with the toughest of privacy policies guarding the data forever. Every mark on every single node or block gets marked and stored as "evidentiary data" for the futuristic purpose of tracing individual corporate personalities. However, policies related to blockchain keeps on changing due to maidenhood stage activities [35].

Key biomedical benefits help healthcare management pacify its system in medical record management, enhanced insurance claim process, research and development, and advanced data ledger. Mitigating circumstances arise with corporate disputes in traceability, confidentiality, speed and scalability of blocks. Artificial Intelligence (AI) poses a threat to the blockchain perspective due to automated features hampering "smart consent". Devices are devoid of consent while collecting sensor-based data, posing a threat to private international law. Jurisdictional limitations may violate laws from one state to another, and the worst-case scenario develops with dispute resolution [47].

16.3.1 LAWS OF THE UNITED KINGDOM AND EUROPEAN UNION

Law-making would rest on differences between private and public blockchain with the differences attached to the same. Block security endures well in personal blocks with pre-selected access but goes rough in general partnerships. But the decentralization is high in a public blockchain, which seems to be the governing factor [3]. Laws may sublime with innovative instrumentation and dependence on technology, but the human intentions are irreversibly true and need a crystallized effort to balance. Inter-block transactions become a question on how to be controlled, verified and approved of as there are no international organizations to regulate it vividly. Application-based laws would be primarily effective for usage options like payments via the interface, public health management, public governance, data management, and so on. Effective and comprehensive, the laws would be easier to frame this way, and some countries have already drafted the same as in the UK. As per the UK Financial Conduct Authority, the "cryptocurrency transactions" come under Financial Services and Markets Act, 2000 (FSMA) [23, 43].

Although there is no specific blockchain-focused law in the UK, the most popular usage level goes up to cryptocurrency trading, Internet of things, security, government tech, healthcare, fintech, entertainment, and so on. All these applications come in concurrence with EU GDPR rules to ensure data accuracy, right to erasure, right to correction, right to retain info and limits of usage. Distributed Ledger Technologies (DLT) passed a difficult test of Financial Conduct Authority (FCA) regulations named "Digital Sandbox" to guarantee fintech via blockchain gateway during the COVID-19 pandemic. The FCA has prohibited derivatives in unregulated crypto assets/tokens. With the application of blockchain technology, UK's implemented the Fifth Money Laundering Directives (MLD5), which supports counter-terrorism financing policies [17].

For government internal procedure affairs, the UK has started an investigation. The COVID-19 is also a challenge for the government; hence the UK came up with blockchain-based technology for supporting this affair. There is a "Her Majesty's Land Registry" (HMLR) has also been investigated the real estate transactions with the help of blockchain technology and this transactions time is less than 10 minutes. HM Treasury launched a consultation on blockchain in 2020 to improve and implement the aspects into the government governance system.

European Union (EU) laws are comparatively more straightforward in the digital environment as the legal codes get a turn down to action if they can't comply with rules. Technical codes must be pitch perfect as promised in a smart contract to seek approval and move forward with the agreement. Regulatory technology should also be enrolled in blockchain technology to make a habitat of authorized nodes to monitor blocks. In line with the Markets in Financial Instruments Directive II (MiFID II), the FCA has confirmed that derivative products referencing either cryptocurrencies or tokens issued through an ICO may be financial instruments, and this means that it may be necessary to apply for authorization to deal in, arrange transactions in, advise, or provide similar services about such derivatives [13].

The GDPR is founded on the premise that, concerning each data item, at least one natural or legal person or the data controller can be contacted by data subjects, to ensure that their rights under EU data protection legislation are upheld. Blockchains, on the other hand, are frequently used to achieve specific goals. Decentralization is the process of replacing a single actor with a large number of distinct participants. As a result, the allocation becomes onerous in terms of accountability and duty, especially given the ambiguous boundaries of, under the rule, the concept of controllership. Another complication in this regard is the fact that is that, in light of current case law developments, determining someone qualifies as a controller can be fraught with a lack of legal certainty. The GDPR is predicated on the idea that data can be changed or destroyed as needed to comply with legal obligations, such as Articles 16 and 17 of the GDPR [5, 6].

On the other hand, blockchains make such data changes intentionally tricky, to guarantee data integrity and network trust. Again, the current uncertainty in EU data protection law adds to the ambiguities in this area of data protection legislation. For example, it is currently unclear how Article 17 GDPR's concept of crasure should be understood. But there are some rights like the right of access by the data subject (Article 15), the right to restriction of processing (Article 18), and the right to data portability (Article 20) which supports the usage in primary and critical healthcare. These rights can accommodate the service providers to use innovative features best under the GDPR compliance [7, 8].

16.3.2 LAWS OF THE UNITED STATES OF AMERICA

The birth of cryptocurrency is considered to be in the US. There have been numerous developments of the cryptocurrency in this land, starting with bitcoin, Litecoin and Ethereum. The paperless digital currency was promoted to the next level with the hope of a "digital economy" with a feeling of Midas touch. It has been a confusing affair to decide who shall control the influx of crypto assets in the US, beginning from the Securities and Exchange Commission (SEC), the Commodities and Futures Trading Commission (CFTC), Internal Revenue Services (IRS), Financial Crimes Enforcement Network (FinCEN), Office of Comptroller of the Currency (OCC) and the Federal Trade Commission (FTC). Six agencies are in the narrow pathway to objectify technology to have a shield of law as complexities derive from the corporate policies on usage, promotion and sharing beyond continents. SEC got into cases where they treated ICOs to be out of the scope of its laws. Still, the Court ruled that the "tokens" would be considered as securities if they pass the Howey test under investment contracts or any interest or instrument is commonly known as security [19].

Public health remains on the serious list with a specific focus on sensitive personal data and management of health at large. Health Insurance Portability and Accountability Act, 1996 (HIPAA) refers to be modern legislation controlling healthcare data privacy in the US. Frauds related to health insurance have damaged the US government around billions of dollars, for which blockchain technology has been adopted to maintain the anti-corruption momentum. Although the non-covered entities (NCEs) like m-health and accessories inclusive of wearables, smartphones, health-tech instruments are not added under federal laws of HIPAA, there is a sharp turn to control the data extraction by individual private manufacturers. Health IT infrastructure is a complex entity that needs to satisfy four measures: centralized, federated, self-sovereign and user-centric. Risk follows up the information stacked above another, but the ultimate solution lies in the blocks used to store data. A shared ledger of data helps maintain the cryptographic rules discharged by the organization's functioning smooth network of data transfer [30].

Apart from data fragmentation, the data itself is diverse. Some information is "typically of high quality, coded and computerized", including diagnostic, procedure, prescription, laboratory and administrative data. On the other hand, most other data is either not available in electronic form or is in free form (doctor's notes), even if it is. Because of the wide variety of availability of specific data, data timeliness is also an issue. Clinical data is nearly always available right away; administrative data that have been coded can take days or weeks to appear, and statistics in government archives can take two or more years to appear. Blockchain technology may erase these obstacles by creating a peer-to-peer repository holding all of this data, decreasing fragmentation. Within the chain, protocols can guarantee that information is uniformly coded and consistent throughout the system, resulting in a homogenous environment favourable to fluid interchange. Finally, using the distributed ledger capability, this data can be instantaneously put onto the blockchain and made available to everyone with an access key. Medical health blended with social media gives a comfortable outlook to customers to connect dots in peer performance. Expansion of HIPAA is going to announce a plethora of new rights and protection with due diligence [11].

In the healthcare business, trust is essential for data, just as it is for financial transactions. Hospitals, health information exchanges, insurance companies, and other intermediaries hold health information and are in a position to abuse that trust while pretending to be trustworthy. The role of these trusted middlemen in safeguarding and sharing individuals' health information is reduced by blockchain technology, changing the power balance in favour of physicians and patients. However, blockchain technology will not address all of the trust issues regarding the security of health data. The US should follow the EU's lead and implement more onerous laws, which would signal a shift in the data ownership paradigm when combined with blockchain technology. Under the new EU model, personal data is defined as "any information connected to an individual, whether it relates to their private, professional, or public life" under the new EU model. The General Data Protection Regulation (GDPR) aims to give individuals control over their data. Ownership is achieved through enforcing substantial penalties for misuse, contesting "automatic individual decision-making", demanding explicit agreement for data collection and usage, and providing persons with an apparent right of erasure [37, 38].

16.3.3 LAWS OF INDIA

Tech hubs begin in Indian land, where they go along the lane towards connecting the healthcare ecosystem with information technology. Indian public health is standardized, wealthy and on the high pitch regarding affordability, connectivity and maintaining the health of a vast population. Therefore,

self-care is the best policy as was evident during the Covid-19 pandemic, which goes parallel to National Health Policy, 2017 (NHP) goals. WHO has promoted universal health coverage for everyone as per "Pradhan Mantri-Jan Arogya Yojana" (PM-JAY) and "Ayushman Bharat Yojana" (ABY)

where technology would make it possible to enforce. The national healthcare information network is promised to be created by the end of 2025, the primary route to manage the data. Blockchain technology can serve India with an integrated healthcare architecture consisting of drug supply management, drug flow reports, personal healthcare management, diagnosis management, and public healthcare data to the greatest extent. As per PM-JAY, 500 million beneficiaries can access healthcare, forming one of the world's most significant government initiatives. Maintenance is a high-profile key with due focus to privacy in hand, is a gruesome task and challenging laws to manipulate human interference instead of technology [25].

Blockchain's overused application, bitcoin, was initially cautioned by the Reserve Bank of India (RBI) in 2013. As per the report from a high-level committee set up by the Government of India (GoI) in 2019, private cryptocurrencies were put on a ban in Indian estate. But the Supreme Court lifted the ban in 2020, as per Article 19(1)(g), or the freedom to practice any profession or carry on any occupation, trade, or business, and the doctrine of proportionality in legit terms. Ultimately, the crypto traders and private token houses benefited from crypto transactions in India, and GoI may soon introduce the "Cryptocurrency and Regulation of Official Digital Currency Bill, 2021". RBI is deeply concerned about the misuse of fintech applications via blockchain, suppressing the energy of the technology. Along with the GoI, RBI is marching towards promoting the "digital currency", which will lift the grey areas of using the private tokens [11].

Since blockchain is immutable, a single source of truth must be established before implementing a process on it. To guarantee the purity of the blockchain network and prevent any post-implementation alterations to previously accepted blocks, all business data must be considered the "single source of truth" once blockchain implementation has taken place. Blockchains expect the asset being monitored to be represented digitally. The process will need to be adjusted to match. A shared vision of success is required to develop that goal. Blockchain use cases that meet the prerequisites are likely to require process adjustments before deployment, making stakeholders hesitant to join [27].

Instead, the deployment of the blockchain eliminates the requirement for conventional intermediaries. Traditionally, certificates and physical verification/presence attestation have been produced in checks and balances (which are issued in the form of certificates or physical verification/presence attestation). Registration of sales deeds at the registrar, for example, during a land transfer process, necessitates the physical presence of witnesses to ensure that transactions are not fraudulent. On the other hand, blockchains provide a way to carry out these tasks in a way that eliminates the need for time-consuming procedures.

Smart contracts may now be framed and deployed at scale because of blockchain technology. Smart contracts result from writing a series of if...then functions to express standard contractual terms in code. Transactions or data on the distributed ledger might activate smart contract provisions that manage real-world assets like real estate, insurance claims, and so forth. Because smart contracts are self-executing and self-enforcing, the parties have no role to play. Whatever result the smart contract accomplishes must be regarded as optimal, regardless of its ridiculousness or practicality. While it is unclear how legal regimes will evolve to incorporate smart contracts, it is evident that computer codes cannot be the entire solution [40].

Machines are incapable of including implicit understandings or tacit agreements due to being both social and legal tools. A fundamental concept is to use a hybrid legal framework, in which contract terms that are easy to understand, and access are built on top of intelligent contract specifications. The traditional contractual instrument takes precedence in a conflict because it more accurately reflects the parties' true intent. At the same time, the importance of establishing which interfaces and processes are contractable and which parties they are contractable with cannot be overstated.

16.3.4 Laws of Singapore

In Singapore, cryptocurrency regulations and laws are in sync. The Monetary Authority of Singapore (MAS) believes in regulating the cryptocurrency ecosystem to ensure that it doesn't hinder innovation while also taking precautions to address possible risks such as money laundering and terrorist financing. The Payment Services Act (PSA), 2019 has arisen for fintech regulations and to streamline the financial transactions (including monetary, digital, and cryptocurrency) under one legislation. The Securities and Futures Act (SFA) was also made relevant for public offers or issues of digital tokens, and a revised Guide to Digital Token Offerings was released in May 2020. If the digital tickets are "capital market goods", MAS will oversee public offers or issuance of digital tokens [28].

Singapore Medical Council (SMC) is empowered by Medical Registration Act to regulate the ethics and guidelines for the medical profession. The body's stability would appreciate some technological achievements, especially in the recent time of the pandemic. The doctor's and patient's discussions about treatment are kept private. SMC cases and ethical norms such as the SMC Code & Guidelines have clearly stated this. The law on this is based on English law, which, while not binding, is regarded as very important in Singapore because no equivalent examples exist. Many of the concepts relating to secrecy, likewise incorporated in the SMC Code & Guidelines, are codified in the Personal Data Protection Act. A patient's right to informational privacy is protected by law. Medical information that identifies a living or deceased person is classified as personal information under the law. Healthcare facilities are mandated by the Personal Data Protection Act to ensure that medical information collected is essential, accurate and complete. They must also adopt appropriate security arrangements to prevent unauthorized access, use, or disclosure of medical information transmitted outside of Singapore and ensure that medical information moved outside of Singapore is similarly protected by a recipient individual or organization. The patient has the right to see their medical records, to have information about how they are used, and to have any inaccurate personal information corrected. Banking is the new challenge as there's a scope of "crypto bank" amid the crypto-friendly nature of the nation [20].

Singapore has created a blockchain-based application aimed at improving the management and security of medical records. The platform, which allows healthcare data to be saved in a digital wallet, was utilized in a pilot where COVID-19 discharge memos were confirmed over 1.5 million times [42]. The "digital health passport" was developed by SGInnovate, a government-owned investment organization, and Accredify, a local start-up, to assist in the control of medical records. Beginning in May, during the height of the global pandemic, SGInnovate called on Accredify to help develop the application. It specializes in managing a company's document lifecycle, which includes document management software [26].

A specific digital wallet has been created with the application of blockchain technology for keeping personal medical history. This wallet will be used for the verification of the newly designed digital health passport. All information will be held in the wallet related to the COVID-19 patient summary and vaccination aspects. It will eliminate the paper formality, which has always fear of misplacing. This facility has always been used and created by an open-source framework [39]. Singapore Government's CIO office has stated that:

> Digital Health Passport leverages blockchain technology to generate tamper-proof cryptographic protections for each medical document. Users can automatically verify the digital records via a mobile app and present it to officials via QR code, for a quick and seamless verification process, SGInnovate said.

In June 2020, Singapore's Ministry of Health and Ministry of Manpower agreed to use a test using the early prototype of the digital health passport, according to SGInnovate. Digital discharge forms for foreign workers, which had recently been introduced as a new feature in the FWMOMCARE app, were used to confirm that they had worked more than 1.5 million times using the Manpower Ministry's health passport. Digital health passports were also used to acquire other medical information, such as the Covid-19 swab findings, immunity proof and vaccination records. Technological advances may be utilized to streamline the application process for "green lane" essential travel for increased safety, such as for airline or bus travel [41].

16.4 DYNAMICS OF BLOCKCHAIN AND TRUST MECHANISM

The biggest obstacle for the blockchain is bridging the trust domains that are currently fragmented. Traditionally, trust stems from a single source and does not apply in a diverse blockchain ecosystem where independent administrative domains own different devices. In parallel to the spectacular volatility and hype of the health sector, the blockchain application boom is fostering something very similar. Because blockchain technology is all about creating one priceless asset – trust – no one can predict what blue-chip industries will be built on it, but people are confident that it will exist. In addition, it is necessary to have a comprehensive understanding of the ethical, trust, rationality, and acceptability issues [44].

16.4.1 ETHICS CODE

Technology is referred to as "neither good nor bad; nor is it neutral". This tells us that technology constantly interacts with society, values and institutions regardless of whether we like it. These interactions may result in both positive and negative outcomes. The Blockchain Code of Ethics attempts to codify a set of ethical business practices for blockchain companies. Codes of ethics that declare companies accountable to values such as humanity, individuals' data, the planet, transparency, and freedom should be outlined in the Declaration of Blockchain Code of Ethics. While it does not include any complete ethical blockchain guideline provisions, it attempts to frame a collection of principles to which firms using the blockchain should adhere. The Blockchain Ethical Design Framework is broader than a set of principles. It incorporates a design and practical framework to address both positive and negative social impacts of blockchain and DLT-based solutions. Emphasizing that designing with intention is crucial, but it believes that implementing blockchain or DLTs can have significant implications for society. As such, intentional design is necessary to achieve positive results [47].

16.4.2   TRUST VS. NATIONALITY

Trust and nationality based on relationship. When you look at the relationship between the members, you see that it is based on hashing and signed exchanged messages. Using the elliptic curve signature algorithm, each member can be confident in the trustworthiness and seamless data integration. While entities distrust each other, entities believe that they can trust other entities. In addition, their framework allows any device to automatically share a transaction without verifying the resource's trustworthiness and validity. This research does not elucidate how members' identity and trust are guaranteed before executing a trusted transaction. Nationality aspects come in when other country entities provide cross-border data flow or blockchain technology. In this situation, it is only trusted which needs to be taken care of [18].

16.4.3   RATIONALITY AND ABSOLUTE 'PUBLIC TRUST'

Blockchain provides a solution to the general trust problem at all public, federated and organizational systems. This is because, while they're essential traits, they are rarely sufficient in and of themselves to supply a complete solution, which is why we frequently see blockchain deployed in tandem with solid cryptographic protocols like zero-knowledge proofs. This cryptographic protocol can build rationality with public trust [34].

16.4.4   ACCEPTANCE OF BLOCKCHAIN

Blockchain technology is ushering in a new approach to safeguarding the information shared with others. It's interesting to think about the potential to bring blockchain technology into existing healthcare infrastructures. The opportunities to realize improved decentralized storage, distributed ledger, interoperability, authentication, trustworthiness, immutability, and more on the healthcare IoT network (i.e., IoHT). In addition, these nodes could be built and managed gradually and efficiently. IoHT enables blockchain technology for various other benefits such as improved system integration, coherence, confidentiality and compliance. All the features of blockchain technology are absolute [38].

16.5 BLOCKCHAIN AND DATA GOVERNANCE

One of the essential facets of the healthcare industry is managing healthcare data governance, which includes storage, access control and sharing of the data. Better care outcomes can be realized when all the patient data is managed correctly. A complete view of the patient can be obtained, the appropriate treatments can be tailored, and effective communication can be established. It is also critical to maintaining the efficacy and efficiency of the healthcare industry. The difficulty in administering healthcare data is due to the sensitive nature of the data and resulting trust issues. These aspects of the healthcare system, including information and services in different silos, are the root causes of the healthcare system's disconnection. This disconnecting system is a significant hindrance to healthcare quality and innovation [44, 45].

By bringing multiple parties into a trusted transaction scheme, the distributed nature of blockchain ensures no single authority is required. However, it is possible to apply several operational models to healthcare organizations. While there are operational models for blockchain-based solutions in which a particular stakeholder assumes the role of a regulator, in some cases, it is imperative to have a regulator enforce order across the entire blockchain network. Most importantly governing model may be required to meet the regulatory standards. Such a governance structure has not yet been demonstrated to be manageable in a system with multiple disparate entities. There is also a connection to the targeted incentive schemes that can be planned. However, a variety of blockchain-based healthcare solutions as blockchain technology evolves within the healthcare sector should be supported by the best governance [46].

16.6 CONCLUSION

Surfacing the best of benefits, every government tries to make work handy and supportive to its public. COVID-19 has been quite evident that the healthcare systems fail for the best of developed nations as well. Therefore, as a collective responsibility, healthcare reforms should be taken in directive ways. Blockchain has served as the key to data management in many nations, and it would help more as well. Throughout this work, we have deciphered the essential facts and the legal challenges in implementing blockchain technologies for public healthcare. Moreover, the governments may have a paradigm shift from human-based solutions to technology-based solutions by the end of 2030. Specifically, the blockchain serves the best of security and purpose of Big Data, data management and secure transactions in every sphere of application in health-tech. Everyone in the world needs improved healthcare options. All citizens, residents, and tourists may be required to sign a worldwide pact for a "health ID" or "health card".

Blockchain is a newer technology for handling electronic data that can help with transparency and accountability. Every computer network participant may see an identical copy of a blockchain. With its little digital footprint and immutability, blockchain is ideally suited for transactions. Blockchains may be particularly beneficial in the health industry for verifying identities, managing medical and pharmaceutical supply chains, and managing dynamic patient consent, data sharing and access rights.

The legal sphere is yet in a nascent stage as the technology has developed shortly, and implementation may take time and effort to find its flaws. Fundamental human rights, privacy laws and existing tech laws are always guiding blockchain-based applications. Compulsory corporate-based policies may restrict malicious usage, but the regulatory bodies should always keep a border check on every transaction. To encourage the use of the technology to advance sustainable development outcomes, known as "blockchain for good", a designation has been adopted.

CONFLICT OF INTEREST

There is no conflict of interests.

FUNDING

There is no funding support.

DATA AVAILABILITY

Not applicable.

REFERENCES

1. Adams, Richard, Kewell, Beth, and Parry, Glenn. 2018. "Blockchain for good? Digital ledger technology and sustainable development goals." In *Handbook of Sustainability and Social Science Research*, pp. 127–140. Springer, Cham.
2. Ahmed, S., Hossain, M.F., Kaiser, M.S., Noor, M.B.T., Mahmud, M., Chakraborty, C. 2021. Artificial intelligence and machine learning for ensuring security in smart cities. In: Chakraborty, C., Lin, J.C.W., Alazab, M. (eds) *Data-Driven Mining, Learning and Analytics for Secured Smart Cities. Advanced Sciences and Technologies for Security Applications.* Springer, Cham. https://doi.org/10.1007/978-3-030-72139-8_2
3. Archives. CoinDesk, https://www.coindesk.com/category/policy-regulation. Accessed 12 July 2021.
4. Arindam, S, Mohammad, Z.A., Moirangthem, M.S., Abdulfattah, N, Chinmay, C., Subhendu, K.P. 2021. Artificial neural synchronization using nature inspired whale optimization. *IEEE Access*, 1–14, doi:10.1109/ACCESS.2021.305288
5. Art. 15 GDPR – Right of Access by the Data Subject. General Data Protection Regulation (GDPR), https://gdpr-info.eu/art-15-gdpr/. Accessed 13 July 2021.

6. Art. 17 GDPR – Right to Erasure ('Right to Be Forgotten'). General Data Protection Regulation (GDPR), https://gdpr-info.eu/art-17-gdpr/. Accessed 13 July 2021.

7. Art. 18 GDPR – Right to Restriction of Processing. General Data Protection Regulation (GDPR), https://gdpr-info.eu/art-18-gdpr/. Accessed 13 July 2021.

8. Art. 20 GDPR – Right to Data Portability. General Data Protection Regulation (GDPR), https://gdpr-info.eu/art-20-gdpr/. Accessed 13 July 2021.

9. Billah, MohdMa'Sum, Amadu, Mohammed Fawzi Aminu. 2019. Shari'ah code of ethics in cryptocurrency. In *Halal Cryptocurrency Management*, pp. 149–163. Palgrave Macmillan, Cham.

10. Casey, Michael J., Vigna, Paul. 2018. In blockchain, we trust. *MIT Technology Review*, 121(3), 10–16.

11. Chakrabarty, S.P., Ghosh, J., Mukherjee, S. 2021. Privacy issues of smart cities: Legal outlook. In: Chakraborty, C., Lin, J.C.W., Alazab, M. (eds) *Data-Driven Mining, Learning and Analytics for Secured Smart Cities. Advanced Sciences and Technologies for Security Applications*. Springer, Cham. doi:10.1007/978-3-030-72139-8_14. Accessed 13 July 2021.

12. Chakraborty, Chinmoy, Sarkar, Chaity, Sinha, Dola. 2021. Design of a priority based local energy market using blockchain technology, pp. 197–201.

13. Chinmay, C., Megha, R. 2021. Smart healthcare systems using big data, Elsevier: Demystifying big data, machine learning and deep learning for healthcare analytics, Ch. 2, 1–16. doi:10.1016/B978-0-12-821633-0.00002-7

14. Collier, R. 2017. NHS ransomware attack spreads worldwide. *CMAJ: Canadian Medical Association journal = journal de l'Associationmedicalecanadienne*, 189(22), E786–E787. doi:10.1503/cmaj.1095434. Accessed 13 July 2021.

15. Cowan, T. A. 1967. Law and technology: Uneasy leaders of modern life. *Case Western Reserve Law Review*, 19(1), 120–124.

16. Cryptocurrency Derivatives. FCA. 2018, April 6. https://www.fca.org.uk/news/statements/cryptocurrency-derivatives. Accessed 13 July 2021.

17. Deo, M. G. 2013. Doctor population ratio for India – the reality. *The Indian Journal of Medical Research*, 137(4), 632–635.

18. Roberto, Di Pietro, Salleras, Xavier, Signorini, Matteo, Waisbard, Erez. 2018. A blockchain-based trust system for the Internet of things. In *Proceedings of the 23rd ACM on Symposium on Access Control Models and Technologies*, pp. 77–83.

19. Digital Sandbox Pilot. https://www.digitalsandboxpilot.co.uk/. Accessed 12 July 2021.

20. Dubai Blockchain Strategy. https://www.smartdubai.ae/initiatives/blockchain. Accessed 9 July 2021.

21. Hammi, Mohamed Tahar, BadisHammi, Patrick Bellot, Serhrouchni, Ahmed. 2018. Bubbles of Trust: A decentralized blockchain-based authentication system for IoT. *Computers & Security*, 78, 126–142.

22. Hasselgren, Anton, Kralevska, Katina, Gligoroski, Danilo, Pedersen, Sindre A., Faxvaag, Arild. 2020. Blockchain in healthcare and health sciences—A scoping review. *International Journal of Medical Informatics*, 134, 104040.

23. HM Land Registry to Explore the Benefits of Blockchain. GOV.UK, https://www.gov.uk/government/news/hm-land-registry-to-explore-the-benefits-of-blockchain. Accessed 12 July 2021.

24. Huang, S. 2021. Crypto assets regulation in the UK: An assessment of the regulatory effectiveness and consistency. *Journal of Financial Regulation and Compliance*, 29(3), 336–351. doi: 10.1108/JFRC-06-2020-0062.

25. IIT-Madras Researchers Develop Blockchain-Based Healthcare Systems. *The New Indian Express*, https://www.newindianexpress.com/cities/chennai/2021/may/08/ iit-madras-researchers-developblockchain-based-healthcare-systems-2299905.html. Accessed 16 July 2021.

26. Joyce, K., Loe, M. 2010. A sociological approach to ageing, technology and health. *Sociology of Health & Illness*, 32(2), 171–180.

27. Katuwal, Gajendra J., Pandey, Sandip, Hennessey, Mark, Lamichhane, Bishal. 2018. Applications of blockchain in healthcare: Current landscape & challenges. arXiv preprint arXiv:1812.02776.

28. Kučera, Jan, Bruckner, Tomáš. 2019. Blockchain and ethics: A brief overview of the emerging initiatives. In *CEUR Workshop Proceedings*, vol. 2443, pp. 129–139.

29. Manpreet, K., Mohammad, Z.K., Shikha, G., Abdulfattah, N., Chinmay, C., Subhendu, K.P. 2021. MBCP: Performance analysis of large-scale mainstream blockchain consensus protocols. *IEEE Access*, 9, 1–14. doi:10.1109/ACCESS.2021.3085187.

30. Leising, Matthew, The ether thief BLOOMBERG. 2017, June 13. https://www.bloomberg.com/features/2017-the-ether-thief/. Accessed 13 July 2021.

31. Mauler, V. 2007. Improving public health: Balancing ethics, culture, and technology. *Georgetown Journal of Legal Ethics*, 20(3), 817–834.

32. McPheat, D. 1996. Technology and life-quality. *Social Indicators Research*, 37(3), 281–301. Retrieved 26 June 2021, from http://www.jstor.org/stable/27522907 Accessed 13 July 2021.

33. Rahman, Md Abdur, Rashid, Md Mamunur, Shamim Hossain, M., Hassanain, Elham, Alhamid, Mohammed F., Guizani, Mohsen. 2019. Blockchain and IoT-based cognitive edge framework for sharing economy services in a smart city. *IEEE Access*, 7, 18611–18621.

34. Reidenberg, J. R. 1997–1998. Lex informatica: The formulation of information policy rules through technology. *Texas Law Review*, 76(3), 553–594.

35. Sachin, D., Chinmay, C., Jaroslav, F., Rashmi, G., Arun, K.R., Subhendu, K.P., 2021. SSII: Secured and high-quality steganography using intelligent hybrid optimization algorithms for IoT. *IEEE Access*, 9, 1–16. doi:10.1109/ACCESS.2021.3089357

36. Salah, K., Rehman, M. H. U., Nizamuddin, N., Al-Fuqaha, A. 2019. Blockchain for AI: Review and open research challenges. *IEEE Access*, 7, 10127–10149.

37. SEC v. C.M. Joiner Leasing Corp, 320 U.S. 344, 351 (1943); Reves v. Ernst & Young, 494 U.S. 56, 61 (1990); SEC v. Telegram.

38. Shuaib, M., Alam, S., Alam, M. S., Nasir, M. S. 2021. Compliance with HIPAA and GDPR in blockchain-based electronic health record. *Materials Today: Proceedings*.

39. Soh, Taylor Vinters Via LLC-Anthony, Feei Sy Tham. 2020, January 14. Why Singapore has become Asia's cryptocurrency and blockchain hub. *Lexology*. https://www.lexology.com/library/detail.aspx?g=ca374a13-ed9f-4705-9a7a-e3fea8901429. Accessed 13 July 2021.

40. Solove, Daniel J., Schwartz, Paul. 2014. *Information Privacy Law*. Wolters Kluwer.

41. The Digital Sandbox Pilot. FCA, 2020, May 4. https://www.fca.org.uk/firms/innovation/digital-sandbox. Accessed 13 July 2021.

42. Topic: Blockchain. Statista, https://www.statista.com/topics/5122/blockchain/. Accessed 10 July 2021.

43. UK Regulatory Approach to Cryptoassets and Stablecoins: Consultation and Call for Evidence. GOV.UK. https://www.gov.uk/government/consultations/uk-regulatory-approach-to-cryptoassets-and-stablecoins-consultation-and-call-for-evidence. Accessed 12 July 2021.

44. Van Rijmenam, Mark, Ryan, Philippa. 2018. *Blockchain: Transforming your business and our world*. Routledge.
45. VitalikButerin, Visions, Part 1: The value of blockchain technology, ETHEREUM BLOG. 2015, April 13. https://blog.ethereum.org/2015/04/13/visions-part-1-the-value-of-blockchain-technology/ Accessed 13 July 2021.
46. Warren, Samuel D., Louis, D. Brandeis, the right to privacy. *4 Harvard Law Review*, 193–220, no. 10.2307 (1890), 1321160.
47. Wright, A., De Filippi, P. 2015. Decentralized blockchain technology and the rise of lex cryptographia. doi:10.2139/ssrn.2580664. Accessed 13 July 2021.

Index

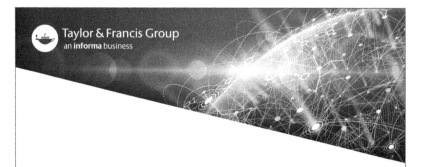